# Ophthalmic Genetic Diseases: A Quick Reference Guide to the Eye and External Ocular Adnexa Abnormalities

# Ophthalmic Genetic Diseases: A Quick Reference Guide to the Eye and External Ocular Adnexa Abnormalities

NATARIO L. COUSER, MD, MS
Assistant Professor of Ophthalmology and Pediatrics
Virginia Commonwealth University School of Medicine
Richmond, Virginia, United States

ELSEVIER

# ELSEVIER

3251 Riverport Lane
St. Louis, Missouri 63043

OPHTHALMIC GENETIC DISEASES: A QUICK REFERENCE GUIDE
TO THE EYE AND EXTERNAL OCULAR ADNEXA ABNORMALITIES     ISBN: 978-0-323-65414-2

*Content Strategist:* Kayla Wolfe
*Content Development Manager:* Kathy Padilla
*Content Development Specialist:* Karen Miller
*Publishing Services Manager:* Jameel Shereen
*Project Manager:* Nadhiya Sekar
*Designer:* Gopalakrishnan Venkatraman

Printed in United States of America

Last digit is the print number: 9 8 7 6 5 4 3 2 1

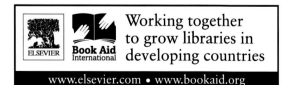

# List of Contributors

**Hind Al Saif, MD, FACMG, FAAP**
Assistant Professor
Department of Human and Molecular Genetics
Clinical Genetics and Metabolism
Virginia Commonwealth University
Richmond, VA, United States

**Tawany Almeida, BS**
Medical Student
Virginia Commonwealth University
 School of Medicine
Richmond, VA, United States

**Kevin Babu**
Virginia Commonwealth University
Richmond, VA, United States

**Gurjas S. Bajaj, BS**
Medical Student
Virginia Commonwealth University
 School of Medicine
Richmond, VA, United States

**Maya Bitar, MD**
Assistant Professor
Department of Ophthalmology
Marshall University
Huntington, WV, United States

**Vikram S. Brar, MD**
Riffenburgh Professor and Program Director
Department of Ophthalmology
Virginia Commonwealth University
Richmond, VA, United States

**Jana Bregman, MD**
Resident Physician
Department of Ophthalmology and Visual Sciences
University of Maryland School of Medicine
Baltimore, MD, United States

**Natario L. Couser, MD, MS**
Assistant Professor of Ophthalmology and Pediatrics
Department of Ophthalmology
Virginia Commonwealth University
Richmond, VA, United States

**Sara Fard, HBSc**
Medical Student
University of Maryland School of Medicine
Baltimore, MD, United States

**Yurika Hara, BA**
Medical Student
Virginia Commonwealth University
 School of Medicine
Richmond, VA, United States

**Jennifer Humberson, MD, FACMG**
Assistant Professor
Department of Pediatrics
Division of Pediatric Genetics
University of Virginia
Charlottesville, VA, United States

**Thomas Hunter, MD**
Assistant Professor
Department of Ophthalmology
Duke University
Durham, NC, United States

**Amy K. Hutchinson, MD**
Professor
Department of Ophthalmology
Emory University
Atlanta, GA, United States

**Mona Kaleem, MD**
Assistant Professor
Department of Ophthalmology and Visual Sciences
University of Maryland School of Medicine
Baltimore, MD, United States

**O'Rese J. Knight, MD**
Assistant Professor
Department of Ophthalmology
University of North Carolina
Chapel HIll, NC, United States

**Scott R. Lambert, MD**
Professor of Ophthalmology and Pediatrics
Stanford University School of Medicine
Stanford, CA, United States

**Eleanor Love, BS**
Medical Student
Virginia Commonwealth University
   School of Medicine
Richmond, VA, United States

**Maheer Masood, BA**
Medical Student
University of North Carolina School of Medicine
Chapel Hill, NC, United States

**Michaela Mathews, MD**
Clinical Assistant Professor
Department of Ophthalmology and Visual Sciences
Neuro-ophthalmology
University of Maryland School of Medicine
Baltimore, MD, United States

**Rakhi Melvani, MD**
Virginia Commonwealth University
   School of Medicine
Richmond, VA, United States

**Payton M. Miller, BS**
Medical Student
Virginia Commonwealth University
   School of Medicine
Richmond, VA, United States

**Mariam Nasir, BS**
Medical Student
Virginia Commonwealth University
   School of Medicine
Richmond, VA, United States

**Harrison Ngo, BS**
Medical Student
Virginia Commonwealth University
   School of Medicine
Richmond, VA, United States

**Chetna Pande, MD, MPH**
Pediatric Critical Care Medicine Fellow
Department of Pediatrics
Baylor College of Medicine
Houston, TX, United States

**Arti Pandya, MD, MBA**
Associate Professor and Division Chief
Department of Pediatrics
Division of Pediatric Genetics and Metabolism
Department of Genetics
University of North Carolina
Chapel Hill, NC, United States

**Adam E. Pflugrath, MD**
Resident Physician
Department of Ophthalmology
Virginia Commonwealth University
Richmond, VA, United States

**Cynthia M. Powell, MD**
Professor
Department of Pediatrics
Division of Pediatric Genetics and Metabolism
Department of Genetics
University of North Carolina
Chapel Hill, NC, United States

**Jessica Randolph, MD**
Assistant Professor
Department of Ophthalmology
Virginia Commonwealth University
Richmond, VA, United States

**Jennifer Rhodes, MD**
Associate Professor of Surgery and Pediatrics
Department of Surgery
Division of Plastic and Reconstructive Surgery
Virginia Commonwealth University
Richmond, VA, United States

**Nikisha Q. Richards, MD**
Assistant Professor
Department of Ophthalmology
Oculoplastics
Virginia Commonwealth University
Richmond, VA, United States

**Dev R. Sahni, BS**
Medical Student
Virginia Commonwealth University
  School of Medicine
Richmond, VA, United States

**Dhruv Sethi, MBA, MPH**
Medical Student
Virginia Commonwealth University
  School of Medicine
Richmond, VA, United States

**Suma P. Shankar, MD, PhD**
Associate Professor
Department of Pediatrics
Division of Genomic Medicine
University of California Davis
Sacramento, CA, United States

**Evan Silverstein, MD**
Assistant Professor
Department of Ophthalmology
Virginia Commonwealth University
Richmond, VA, United States

**Laurie D. Smith, PhD, MD**
Associate Professor
Department of Pediatrics
Division of Pediatric Genetics and Metabolism
University of North Carolina
Chapel Hill, NC, United States

**Janine Smith-Marshall, MD**
Director of Pediatric Ophthalmology and Strabismus
Department of Ophthalmology
Howard University
Washington, DC, United States

**Daniela Toffoli, MDCM**
Assistant Professor
Paediatric Ophthalmology and Neuro-
  Ophthalmology
Montreal Children's Hospital
McGill University and Centre Hospitalier
  de l'Université de Montréal (CHUM)
Montreal, QC, Canada

# Biography

Natario L. Couser MD, MS, is an ophthalmic geneticist, pediatric ophthalmologist, and adult strabismus specialist. He has a clinical and research interest in genetic diseases that affect the eye, eyelids, and external ocular adnexa structures and has uniquely received formal training in ophthalmology, clinical genetics, and biotechnology.

Dr. Couser received his undergraduate degree in biochemistry from the University of Virginia and completed his medical education and internship in Internal Medicine at the Virginia Commonwealth University (VCU) School of Medicine. He completed his ophthalmology residency at Howard University, serving as co-chief resident in his final year. He received fellowship training in pediatric ophthalmology and adult strabismus at Emory University. He then completed a Master of Science degree in biotechnology from Johns Hopkins University and subspecialty training in clinical genetics at the University of North Carolina at Chapel Hill. Dr. Couser has served as the medical director for a pioneer Prevent Blindness America pediatric vision screening program, participated as a consultant and principal investigator for several clinical trials, presented invited lectures, won awards for research, has published numerous research papers and book chapters in the fields of ophthalmology and genetics, and serves as a reviewer for multiple medical journals. He is currently an Assistant Professor with the Department of Ophthalmology at the Virginia Commonwealth University School of Medicine in Richmond, Virginia, where he initiated the first dedicated ophthalmic genetics specialty service in the state. He is a Fellow of the American Academy of Ophthalmology, and a member on the Genetic Eye Disease Committee of the American Association for Pediatric Ophthalmology and Strabismus.

# Preface

An ophthalmic genetic disorder defined broadly is any genetic disease involving an abnormality in the bulbus oculi or eyeball, eyelids, external ocular adnexa, or visual pathway from the retina to the brain. Many of the conditions in this heterogeneous group are exceedingly rare, although collectively they account for the leading cause of childhood blindness and are a major cause of visual impairment in adults. Some genetic eye diseases are known for their abnormal ocular manifestation leading to significant visual limitation, while others may have no associated visual compromise but have eye or ocular adnexa characteristics that represent a diagnostic clue. The techniques in molecular genetics and subsequent ability to use these tools to describe the underlying genetic etiology of ophthalmic genetic disorders have rapidly advanced within the past few years. The discovery of specific genes associated with conditions has allowed for the development of sequencing panels that can interrogate multiple genes at the same time allowing for earlier diagnosis and interventions. Whole exome sequencing and whole genome sequencing have been instrumental in identifying new causative genes as well.

An ophthalmologist, primary care practitioner, or optometrist who may frequently encounter patients with genetic eye diseases often has a varying level of experience and comfort with the clinical genetic aspects that help reach a diagnosis. Similarly, the geneticist or genetic counselor may be unfamiliar with the ocular pathology associated with these conditions. An up-to-date guidebook with diseases listed in a concise and easy to find manner available as a resource to the busy practitioner is indispensable. *Ophthalmic Genetic Diseases: A Quick Reference Guide to the Eye and External Ocular Adnexa Abnormalities* is a comprehensive up-to-date reference and clinical guide to genetic eye diseases. The clinical eye findings and essential genetic information on approximately 500 diseases are described. The conditions listed are grouped by ocular anatomical location most often affected for easy accessibility, and each is presented in a clear and concise manner. Topics covered include the eye abnormalities in patients with chromosomal disorders, craniofacial syndromes, corneal dystrophies, hereditary optic neuropathies, congenital cataracts, inherited retinal diseases, and the phakomatoses. A handy list of relevant resources, a glossary, and a section that lists disorders by select clinical features are additionally included. This reference book is a necessity for the researcher, medical student, resident, or fellow in training; it will be of equal value to the practicing ophthalmologist, geneticist, genetic counselor, pediatrician, optometrist, and any other health professional who encounters patients with genetic eye diseases. Staying up-to-date with the rapid advances in molecular genetics is challenging. This book serves as a resource on a spectrum of inherited eye diseases from the relatively common to the exceptionally rare. Easy access to the clinical features and essential genetic information is provided in an organized and concise manner by chapter for hundreds of genetic diseases of the eye. It is essential that clinicians involved in managing patients with ophthalmic genetic disorders have an understanding of the nature of these conditions and advances in genomic research.

*To my wife, Deanna, thank you for your love, companionship, support, and encouragement through my endless pursuit of learning and achievement. I cherish the growing faith we share, our unbreakable bond we hold steady through life's countless adversities, and the loving family we have created together.*

*To my children, Tyce, Jase, and Emerson, who have all led me to a deeper understanding of unconditional love. I admire your inner joy, boundless energy, exceptional imagination, and kind heart.*

# Contents

# CHAPTER 1

# Eye Abnormalities in Patients With Chromosomal Disorders

CYNTHIA M. POWELL • ARTI PANDYA • HIND AL SAIF • KEVIN BABU •
NATARIO L. COUSER

The estimated prevalence of congenital eye malformations is approximately 3.68—7.50 in 10,000 births.[1,2,3,4] Chromosomal abnormalities are present 1 in 200 live births[5] and are the third most common cause of eye malformations at about 17%; unknown cause and monogenic causes are 58% and 22%, respectively.[1] Eye malformations are present in approximately 24.88 per 10,000 stillbirths.[1] There are few large epidemiological studies focused on congenital eye malformations, and many ocular manifestations may not be identified before the end of the neonatal period. In addition, minor eye anomalies or abnormal ocular adnexa features may not cause visual problems or be readily apparent and only be incidentally observed upon careful inspection.

The most common type of chromosome abnormality is aneuploidy, or a numerical change, meaning missing (monosomy) or extra (trisomy) whole chromosomes. It is also possible for more than one chromosome to be missing or duplicated. Autosomal (non-sex chromosome) aneuploidies are the most common type of aneuploidy. Structural aberrations involve an incorrect rejoining of chromosomal segments after a breakage; these may result in a deletion or duplication of a portion of the chromosome, or the formation of inversions, translocations, ring, or isochromosomes.

Abnormal eye and ocular adnexa features may be present in sex and autosomal chromosomal aberrations, whether numerical or structural, throughout the genome. Disorders of the sex chromosomes tend to have less phenotypic effect than autosomal disorders due to X-inactivation compensating for X chromosome aneuploidy. Common sex chromosome disorders include Turner syndrome in females with a single X chromosome and Klinefelter syndrome in males with an extra X chromosome. Common autosomal chromosome abnormalities include trisomy 21 (Down syndrome), trisomy 18 (Edward syndrome), and trisomy 13 (Patau syndrome) (Table 1.1).[5] Detection and diagnosis of these abnormalities is done using conventional chromosome analysis (karyotype), fluorescent in situ hybridization, or cytogenetic microarray technology.

Common eye abnormalities in chromosomal disorders include hypertelorism, epicanthal folds, aberrant orientation of the palpebral fissures, and colobomas and strabismus (Table 1.2). In certain disorders, the ocular abnormality is one of the defining features of the genetic condition. For example, in cat eye syndrome, associated with partial tetrasomy (four copies) of chromosome 22, affected individuals often have a coloboma of the iris giving the appearance of elongated, cat-like pupils.[6] Likewise, individuals with Williams syndrome, associated with microdeletions on the long arm of chromosome 7, often have a star-shaped or stellate pattern of the iris.[7] Unique eye findings in specific deletion or duplication syndromes include the morning glory disc anomaly with trisomy 4q; aniridia and retinoblastoma with 11p13 deletion and 13q14 deletion, respectively.[8–10] This chapter provides an overview of the most common chromosomal abnormalities and their related ophthalmic features; commonly reported eye and ocular adnexa findings in deletion and duplication aberrations in the chromosomal autosomes, listed by chromosome number and arm (p or short arm, and q or long arm) are included (Table 1.3).[5,11–30] It should be noted that deletions and duplications may involve any region on the short or long arm of a chromosome and vary in size. The specific region involved and the size of the deletion or duplication will influence the phenotype, at least in part due to the specific genes that are missing or duplicated.

| TABLE 1.1 Most Common Chromosomal Disorders | |
|---|---|
| **Disorder** | **Incidence** |
| **AUTOSOMAL CHROMOSOME ABNORMALITIES** | |
| Trisomy 21 (Down syndrome) | 1 in 700 |
| Trisomy 18 (Edward syndrome) | 1 in 5000 |
| Trisomy 13 (Patau syndrome) | 1 in 5000 |
| **SEX CHROMOSOME ABNORMALITIES** | |
| 45, X (Turner syndrome)—females | 1 in 2500 |
| 47, XXX (Trisomy X)—females | 1 in 1000 |
| 47, XXY (Klinefelter syndrome)—males | 1 in 500–1 in 1000 |
| 47, XYY—males | 1 in 1000 |

| TABLE 1.2 Common Eye and Ocular Adnexa Findings in Chromosomal Disorders |
|---|
| **Ophthalmic Finding** |
| Upslanting/downslanting palpebral fissures |
| Epicanthal folds |
| Hypertelorism |
| Iris coloboma |
| Ptosis |
| Strabismus |

## GENETIC DISORDERS

### Angelman Syndrome[31,32]

*OMIM*: #105830.

*Description*: Angelman syndrome is a neurodevelopmental disorder characterized by intellectual disability, movement or balance disorder, typical abnormal behaviors, and severe limitations in speech and language. Most cases arise from maternal de novo deletions.

*Epidemiology*: incidence of 1/12,000–1/20,000.

*Eye Findings*: refractive errors, strabismus, and iris and choroidal hypopigmentation.

*Inheritance*: most cases are de novo.

*Chromosomal Abnormality*: 15q11.2-q13 deletion (maternal), uniparental disomy (paternal), imprinting defects, mutations in *UBE3A*.

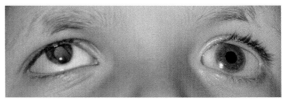

FIG. 1.1  Cat eye syndrome. Iris coloboma of the right eye. (Courtesy Meier, Petra, Wiedemann, Peter. Surgery for pediatric vitreoretinal disorders. In: *Ryan's Retina*. January 1, 2018:2170–2193. © 2018.)

### Cat Eye Syndrome[6,33,34,35]

*OMIM*: #115470.

*Description*: Features of cat eye syndrome include anal atresia with fistula, coloboma of the iris, downslanting palpebral fissures, preauricular pits or tags, and often normal mental state. Heart and renal malformations are often present in those affected.

*Epidemiology*: incidence of 1/50,000–1/150,000.

*Eye Findings*: coloboma of the iris (Fig. 1.1), downslanting palpebral fissures, hypertelorism, epicanthal folds, microphthalmia, and strabismus.

*Inheritance*: most cases are de novo.

*Chromosomal Abnormality*: trisomy/tetrasomy 22pter→q11, inverted dicentric duplication.

### Cri Du Chat Syndrome[36,37,38]

*OMIM*: #123450.

*Description*: Cri du chat syndrome is recognized at birth by a high-pitched, cat-like cry, accompanied by microcephaly, hypotonia in infancy, a distinct rounded face with hypertelorism and low-set ears, and severe intellectual disability.

*Epidemiology*: incidence of 1/15,000–1/50,000.

*Eye Findings*: downslanting palpebral fissures, epicanthal folds, and hypertelorism.

*Inheritance*: most cases are de novo.

*Chromosomal Abnormality*: 5p deletion, translocation, mosaic.

### DiGeorge Syndrome[21,39,40,41]

*OMIM*: #188400.

*Description*: 22q11.2 deletion syndrome, also known as velocardiofacial syndrome or DiGeorge syndrome, is the most common microdeletion syndrome and presents with involvement of multiple body systems. The condition is also known by the acronym CATCH 22 (Cardiac defects, Abnormal facies, Thymic hypoplasia, Cleft palate, Hypocalcemia, 22q11 deletions) that highlights some of the main features of the deletion

**TABLE 1.3**

**General Compilation of Common Eye and Ocular Adnexa Abnormalities Reported With Any Deletion and Duplication Aberrations in the Chromosomal Autosomes (Chromosomes 1–22); to Note, Specific Region Involved and the Size of the Deletion or Duplication Will Influence the Phenotype**

| Chromosome No. | p Deletions | q Deletions | p Duplications | q Duplications |
|---|---|---|---|---|
| 1 | Cataracts, cranial nerve VI palsy, colobomas (choroid, iris, optic nerve), epicanthal folds, eyelashes abnormal (long), hypertelorism, microphthalmia, nystagmus, optic atrophy, orbit deep-set, palpebral fissures abnormal (almond-shaped, short, upslanting), refractive errors (hyperopia), retina hypopigmented, strabismus, synophrys | Cataracts, colobomas (iris), Duane syndrome, epicanthal folds, hypertelorism, microphthalmia, palpebral fissures abnormal (upslanting), ptosis, strabismus | Blue sclera, epicanthal folds, euryblepharon, eyelashes abnormal (long), ptosis | Blue sclera, cataracts, coloboma (iris, optic nerve), epicanthal folds, eyebrows arched, eyelashes abnormal (long), glaucoma, hypertelorism, optic disc hypoplasia, palpebral fissures abnormal (downslanting, short), ptosis, refractive error (myopia) |
| 2 | Blepharophimosis, cyclopia, epicanthal folds, eyebrows arched, palpebral fissures abnormal (long), ptosis, telecanthus | Blepharophimosis, cataracts, coloboma (choroid, iris, retina), corneal opacities, eyebrows thick, hypertelorism, keratoconus, microphthamia, optic nerve hypoplasia, palpebral fissures abnormal (downslanting, short), proptosis, ptosis, supraorbital ridges prominent, synophrys | Hypertelorism, nasolacrimal duct obstruction, palpebral fissures abnormal (short) | Blue sclera, epicanthal folds, hypertelorism, orbits shallow, palpebral fissures abnormal (upslanting), strabismus |
| 3 | Blepharophimosis, coloboma (iris), epicanthal folds, hypertelorism, microphthalmia, nasolacrimal duct stenosis, orbit deep-set, abnormal palpebral fissures (almond-shaped, downslanting, short, upslanting), ptosis, synophrys | Blepharophimosis, epicanthus inversus, ptosis, telecanthus | Hypertelorism, ptosis | Anophthalmia, cataract, coloboma (iris), corneal opacity, epicanthal folds, eyelashes long, glaucoma, microphthalmia, nasolacrimal duct obstruction, palpebral fissures abnormal (downslanting, upslanting), strabismus, synophrys |

Continued

**TABLE 1.3**
General Compilation of Common Eye and Ocular Adnexa Abnormalities Reported With Any Deletion and Duplication Aberrations in the Chromosomal Autosomes (Chromosomes 1–22); to Note, Specific Region Involved and the Size of the Deletion or Duplication Will Influence the Phenotype—cont'd

| Chromosome No. | p Deletions | q Deletions | p Duplications | q Duplications |
|---|---|---|---|---|
| 4 | Blue sclera, cataracts, coloboma (choroid, eyelid, iris, retina), epicanthal folds, eyebrows arched, and defect medial half, exophthalmos, foveal hypoplasia, glaucoma, hypertelorism, iris heterochromia, microcornea, microphthalmia, nasolacrimal duct obstruction, nystagmus, palpebral fissures abnormal (downslanting, upslanting), Peters anomaly, ptosis, Rieger anomaly, strabismus | Epicanthal folds, Duane syndrome, dystopia canthorum, hypertelorism, microphthalmia, palpebral fissures abnormal (short, upslanting), pigmentary retinopathy, ptosis, refractive errors, strabismus | Coloboma, microphthalmia | Epicanthal folds, microphthalmia, morning glory disc anomaly (trisomy 4q) |
| 5 | Epicanthal folds, hypertelorism, optic atrophy, palpebral fissures abnormal (downslanting, upslanting), refractive errors (myopia), strabismus | Epicanthal folds, exophthalmos, palpebral fissures abnormal (upslanting) ptosis, synophrys | Coloboma, epicanthal folds, hypertelorism, microphthalmia, palpebral fissures abnormal (downslanting), Peter's anomaly, strabismus, telecanthus | Coloboma (choroid, retina), epicanthal folds, hypertelorism, palpebral fissures abnormal (almond shaped, downslanting) |
| 6 | Anterior segment dysgenesis, blepharophimosis, blue sclera, coloboma (iris), epicanthal folds, hypertelorism, microphthalmia, nystagmus, optic atrophy, optic nerve hypoplasia, Peters anomaly, refractive errors (hyperopia), pigmentary retinopathy, strabismus, synophrys, telecanthus | Blue sclera, cataract, epicanthal folds, hypertelorism, hypotelorism, macular hypoplasia, microphthalmia, nasolacrimal duct obstruction, nystagmus, palpebral fissures abnormal (downslanting, short), strabismus, synophrys | Blepharophimosis, corneal clouding, eyelashes long, palpebral fissures abnormal (downslanting) | Blue sclera, epicanthal folds, glaucoma, hypertelorism, palpebral fissures abnormal (almond-shaped, downslanting, upslanting) |
| 7 | Epicanthal folds, eyelashes long, nasolacrimal duct obstruction, palpebral fissures abnormal (downslanting), ptosis | Anophthalmia, coloboma (retinal), hypertelorism, microphthalmia, palpebral fissures abnormal (downslanting), strabismus | Eyebrows arched, glaucoma, hypertelorism, palpebral fissures abnormal (downslanting) | Hypertelorism, palpebral fissures abnormal (downslanting, short) |

| | | | | |
|---|---|---|---|---|
| 8 | Coloboma (choroid, iris), epicanthal folds, eyebrows long, hypertelorism, optic atrophy, microcornea, nystagmus, retinal dysplasia, strabismus, synophrys | Hypertelorism, orbit deep-set, palpebral fissures abnormal (upslanting) | Epicanthal folds, glaucoma, hypertelorism, palpebral fissures abnormal (upslanting) telecanthus | Epicanthal folds, hypertelorism, strabismus |
| 9 | Epicanthal folds, eyebrows arched, glaucoma, palpebral fissures abnormal (short, upslanting), ptosis, supraorbital ridges hypoplastic | Epicanthal folds, hypotelorism, eyebrows arched, eyelashes long, hypertelorism, hypotelorism, palpebral fissures abnormal (downslanted, short, upslanted) ptosis, sclerocornea, strabismus, supraorbital ridge hypoplasia, synophrys, telecanthus | Hypertelorism, orbit deep-set, palpebral fissures abnormal (downslanting) | Epicanthal folds, hypotelorism, microphthalmia, orbit deep-set, palpebral fissure abnormal (downslanted, short), strabismus, synophrys |
| 10 | Epicanthal folds, hypertelorism, orbit deep-set, optic nerve hypoplasia, palpebral fissures abnormal (downslanting, short), refractive error (myopia) | Hypertelorism, palpebral fissures abnormal (downslanting) pseudopapilledema, strabismus, | Epicanthal folds, hypertelorism, microphthalmia, palpebral fissures abnormal (downslanting, upslanting) | Blepharophimosis, coloboma (iris), epicanthal folds, eyebrows arched, microphthalmia, palpebral fissures abnormal (downslanting, short, upslanting), ptosis, retinal dysplasia, strabismus |
| 11 | Aniridia (11p13 deletion), cataracts, glaucoma, keratopathy, macular hypoplasia, optic atrophy, nystagmus, ptosis, refractive errors (myopia), strabismus | Cataracts, coloboma (choroid, eyelid, optic nerve, retina), corectopia, ectropion, epicanthal folds, eyelashes short or long, glaucoma, hypertelorism, hypotelorism, microphthalmia, optic atrophy, palpebral fissures abnormal (downslanting, upslanting), Peters anomaly, ptosis, refractive errors (hyperopia, myopia), retinal dysplasia, strabismus, telecanthus, vitreoretinopathy | Conjunctival telangiectasia, epicanthal folds, hypertelorism, microphthalmia, nystagmus, palpebral fissures abnormal (downslanting), pupils eccentric, refractive errors (hyperopia, myopia), retinal detachment, strabismus | Blue sclera, coloboma (iris), epicanthal folds, eyebrows arched, hypertelorism, nystagmus, palpebral fissures abnormal (short), ptosis, refractive error (myopia), strabismus |
| 12 | Orbit deep-set, palpebral fissures abnormal (downslanting), strabismus | Epicanthal folds, eyebrows arched, hypertelorism, palpebral fissures abnormal (downslanting, short, upslanting), ptosis, strabismus | Coloboma, corneal opacity, entropion, epicanthal folds, eyebrows sparse, hypertelorism, nystagmus, palpebral fissures abnormal (downslanting, upslanting), ptosis, refractive errors (myopia), strabismus, supraorbital ridges depressed | Epicanthal folds, eyebrows arched, hypertelorism, palpebral fissures abnormal (wide) |

Continued

**TABLE 1.3**
General Compilation of Common Eye and Ocular Adnexa Abnormalities Reported With Any Deletion and Duplication Aberrations in the Chromosomal Autosomes (Chromosomes 1–22); to Note, Specific Region Involved and the Size of the Deletion or Duplication Will Influence the Phenotype—cont'd

| Chromosome No. | p Deletions | q Deletions | p Duplications | q Duplications |
|---|---|---|---|---|
| 13 | — | Coloboma (retina), epicanthal folds, hypertelorism, iris heterochromia, microphthalmia, nasolacrimal duct obstruction, orbit deep-set, optic atrophy, optic nerve hypoplasia, palpebral fissures abnormal (downslanting), refractive errors (hyperopia), retinal dysplasia, retinoblastoma (13q14 deletions), strabismus | — | Palpebral fissures abnormal (wide) |
| 14 | — | Anophthalmia, blepharophimosis, cataract, epicanthal folds, hypertelorism, palpebral fissures abnormal (downslanting), ptosis | Orbit deep-set | Coloboma (iris), epicanthal folds, hypertelorism, optic atrophy, palpebral fissures abnormal (downslanting), refractive errors (astigmatism, hyperopia) |
| 15 | — | Oculocutaneous albinism, palpebral fissures abnormal (almond-shaped) | — | Palpebral fissures abnormal (downslanted, short), ptosis |
| 16 | Blepharophimosis, epicanthal folds, hypertelorism, orbits shallow, palpebral fissures abnormal (downslanting) | Cataracts, coloboma (iris), eyelashes long, hypertelorism, microphthalmia, palpebral fissures abnormal (short, upslanting), ptosis, strabismus, synophrys | Epicanthal folds, eyebrows sparse, hypertelorism, microphthalmia, palpebral fissures abnormal (short), strabismus | Palpebral fissures abnormal (upslanting) |
| 17 | Anisocoria, cataracts, coloboma (iris), epicanthal folds, iris dysgenesis, microcornea, nystagmus, optic nerve hypoplasia, palpebral fissures abnormal (upslanting), refractive errors (myopia), retinal detachment, strabismus | Palpebral fissures abnormal (short), refractive errors (hyperopia), strabismus | Iris transillumination, palpebral fissures abnormal (downslanting), pupils eccentric | Nystagmus, strabismus |

| | | | | |
|---|---|---|---|---|
| 18 | Cataracts, epicanthal folds, hypertelorism, strabismus | Cataracts, coloboma (choroid), corectopia, corneal opacities, epicanthal folds, exophthalmos, iris hypoplasia, hypertelorism, microcornea, microphthalmia, nystagmus, optic atrophy, ptosis, refractive errors (myopia), retinal degeneration, staphylomas, strabismus | Palpebral fissures abnormal (downslanting) | Epicanthal folds, eyebrows sparse and lateral, hypertelorism, palpebral fissures abnormal (downslanting) nystagmus, strabismus |
| 19 | — | — | Blue sclera, eyebrows scant, palpebral fissures abnormal (upslanting), strabismus | Hypertelorism, palpebral fissures abnormal (downslanting) |
| 20 | Coloboma (iris), epicanthal folds, hypertelorism, iris adhesions, orbit deep-set, palpebral fissures abnormal (downslanting, short), posterior embryotoxon, pupils irregular, retinal dystrophy, strabismus | Duane anomaly, microphthalmia, refractive errors (astigmatism, hyperopia), strabismus | — | Hypertelorism, strabismus |
| 21 | — | Corneal opacity, hypertelorism, microphthalmia, palpebral fissures abnormal (downslanting) | — | — |
| 22 | — | Optic nerves tilted, outer canthi lateral displacement, posterior embryotoxon, ptosis, retinal vessels tortuous, strabismus, upper eyelid hooding | — | Coloboma (iris), hypertelorism, pupils triangular shaped |

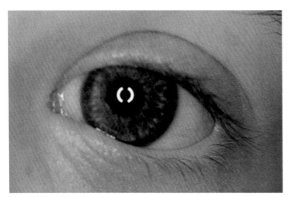

FIG. 1.2 Brushfield spots in the iris in a patient with Down syndrome. (Courtesy Caluseriu, Oana, Reardon, William. Malformation syndromes. In: *Rennie and Roberton's Textbook of Neonatology*. January 2, 2012:791–817. © 2012.)

syndrome. Clinical features present may vary extensively even among related individuals; phenotype may include thymic hypoplasia, congenital heart defects, immunodeficiency, hearing problems, cleft palate, craniofacial abnormalities, scoliosis, learning problems, developmental delays, seizures, bipolar disorder, schizophrenia, and parathyroid hypoplasia, which results in hypocalcemia.

*Epidemiology*: incidence of 1/4000.

*Eye Findings*: hypertelorism, and upslanting/downslanting palpebral fissures.

*Inheritance*: most cases are de novo, AD.

*Chromosomal Abnormality*: deletion of chromosome 22q11.2; *TBX1* haploinsufficiency.

## Down Syndrome[21,33,42,43,44,45]

OMIM: #190685.

*Description*: Down syndrome is the most common chromosomal aneuploidy disorder that is associated with characteristic facial features, hypotonia, single transverse palmar creases, congenital cardiac anomalies, and intellectual disability. Advanced maternal age (defined as 35 years of age and older at delivery) increases the risk to have a baby with Down syndrome due to chromosomal nondisjunction.

*Epidemiology*: incidence of 1/700.

*Eye Findings*: epicanthal folds, iris Brushfield spots (Fig. 1.2), increased likelihood for refractive errors, upslanting palpebral fissures, and strabismus.

*Inheritance*: most cases are de novo.

*Chromosomal Abnormality*: full trisomy 21 secondary to nondisjunction (Fig. 1.3), mosaic trisomy 21, translocation.

## Edwards Syndrome[21,33,44,46,47,48]

OMIM: −

*Description*: Edwards syndrome is marked by intrauterine growth restriction, micrognathia, low-set ears, facial asymmetry, abnormal organ development, heart defects, clenched hands, and polydactyly. It is caused by meiotic nondisjunction resulting in an extra copy of chromosome 18, usually in the mother, and as such, the risk of having a child with Edwards syndrome increases with maternal age.

*Epidemiology*: incidence of 1/5000.

*Eye Findings*: hypertelorism, epicanthal folds, short palpebral fissures, microphthalmia, and ptosis.

*Inheritance*: most cases are de novo.

*Chromosomal Abnormality*: full trisomy 18 secondary to nondisjunction, mosaic trisomy 18, translocation.

## Jacobsen Syndrome[49,50]

OMIM: #147791.

*Description*: A wide range of malformations are associated with Jacobsen syndrome, including stunted development, psychomotor retardation, congenital cardiac anomalies, thrombocytopenia, trigonocephaly, and an increased likelihood of behavioral issues such as attention-deficit hyperactivity disorder and compulsiveness.

*Epidemiology*: incidence of 1/100,000.

*Eye Findings*: abnormal retinal development, anomalous extraocular muscles, coloboma of the iris and chorioretina, ptosis, epicanthal folds (Fig. 1.4), hypertelorism (Fig. 1.4), microcornea, microphthalmia, optic atrophy, and strabismus.

*Inheritance*: most cases are de novo.

*Chromosomal Abnormality*: 11q terminal deletion.

## Klinefelter Syndrome[21,51,52,53,54]

OMIM: −

*Description*: Individuals with Klinefelter syndrome, one of the more common sex chromosomal abnormalities, have small testes, lower testosterone production, gynecomastia, and delayed or incomplete puberty; are more likely to have behavioral and psychosocial problems; and are often infertile and taller than normal.

*Epidemiology*: incidence of 1/500−1/1000 males.

*Eye Findings*: colobomas of iris, choroid, optic nerve, glaucoma, microphthalmia, and strabismus.

*Inheritance*: most cases are de novo.

*Chromosomal Abnormality*: 47, XXY, occasional mosaicism.

## Nablus Mask-Like Facial Syndrome[86−88]

OMIM: #608156.

*Description*: Nablus mask-like facial syndrome, also called chromosome 8q22.1 deletion syndrome, is a rare

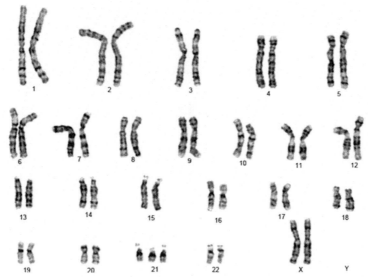

FIG. 1.3  A human karyotype (47, XX), consistent with a female patient with trisomy 21 (Down syndrome). (Courtesy Trent, Ronald J. Genes to Personalized Medicine. In: *Molecular Medicine*. January 1, 2012:1—37. © 2012; Karyotype provided by Dr. Melody Caramins, Genetics Laboratory Services, Prince of Wales Hospital, Sydney, Australia.)

microdeletion syndrome characterized by having a mask-like facial appearance. Features include having a long face, tight glistening appearance of the facial skin, upswept frontal hairline, and sparse eyebrows and eyelashes.

*Epidemiology*: unknown.

*Eye Findings*: blepharophimosis, hypertelorism, narrow palpebal fissures, and sparse eyebrows and eyelashes.

*Inheritance*: de novo, AD.

*Chromosomal Abnormality*: 8q22.1 deletion.

## Patau Syndrome[21,33,44,46,48,55]

*OMIM*: —

*Description*: Patau syndrome results in severe intellectual disability, midline field defects including holoprosencephaly, congenital cardiac abnormalities, polydactyly, cleft lip/palate, and cutis aplasia.

*Epidemiology*: incidence of 1/5000.

*Eye Findings*: anopthalmia/microphthalmia, coloboma of iris, orbital hypotelorism, and retinal dysplasia.

*Inheritance*: most cases are de novo.

*Chromosomal Abnormality*: full trisomy 13 secondary to nondisjunction, translocation.

## Phelan-McDermid Syndrome[56—58]

*OMIM*: #606232.

*Description*: Phelan-McDermid syndrome (PHMDS), also called chromosome 22q13.3 deletion syndrome, is a developmental disorder with developmental delays, hypotonia, delayed speech, autistic behaviors, and intellectual disability. PHMDS has a

wide variety of clinical features and body systems involved.

*Epidemiology*: unknown; about 500 cases reported.

*Eye Findings*: epicanthal folds and ptosis.

*Inheritance*: most cases are de novo.

*Chromosomal Abnormality*: 22q13.3 deletion, mutations in *SHANK3*.

## Prader—Willi Syndrome[59—61]

*OMIM*: #176270.

*Description*: Prader—Willi syndrome is characterized by diminished fetal activity, extreme obesity, muscular hypotonia, intellectual disability, short stature, hypogonadotropic hypogonadism, and small hands and feet. Commonly due to a microdeletion of the paternally inherited allele.

*Epidemiology*: incidence of 1/10,000—30,000.

*Eye Findings*: almond-shaped eyes, refractive errors, strabismus, upslanting palpebral fissures, and glaucoma.

*Inheritance*: most cases are de novo.

*Chromosomal Abnormality*: 15q11-q13 deletion (paternal), uniparental disomy (maternal), mutation in the imprinting center (deletion of paternal copies of *NDN*, *SNRPN*).

## Smith-Magenis Syndrome (Chromosome 17p11.2 Deletion Syndrome)[62,63]

*OMIM*: #182290.

*Description*: Smith-Magenis syndrome is a complex developmental disorder that affects multiple organ

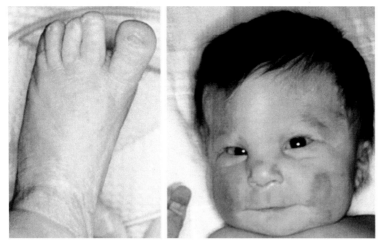

FIG. 1.4 Jacobsen syndrome. Note the broad thumbs and great toes (left photo), and the epicanthal folds and hypertelorism (right photo). (Courtesy Graham, John M., Sanchez-Lara, Pedro A. Metopic craniosynostosis. In: *Smith's Recognizable Patterns of Human Deformation*. January 1, 2016:218–224. © 2016.)

systems of the body. The disorder is characterized by a pattern of abnormalities that are present at birth, as well as behavioral and cognitive problems.

*Epidemiology*: prevalence of 1/15,000.

*Eye Findings*: microcornea, strabismus, iris anomalies, and myopia.

*Inheritance*: AD (sporadic unless secondary to a parental balanced translocation).

*Chromosomal Abnormality*: most cases caused by a 3.7-Mb interstitial deletion in chromosome 17p11; also caused by mutations in *RAI1*.

### Triple X Syndrome[52,64,65]

*OMIM*: —

*Description*: The most common chromosomal anomaly affecting females, triple X syndrome results in subtle physical abnormalities; affected females tend to be taller than normal and are more likely to have intellectual disabilities, delayed language and motor skills, seizures, and kidney problems.

*Epidemiology*: incidence of 1/1000 females.

*Eye Findings*: epicanthal folds, hypertelorism, and upslanting palpebral fissures.

*Inheritance*: most cases are de novo.

*Chromosomal Abnormality*: trisomy X (47, XXX) secondary to nondisjunction, mosaicism.

### Triploidy[21,33,66,67,68]

*OMIM*: —

*Description*: Triploidy affects 1% of recognized pregnancies; however, most fetuses with triploidy

are spontaneously aborted, with very few surviving at birth. The syndrome is most often caused by dispermy and is characterized by growth retardation and asymmetric growth, 3—4 syndactyly, abnormal skull structure, cardiac and brain anomalies, genital ambiguity, and hydatidiform changes of the placental mole.

*Epidemiology*: incidence of 1/100,000.

*Eye Findings*: absent or underdeveloped eyes, coloboma of iris or choroid, hypertelorism, iris heterochromia, and microphthalmia.

*Inheritance*: de novo.

*Chromosomal Abnormality*: three sets of chromosomes (69 total) instead of the usual pair; occasional diploid/triploid mosaicism.

### Turner Syndrome[21,52,69,70,71,72,73]

*OMIM*: —

*Description*: Turner syndrome is a sex chromosome abnormality where females have only a single X chromosome. It is characterized by short stature, broad chest, ovarian dysgenesis, webbed neck, cubitus valgus, low posterior hairline, and delayed pubertal development in affected females. Most (99%) of the 45, X conceptions are not viable and are lost early in pregnancy.

*Epidemiology*: incidence of 1/2500 females.

*Eye Findings*: amblyopia, downslanting palpebral fissures, blue sclera, cataracts, epicanthal folds, hypertelorism, ptosis, and strabismus.

*Inheritance*: most cases are de novo.

*Chromosomal Abnormality*: 45, X, *SHOX* haploinsufficiency, X-isochromosome Xq, mosaicism, ring X chromosome.

## Williams Syndrome[21,74,75,76,77]

*OMIM*: —

*Description*: Williams syndrome often presents with moderate intellectual disability, microcephaly, cardiovascular abnormalities, outgoing and friendly personality, and hypersensitivity to sound. In addition, individuals with this disorder have distinct facial characteristics including a large mouth, long philtrum, prominent lips, depressed nasal bridge, and hypodontia.

*Epidemiology*: prevalence of 1/7500.

*Eye Findings*: epicanthal folds, hypotelorism, refractive errors, short palpebral fissures, stellate pattern in iris, and strabismus.

*Inheritance*: most cases are de novo, AD.

*Chromosomal Abnormality*: 7q11.23 deletion.

## Wolf-Hirschhorn Syndrome (Wittwer Syndrome)[40,78–82]

*OMIM*: #194190.

*Description*: Wolf-Hirschhorn syndrome, also known as Wittwer syndrome, chromosome 4p16.3 deletion syndrome, Pitt-Rogers-Danks syndrome or Pitt syndrome, is characterized by "Greek warrior helmet" facies, microcephaly, seizure disorder, and closure defects (coloboma, cleft lip or palate, and cardiac defects). Growth and intellectual disability are both common. There is a wide variation in phenotypic expression which can be explained by the size of the deletion.

*Epidemiology*: prevalence of 1/20,000–1/50,000.

*Eye Findings*: coloboma, epicanthal folds, downslanting palpebral fissures, hypertelorism, megalocornea, microphthalmia, nystagmus, optic atrophy, proptosis, ptosis, retinal hypoplasia, Rieger anomaly, and telecanthus.

*Inheritance*: de novo.

*Chromosomal Abnormality*: 4p16.3 deletion.

## XYY Syndrome[33,52,54,83,84]

*OMIM*: —

*Description*: Individuals with 47, XYY may have varied yet subtle dysmorphic features, presenting in affected males in taller than normal stature, increased risk for behavior issues, mild tremors, and learning disabilities, hypotonia, and severe acne. XYY syndrome is underdiagnosed, and most males with this disorder have normal lives.

*Epidemiology*: incidence of 1/1000 males.

*Eye Findings*: mild hypertelorism.

*Inheritance*: de novo.

*Chromosomal Abnormality*: 47, XYY; mosaicism possible.

## REFERENCES

1. Bermejo E, Martínez-Frías ML. Congenital eye malformations: clinical-epidemiological analysis of 1,124,654 consecutive births in Spain. *Am J Med Genet*. 1998;75(5):497–504.
2. Källén B. Severe eye malformations. In: *Epidemiology of Human Congenital Malformations*. Cham: Springer; 2014.
3. Stoll C, Alembik Y, Dott B, Roth MP. Epidemiology of congenital eye malformations in 131,760 consecutive births. *Ophthalmic Paediatr Genet*. 1992;13(3):179–186.
4. Stoll C1, Alembik Y, Dott B, Roth MP. Congenital eye malformations in 212,479 consecutive births. *Ann Genet*. 1997;40(2):122–128.
5. Nussbaum RL, McInnes RR, Willard HF. Chapter 6, clinical cytogenetics: disorders of the autosomes and the sex chromosomes. In: *Thompson & Thompson, Genetics in Medicine*. 7th ed. Saunders Elsevier; 2007:89–113.
6. Rosa RF, Mombach R, Zen PR, Graziadio C, Paskulin GA. Clinical characteristics of a sample of patients with cat eye syndrome. *Rev Assoc Med Bras (1992)*. 2010;56(4):462–465.
7. Halás M, Bzdúch V. Ocular changes in the Williams-Beuren syndrome. *Cesk Oftalmol*. 1991;47(3):178–182.
8. Nucci P, Mets MB, Gabianelli EB. Trisomy 4q with morning glory disc anomaly. *Ophthalmic Paediatr Genet*. 1990;11(2):143–145.
9. Hingorani M, Moore A. Aniridia. In: Adam MP, Ardinger HH, Pagon RA, et al., eds. *GeneReviews® [Internet]*. Seattle (WA): University of Washington, Seattle; May 20, 2003, 1993–2018. [Updated 2013 November 14].
10. Lohmann DR, Gallie BL. Retinoblastoma. In: Adam MP, Ardinger HH, Pagon RA, et al., eds. *GeneReviews® [Internet]*. Seattle (WA): University of Washington, Seattle; July 18, 2000, 1993–2018. [Updated 2015 November 19].
11. Abu-Amero KK, Kondkar AA, Khan AO. Molecular karyotyping of a dysmorphic girl from Saudi Arabia with CYP1B1-negative primary congenital glaucoma. *Ophthalmic Genet*. 2016;37(1):98–101.
12. Atack E, Fairtlough H, Smith K, Balasubramanian M. A novel (paternally inherited) duplication 13q31.3q32.3 in a 12-year-old patient with facial dysmorphism and developmental delay. *Mol Syndromol*. 2014;5(5):245–250.
13. Battaglia A, Gurrieri F, Bertini E, et al. The inv dup(15) syndrome: a clinically recognizable syndrome with altered behavior, mental retardation, and epilepsy. *Neurology*. 1997;48:1081–1086.
14. Cartwright MJ, Hassan TS, Frueh BR. Microdeletion of chromosome 7P syndrome ocular manifestations. *Ophthal Plast Reconstr Surg*. 1995;11(2):139–141.
15. Ceccarini C, Sinibaldi L, Bernardini L, et al. Duplication 18q21.31-q22.2. *Am J Med Genet A*. 2007;143A:343–348.
16. Chen CP, Lin SP, Chern SR, et al. De novo satellited 21q associated with corpus callosum dysgenesis, colpocephaly, a concealed penis, congenital heart defects, and developmental delay. *Genet Couns*. 2004;15(4):437–442.

17. Goitia V, Oquendo M, Stratton R. Case of 7p22.1 microduplication detected by whole genome microarray (REVEAL) in workup of child diagnosed with autism. *Case Rep Genet.* 2015;2015:212436.

18. Iglesias A, Rauen KA, Albertson DG, Pinkel D, Cotter PD. Duplication of distal 20q: clinical, cytogenetic and array CGH. Characterization of a new case. *Clin Dysmorphol.* 2006;15(1):19−23.

19. Jamsheer A, Sowińska A, Simon D, Jamsheer-Bratkowska M, Trzeciak T, Latos-Bieleńska A. Bilateral radial agenesis with absent thumbs, complex heart defect, short stature, and facial dysmorphism in a patient with pure distal microduplication of 5q35.2-5q35.3. *BMC Med Genet.* 2013;14:13.

20. Johansson B, Mertens F, Palm L, Englesson I, Kristoffersson U. Duplication 18p with mild influence on the phenotype. *Am J Med Genet.* 1988;29(4):871−874.

21. Jones KL. Chapter 1, recognizable patterns of malformation. In: *Smith's Recognizable Patterns of Human Malformation.* 5th ed. Philadelphia, PA: W.B. Saunders Company; 1997:7−117.

22. Klein F, Schuck D, Noël B, Stoessel J, Vibert M. Proximal trisomy 19q. Interstitial deletion and ring chromosome derived from 19q. *Pediatrie.* 1989;44(9):717−720.

23. Lukusa T, Fryns JP. Syndrome of facial, oral, and digital anomalies due to 7q21.2->q22.1 duplication. *Am J Med Genet.* 1998;80(5):454−458.

24. Magnelli NC, Therman E. Partial 12p deletion: a cause for a mental retardation, multiple congenital abnormality syndrome. *J Med Genet.* 1975;12(1):105−108.

25. McMorrow LE, Toth IR, Gluckson MM, Leff A, Wolman SR. A lethal presentation of de novo deletion 7q. *J Med Genet.* 1987;24(10):629−631.

26. Reynolds JD, Golden WL, Zhang Y, Hiles DA. Ocular abnormalities in terminal deletion of the long arm of chromosome seven. *J Pediatr Ophthalmol Strabismus.* 1984;21(1):28−32.

27. Ryan AK, et al. Spectrum of clinical features associated with interstitial chromosome 22q11 deletions: a European collaborative study. *J Med Genet.* 1997;34:798.

28. Stratakis CA, Lafferty A, Taymans SE, Gafni RI, Meck JM, Blancato J. Anisomastia associated with interstitial duplication of chromosome 16, mental retardation, obesity, dysmorphic facies, and digital anomalies: molecular mapping of a new syndrome by fluorescent in situ hybridization and microsatellites to 16q13 (D16S419-D16S503). *J Clin Endocrinol Metab.* 2000;85(9):3396−3401.

29. Traboulsi EI. Section one malformations, chapter 13, ocular manifestations of chromosomal abnormalties. In: *Genetic Diseases of the Eye.* 2nd ed. Oxford University Press; 2012:190−235.

30. Wang C, Maynard S, Glover TW, Biesecker LG. Mild phenotypic manifestation of a 7p15.3p21.2 deletion. *J Med Genet.* 1993;30(7):610−612.

31. Michieletto P, Bonanni P, Pensiero S. Ophthalmic findings in Angelman syndrome. *J AAPOS.* 2011;15:158−161.

32. Saitoh S, Harada N, Jinno Y, et al. Molecular and clinical study of 61 Angelman syndrome patients. *Am J Med Genet.* 1994;52:158−163.

33. Chen H. *Atlas of Genetic Diagnosis and Counseling.* Totowa, NJ: Humana Press; 2006:136−137, 295-298, 976-977, 985-986,990, 1075.

34. Karcaaltincaba D, Ceylaner S, Ceylaner G, Dalkilic S, Karli-Oguz K, Kandemir O. Partial trisomy due to a de novo duplication 22q11.1-22q13.1: a cat-eye syndrome variant with brain anomalies. *Genet Couns.* 2010;21(1):19−24.

35. Rosias PPR, et al. Phenotypic variability of the cat-eye syndrome, case report and review of the literature. *Genet Counsel.* 2001;12:273.

36. Kajii T, Homma T, Oikawa K, Furuyama M, Kawarazaki T. Cri du chat syndrome. *Arch Dis Child.* 1966;41:97−101.

37. Mainardi PC. Cri du chat syndrome. *Orphanet J Rare Dis.* 2006;1:33.

38. Mainardi PC, et al. The natural history of cri du chat syndrome. A report from the Italian register. *Eur J Med Genet.* 2006;49:363.

39. Goldberg R, et al. Velo-cardio-facial: a review of 120 patients. *Am J Med Gent.* 1993;45:313.

40. Korf BR. *Human Genetics: A Problem-based Approach.* 2nd ed. Cambridge, MA: Blackwell Science Ltd; 2000:183−208.

41. Chieffo C, Garvey N, Gong W, et al. Isolation and characterization of a gene from the DiGeorge chromosomal region homologous to the mouse Tbx1 gene. *Genomics.* 1997;43:267−277.

42. Caputo AR, Wagner RS, Reynolds DR, Guo S, Goel AK. Down syndrome: clinical review of ocular features. *Clin Pediatr.* 1989;28:355−358.

43. DaCunha RP, Moreira JB. Ocular findings in Down's syndrome. *Am J Ophthal.* 1996;122:236−244.

44. De Souza E, et al. Recurrence risks for trisomies 13, 18, and 21. *Am J Med Genet.* 2009;149A:2716.

45. Pueschel SM. Atlantoaxial instability and Down syndrome. *Pediatrics.* 1988;81:879.

46. Baty BJ, et al. Natural history of trisomy 18 and trisomy 13: I: growth, physical assessment, medical histories, survival and recurrence risk. *Am J Med Genet.* 1994;49:175.

47. Edwards M, Mulcahy D, Turner G. X-linked recessive inheritance of an orofaciodigital syndrome with partial expression in females and survival of affected males. *Clin Genet.* 1988;34:325−332.

48. Rasmussen SA, et al. Population-based analysis of mortality in trisomy 13 and trisomy 18. *Pediatrics.* 2003;111:777.

49. Mattina T, Perrotta CS, Grossfeld P. Jacobsen syndrome. *Orphanet J Rare Dis.* 2009;4:9.

50. Miller GL, Somani S, Nowaczyk MJM, et al. The ocular manifestations of Jacobsen syndrome: a report of four cases and a review of the literature. *Ophthal Genet.* 2006;27:1−7.

51. Chopra R, Chander A, Jacob JJ. The eye as a window to rare endocrine disorders. *Indian J Endocrinol Metab.* 2012;16:331−338.

52. Ottesen AM, et al. Increased number of sex chromosomes affects height in a nonlinear fashion: a study of 305 patients with sec chromosome aneuploidy. *Am J Med Genet.* 2010;152A:1206.

53. Ross JL, et al. Cognitive and motor development during childhood in boys with Klinefelter syndrome. *Am J Med Genet.* 2008;146A:708.

54. Ross JL, et al. Behavioral and social phenotypes in boys with 47, XYY syndrome or 47, XXY Klinefelter syndrome. *Pediatrics*. 2012;129:769.

55. Bruns D, et al. Birth history, physical characteristics, and medical survivors with full trisomy 13. *Am J Med Genet*. 2011;155A:2634.

56. Soorya L, Kolevzon A, Zweifach J, et al. Prospective investigation of autism and genotype-phenotype correlations in 22q13 deletion syndrome and SHANK3 deficiency. *Mol Autism*. 2013;4:18.

57. Phelan MC, Rogers RC, Saul RA, et al. 22q13 deletion syndrome. *Am J Med Genet*. 2001;101:91—99.

58. Moessner R, Marshall CR, Sutcliffe JS, et al. Contribution of SHANK3 mutations to autism spectrum disorder. *Am J Hum Genet*. 2007;81:1289—1297.

59. Buiting K. Prader-Willi syndrome and Angelman syndrome. *Am J Med Genet C Seminars Med Genet*. 2010;154:365—376.

60. Cassidy SB, Driscoll DJ. Prader-Willi syndrome. *Eur J Hum Genet*. 2009;17:3—13.

61. Cassidy SB, Schwartz S, Miller JL, Driscoll DJ. Prader-Willi syndrome. *Genet Med*. 2012;14:10—26.

62. Barnicoat AJ, Moller HU, Palmer RW, Russell-Eggitt I, Winter RM. An unusual presentation of Smith-Magenis syndrome with iris dysgenesis. *Clin Dysmorph*. 1996;5:153—158.

63. Girirajan S, Elsas 2nd LJ, Devriendt K, Elsea SH. RAI1 variations in Smith-Magenis syndrome patients without 17p11.2 deletions. *J Med Genet*. 2005;42:820.

64. Otter M, Schrander-Stumpel CT, Curfs LM. Triple X syndrome: a review of the literature. *Eur J Hum Genet*. 2010;18:265—271.

65. Tartaglia NR, Howell S, Sutherland A, Wilson R, Wilson L. A review of trisomy X (47,XXX). *Orphanet J Rare Dis*. 2010;5:1—9.

66. Graham JM, et al. Diploid-triploid mixoploidy: clinical and cytogenic aspects. *Pediatrics*. 1981;68:23.

67. Wulfsberg EA, et al. Monozygotic twin girls with diploid/triploid chromosome mosaicism and cutaneous pigmentary dysplasia. *Clin Genet*. 1991;39:370.

68. Zaragoza MV, et al. Parental origin and phenotype of triploidy in spontaneous abortions: predominance of diandry and association with the partial hydatidiform mole. *Am J Hum Genet*. 1807;66:2000.

69. Al Alwan I, Khadora M, Amir I, et al. Turner syndrome genotype and phenotype and their effect on presenting features and timing of diagnosis. *Int J Health Sci*. 2014;8:195—199.

70. Bondy CA, et al. Care of girls and women with Turner syndrome: a guideline of the Turner syndrome study group. *J Clin Endocrinol Metab*. 2007;92:10.

71. Dacou Voutetakis C, Kakourou T. Psoriasis and blue sclerae in girls with Turner syndrome. *J Am Acad Dermatol*. 1996;35:1002—1004.

72. Pinsker JE. Clinical review: Turner syndrome: updating the paradigm of clinical care. *J Clin Endocrinol Metab*. 2012;97: e994.

73. Ganguly BB, Sahni S. X chromosomal abnormalities in Indian adolescent girls. *Teratog Carcinog Mutagen*. 2003; (suppl 1):245—253.

74. Donnai D, Karmiloff-Smith A. William syndrome: from genotype through to the cognitive phenotype. *Am J Med Genet*. 2000;97:164.

75. Holmstrom G, Almond G, Temple K, Taylor D, Baraitser M. The iris in Williams syndrome. *Arch Dis Child*. 1990;65:987—989.

76. Morris CA. Williams syndrome. In: Adam MP, Ardinger HH, Pagon RA, et al., eds. *GeneReviews®* [Internet]. Seattle (WA): University of Washington, Seattle; April 9, 1999, 1993—2018. [Updated 2017 March 23].

77. Strømme P, Bjørnstad PG, Ramstad K. Prevalence estimation of Williams syndrome. *J Child Neurol*. 2002;17(4):269—271.

78. Bergemann AD, Cole F, Hirschhorn K. The etiology of Wolf-Hirschhorn syndrome. *Trends Genet*. 2005;21: 188—195.

79. Dickmann A, Parrilla R, Salerni A, et al. Ocular manifestations in Wolf-Hirschhorn syndrome. *J AAPOS*. 2009;13: 264e7.

80. Wolf-hirschhorn syndrome. In: Chen H, ed. *Atlas of Genetic Diagnosis and Counseling*. 2nd ed. New York, NY; USA: Springer; 2012:2165—2177.

81. Maas N. Genotype-phenotype correlation in 21 patients with Wolf-Hirschhorn syndrome using high resolution array comparative genome hybridisation (CGH). *J Med Genet*. 2008;45:71—80.

82. Wieland I. A cryptic unbalanced translocation der(4)t(4; 17)(p16.1;q25.3) identifies Wittwer syndrome as a variant of Wolf-Hirschhorn syndrome. *Am J Med Genet A*. 2014; 164:3213—3214.

83. Lalatta F, Folliero E, Cavallari U, et al. Early manifestations in a cohort of children prenatally diagnosed with 47, XYY. Role of multidisciplinary counseling for parental guidance and prevention of aggressive behavior. *Ital J Pediatr*. 2012; 3:38—52.

84. Stochholm K, et al. Diagnosis and mortality in 47, XYY persons: a registry study. *Orphanet J Rare Dis*. 2010;5:15.

85. Jain S, Yang P, Farrell SA. A case of 8q22.1 microdeletion without the Nablus mask-like facial syndrome phenotype. *Europ J Med Genet*. 2010;53:108—110.

86. Raas-Rothschild A, Dijkhuizen T, Sikkema-Raddatz B, Werner M, Dagan J, Abeliovich D, Lerer I. The 8q22.1 microdeletion syndrome or Nablus mask-like facial syndrome: report on two patients and review of the literature. *Europ J Med Genet*. 2009;52:140—144.

87. Salpietro CD, Briuglia S, Rigoli L, Merlino MV, Dallapiccola B. Confirmation of Nablus mask-like facial syndrome. *Am J Med Genet*. 2003;121A:283—285.

88. Teebi AS. Nablus mask-like facial syndrome. *(Letter) Am J Med Genet*. 2000;95:407—408.

# CHAPTER 2

# Genetic Abnormalities of the Anterior Segment, Eyelids, and External Ocular Adnexa

LAURIE D. SMITH • MAHEER MASOOD • GURJAS S. BAJAJ • NATARIO L. COUSER

Genetic disorders that involve the anterior segment of the eye, the eyelids, or external ocular adnexa are as heterogeneous as they are numerous. These disorders are generally grouped by their anatomical locations.[1] The anterior segment of the eye is defined as structures anterior to the vitreous humor, which include the aqueous humor, cornea, ciliary body, iris, lens, pupil, and trabecular network (Figs. 2.1 and 2.2). Abnormalities of the iris include absence of the iris (aniridia),[2] iris hypoplasia and dysplasia, iris coloboma (missing tissue), and complete or segmental heterochromia iridis. The pupil may be affected by displacement from the normal central position (corectopia), being poorly reactive or having a diminished size (microcoria).[3] Descriptions for an abnormal cornea include megalocornea or microcornea,[4] corneal thinning,[5] a flattened cornea (cornea plana),[6] corneal hypoplasia and dysplasia, coloboma of the cornea, clouding, perforation, or scarring. Lens abnormalities include microphakia (abnormally small), spherophakia (small and abnormally round), and/or opacification. Furthermore, the orbit itself may be diminished in size, referred to as microphthalmia.[7,8]

The external ocular adnexa refers to the eyebrows, eyelashes, eyelids, and lacrimal system; these structures function to lubricate and protect the eye. There are several abnormalities specific to the eyelids. Ablepharon refers to absent eyelids. Microablepharon refers to vertical shortening of the eyelids, whereas euryblepharon is an increase in the vertical palpebral fissure.[9] Blepharoptosis, or simply ptosis, refers to abnormal relaxation of the upper eyelid. Ectropion and entropion are outward and inward turned eyelids, respectively. Each component of the external ocular adnexa can have several abnormalities. The lacrimal system may have a deficiency of tear production (alacrima), or excessive tearing (epiphora). The eyelashes may be absent (madarosis), may have abnormal growth of a second set (distichiasis),[10,11] or turn inward (epiblepharon). The eyebrows may be absent or abnormal in shape, or may be present as a unibrow (synophrys).

Many of the disorders listed below are rare with unknown disease epidemiology data, however, there are a few that are relatively common in the population. Aniridia, a disorder characterized by a partial or complete absence of iris tissue, affects 1 in 40,000−100,000 births and can occur with other ocular manifestations.[12] This is a bilateral condition, which can be familial or sporadic, that is characterized by having a nearly absent or mildly hypoplastic iris. Additional clinical features include nystagmus, decreased vision, foveal or optic nerve hypoplasia, cataracts, glaucoma, or corneal clouding. The disorder is caused by mutations in the *PAX6* gene located on chromosome 11p13.[13] Wilms tumor is a risk associated with sporadic causes of aniridia. WAGR complex refers to the presence of *W*ilms tumor, *A*niridia, *G*enitourinary malformations, and intellectual disability (formerly referred to as mental *R*etardation), the result of mutations in the *WT1* gene; this condition has been diagnosed in as early as the prenatal period.[14]

Albinism refers to a group of disorders characterized by an abnormal production of melanin in the skin, hair and/or eyes. The ocular clinical features include iris transillumination defects, nystagmus, decreased vision, sensitivity to light, foveal hypoplasia, and hypopigmentation of the retina.[15] X-linked ocular albinism, which predominantly involves the eyes, affects 1 in 50,000 individuals worldwide.[15] Oculocutaneous albinism (OCA), inherited in an autosomal recessive pattern, may be associated with Hermansky-Pudlak syndrome, a platelet bleeding disorder, or Chediak-Higashi syndrome, a lysosomal trafficking disorder that results in

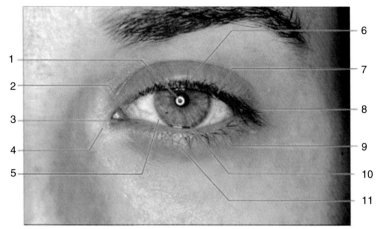

FIG. 2.1 The eyelids and anterior aspect of the eyeball. Key: 1, pupil; 2, plica semilunaris; 3, lacrimal caruncle; 4, medial canthus; 5, conjunctiva; 6, upper eyelid; 7, eyelashes; 8, lateral canthus; 9, lid margin; 10, iris; 11, lower eyelid. (Courtesy Standring S, MBE, PhD, DSc, FKC, Hon FAS, *Hon FRCS Gray's Anatomy*; January 1, 2016:666–685.e1. © 2016. With permission from Berkovitz BKB, Moxham BJ. *Head and Neck Anatomy*. London: Martin Dunitz; 2002.)

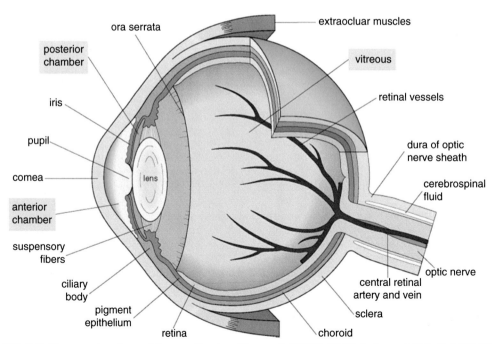

FIG. 2.2 The normal anatomy of the eye. (Courtesy Stevens A, MB BS, FRCPath, Lowe J, BMedSci, BM BS, DM, FRCPath, Scott I, BSc, MB BS, MD, DPhil, FRCPath. *Ophthalmic pathology, Core Pathology*; January 1, 2009:495–504. © 2009.)

increased susceptibility to infection. There are many types of OCA, and genes that have been recently identified to cause OCA are SLC24A5 (OCA6) and C10orf11 (OCA7).[16]

Other relatively common disorders include the overgrowth syndrome Beckwith-Wiedemann syndrome, which affects 1 in 13,700 individuals; ocular features may include epicanthal folds, hypertelorism, and synophrys.[17] Blepharophimosis, ptosis, and epicanthus inversus (BPES) affect 1 in 50,000 births and can present with a variety of ocular abnormalities.[18] Branchiootorenal syndrome affects 1 in 40,000 individuals and can lead to absent eyes and iris atrophy, along with ear and renal defects.[19] Cornelia De Lange syndrome is a multisystem disorder that affects 1 in 10,000 births, ocular features include long eyelashes and synophrys.[20] Gilbert syndrome is an unconjugated hyperbilirubinemia that affects 5%—10% Caucasians and may present with jaundice affecting the eyes.[21] Hereditary hemorrhagic telangiectasia is quite frequent, with an incidence of 1 in 5000 individuals and is defined by vascular abnormalities that may impact the eye.[22] Kabuki syndrome, another multisystem cognitive disorder seen in 1 per 32,000 births, can present with ptosis, thick eyelashes, and long palpebral fissures.[23] Noonan syndrome is a genetic disorder that affects 6—9 in 10,000 individuals, which has distinct phenotypic features including the ocular manifestations of downslanting palpebral fissures, epicanthal folds, hypertelorism, myopia, and ptosis.[24] Osteogenesis imperfecta, with an incidence of 6—7 per 100,000 births, is a genetic disorder mainly affecting the skeletal system, however, individuals may present initially with a blue sclera.[25]

## GENETIC DISORDERS
### Ablepharon Macrostomia Syndrome[9,26—28]
*OMIM*: #200110

*Description*: Ablepharon macrostomia syndrome is a rare congenital ectodermal dysplasia caused by mutations in the basic domain of the *TWIST2* gene, affecting its DNA-binding activity. This syndrome is characterized by abnormal physical growth including macrostomia; absent or hypoplastic eyelids; microtia; abnormal nose, ears, nipples, genitalia, and hands; excess skin; and sparse hair.

*Epidemiology*: unknown; fewer than 20 cases in literature

*Eye findings*: ablepharon or microablepharon, absent eyelashes and eyebrows, corneal clouding, ectropion. Persistent visual problems and corneal opacities due to early corneal exposure.

*Inheritance*: AD

*Known genes or gene locus*: TWIST2

*Special note*: Similar genotypic and phenotypic findings as Barber Say syndrome; may represent a continuum.

### ADULT Syndrome[29—32]
*OMIM*: #103285

*Description*: ADULT syndrome, also known as acrodermato-ungual-lacrimal-tooth syndrome, is a rare syndrome characterized by ectrodactyly, excessive freckling, nail dysplasia, lacrimal duct obstruction, and hypodontia. Other findings can include sparse hair, hypoplastic breast and nipples, various digital abnormalities, and imperforate anus.

*Epidemiology*: unknown

*Eye findings*: lacrimal duct atresia or stenosis, lacrimal mucoceles leading to tearing and conjunctivitis, periorbital darkening

*Inheritance*: AD

*Known genes or gene locus*: TP63

*Special notes*: May have considerable phenotypic and genotypic overlap with EEC syndrome, Hays—Wells syndrome, and Limb-Mammary syndrome.

### Alagille Syndrome[33—35]
*OMIM*: #118450, #610205

*Description*: Alagille syndrome is a neonatal cholestatic jaundice characterized by hepatic duct dysplasia, skeletal abnormalities, pulmonic valve and peripheral arterial stenosis, and ocular abnormalities. Characteristic facies defined by broad forehead, deep-set eyes, upslanting palpebral fissures, hypertelorism, bulbous nose and pointed chin.

*Epidemiology*: prevalence of 1/70,000

*Eye findings*: anomalous optic disc, band keratopathy, cataracts, chorioretinal atrophy, choroidal folds, deep-set eyes, diffuse fundus hypopigmentation, ectopic pupils, hypertelorism, microcornea, myopia, posterior embryotoxon, retinal pigment clumping, strabismus, upslanting palpebral fissures.

*Inheritance*: AD; 50%—70% de novo

*Known genes or gene locus*: JAG1 (Type 1), NOTCH2 (Type 2)

### Alkaptonuria[36—39]
*OMIM*: #203500

*Description*: Alkaptonuria is a metabolic disorder in processing phenylalanine and tyrosine caused by mutations in homogentisate 1,2-dioxygenase gene, resulting in accumulation of homogentisic acid. Phenotypic findings include pigmented urine, ochronosis, cardiac valve destruction, arthritis, and calcifications of vertebral discs.

*Epidemiology*: incidence of 1/250,000—1,000,000

*Eye findings*: astigmatism; central vein occlusion; chamber angle hyperpigmentation; elevated intraocular pressure; pigmentation of bulbar conjunctiva, cornea, optic disk, retina, sclera, and vitreous.

*Inheritance*: AR

*Known genes or gene locus*: HGD

## Aniridia[2,12,40]

OMIM: #106210

*Description*: Aniridia is a panocular disorder that is frequently defined by hypoplasia of iris and can be present as minor iris abnormalities to complete loss of the iris. Other manifestations include cataract, glaucoma, nystagmus, and aniridia-associated keratopathy.

*Epidemiology*: prevalence of 1/40,000—100,000

*Eye findings*: iris hypoplasia (Fig. 2.3), aniridia-associated keratopathy, aniridic fibrosis syndrome, astigmatism, cataract, corneal clouding, elevated intraocular pressure, foveal hypoplasia, glaucoma, hypermetropia, microphthalmia, myopia, nystagmus, optic nerve hypoplasia, Peter's anomaly

*Inheritance*: AD

*Known genes or gene locus*: PAX6, ELP4

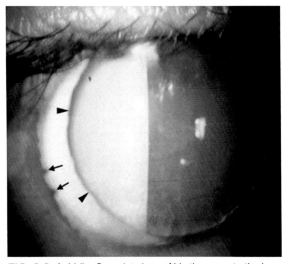

FIG. 2.3 Aniridia. Complete loss of iris tissue; note the lens edge (*black arrowheads*) and visible ciliary processes (*black arrows*). (Courtesy Liu Y, Allingham RR. *Genetics of Glaucoma, Glaucoma*; January 1, 2015:291–299. © 2015.)

## Anterior Segment Mesenchymal Dysgenesis[41—45]

OMIM: #107250, #610256, #601631, #137600, #604229, #617315, #269400, #617319

*Description*: Anterior segment mesenchymal dysgeneses are a series of rare developmental disorders affecting the anterior portion of the eye. Ocular findings may occur with other systemic developmental disorders.

*Epidemiology*: unknown

*Eye findings*: cataract, corectopia, corneal opacity and vascularization, dysgenesis of ocular anterior segment, ectopia lentis, ectropion uveae, elevated intraocular pressure, iris hypoplasia, microphakia, nystagmus, optic nerve dysplasia, polycoria, posterior embryotoxon, trabecular network, and ciliary body abnormalities

*Inheritance*: AD, AR

*Known genes or gene locus*: PITX3 AD (type 1), FOXE3 AR (type 2), FOXC1 AD (type 3), PITX2 AD (type 4), PAX6 AD (type 5), CYP1B1 (type 6), PXDN AR (type 7), CPAMD8 AR (type 8)

## Axenfeld-Rieger Syndrome[46—48]

OMIM: #180500, %601499, #602482

*Description*: Axenfeld-Rieger syndrome refers to a series of developmental disorders characterized by abnormalities of the anterior portion of the eye, which carry a 50% chance of resulting in glaucoma and blindness. Systemic effects, including dental, maxillary, facial, umbilical, and cardiac abnormalities can also occur.

*Epidemiology*: incidence of 1/200,000

*Eye findings*: blue sclera, choroidal hypoplasia, conjunctival xerosis, corectopia, corneal opacities, glaucoma, hypertelorism, iridocorneal angle abnormalities, iris dysplasia, iris hypoplasia, iris strands, lens defects, persistent papillary membrane, polycoria, posterior embryotoxon, prominent Schwalbe line, retinal detachment, strabismus, telecanthus

*Inheritance*: AD, 30% sporadic

*Known genes or gene locus*: PITX2, FOXC1, 13q14

## Baraitser-Winter Syndrome[49—51]

OMIM: #243310

*Description*: Baraitser-Winter syndrome is a rare developmental disorder caused by mutation of actin-encoding genes. This syndrome is characterized by craniofacial abnormalities, intellectual disability, anterior neural migration disorders, and ocular coloboma. Other features include microcephaly, short stature, epilepsy, metopic ridging, pachygyria, and lissencephaly.

*Epidemiology*: unknown

*Eye findings*: arched eyebrows, bilateral congenital nonmyopathic ptosis, coloboma of iris or retina, downslanting palpebral fissures, epicanthal folds, hypertelorism, microphthalmia

*Inheritance*: AD, often de novo

*Known genes or gene locus*: ACTB (Baraitser-Winter syndrome 1), ACTG1 (Baraitser-Winter syndrome 2)

## Barber Say Syndrome[26,27,52,53]

*OMIM*: #209885

*Description*: Barber Say syndrome is a rare mutation in the basic domain of the *TWIST2* gene, affecting its DNA-binding activity. It is characterized by hypertrichosis, macrostomia, atrophic and redundant skin, nipple abnormalities, characteristic facial changes, and eyelid agenesis.

*Epidemiology*: unknown; less than 20 cases in literature

*Eye findings*: corneal clouding, ectropion, exophthalmia, hypertelorism, periorbital fullness, telecanthus, underdeveloped or absent eyelids

*Inheritance*: AD

*Known genes or gene locus*: TWIST2

*Special note*: Similar genotypic and phenotypic findings as ablepharon macrostomia, which may represent a continuum.

## Barth Syndrome[54,55]

*OMIM*: #302060

*Description*: Barth syndrome is caused by mutations in the *TAZ* gene at Xq28, which lead to changes in cardiolipin composition and mitochondrial function. It is characterized by cardiomyopathy and other cardiac abnormalities, skeletal myopathy, prepubertal growth delay, neutropenia, and 3-methylglutaconic aciduria.

*Epidemiology*: prevalence of 1/300,000

*Eye findings*: deep set eyes

*Inheritance*: XLR, 13% de novo

*Known genes or gene locus*: TAZ

## Basal Cell Nevus Syndrome[56–59]

*OMIM*: #109400

*Description*: Basal cell nevus syndrome, also known as Gorlin syndrome, causes increased risk of various neoplasms and developmental abnormalities by mutations in the sonic hedgehog pathway. This syndrome is characterized by multiple basal cell carcinomas, jaw keratocyst, and bifid ribs. Other manifestations include palmar or plantar pits, calcification of falx cerebri, macrocephaly, congenital malformations, polydactyly, skeletal, reproductive, and ocular abnormalities.

*Epidemiology*: prevalence of 1/57,000

*Eye findings*: cataract, coloboma of iris, choroid, and optic nerve, chalazions, exophthalmos, glaucoma, hypertelorism, lateral displacement of inner canthi, medullated retinal nerve fibers, microphthalmia, nystagmus, strabismus, subconjunctival epithelial cysts

*Inheritance*: AD, 40% de novo

*Known genes or gene locus*: PTCH1, PTCH2, SUFU

## Bazex-Dupre-Christol Syndrome[60–62]

*OMIM*: %301845

*Description*: Bazex-Dupre-Christol syndrome is a rare disorder linked to Xq24-q27 that is defined by congenital hypotrichosis; follicular atrophoderma; and hypohidrosis affecting the dorsa of hands and feet, extensor surfaces of elbows and knees and face. With age, basal cell neoplasms develop primarily on the face.

*Epidemiology*: unknown; largely affects individuals of Caucasian descent

*Eye findings*: hypotrichosis of eyebrows, periorbital milia

*Inheritance*: XLD

*Known genes or gene locus*: Xq24-q27. UBE2A is a candidate gene.

## Beckwith-Wiedemann Syndrome[17,63]

*OMIM*: #130650

*Description*: Beckwith-Wiedemann syndrome, caused by a dysregulation of the expression of imprinted genes on chromosome 11p15.5, is a disorder characterized by abnormal prenatal and postnatal overgrowth; macroglossia, omphalocele, and neonatal hypoglycemia may be present, and an associated increase risk of Wilms tumor and hepatoblastoma exist.

*Epidemiology*: incidence of 1/13,700

*Eye findings*: deep-set eyes, downslanting palpebral fissures, epicanthal folds, hypertelorism, synophrys

*Inheritance*: Sporadic (majority of cases), rarely AD

*Known genes or gene locus*: NSD1, H19, KCNQ1OT1, CDKN1C

*Special note*: Abdominal ultrasound exams every 3 months to the age of 8 years (screening for abdominal tumors) and serum α-fetoprotein (AFP) measured every 2–3 months to the age of 4 years (screening for hepatoblastoma) should be part of the tumor surveillance in patients diagnosed or suspected to have the syndrome.

## Blau Syndrome[64–66]

*OMIM*: #186580

*Description*: Blau syndrome is a rare disorder caused by a mutation of *NOD2* at 16q12 and is characterized by granulomatous arthritis, uveitis, and dermatitis. Other manifestations include fever, erythema nodosum, neuropathies, lymphadenopathy, pulmonary, cardiovascular and renal involvement.

*Epidemiology*: unknown

*Eye findings*: band keratopathy, cataract, cystoid macular edema, glaucoma, granulomatous uveitis, hyalitis, iritis, multifocal choroiditis, peripheral synechiae, optic disk edema

*Inheritance*: AD

*Known genes or gene locus*: NOD2

*Special note*: Referred to as early-onset sarcoidosis when de novo mutation.

### Blepharophimosis, Ptosis, and Epicanthus Inversus[18,67,68]

OMIM: #110100

*Description*: BPES syndrome is a dysplasia of the eyelids caused by mutations in *FOXL2* on 3q22 and is characterized by blepharophimosis, bilateral ptosis, epicanthus inversus, telecanthus, and a characteristic backward-tilted head to compensate for visual field defects. Extraocular presentation includes broad nasal bridge, high-arched palate, and cup-shaped ears. BPES type 1 presents with premature ovarian failure, and BPES type 2 presents with normal ovarian function.

*Epidemiology*: prevalence of 1/50,000

*Eye findings*: amblyopia, Axenfeld-Rieger syndrome, blepharophimosis (Fig. 2.4), epicanthus inversus (Fig. 2.4), euryblepharon, hypermetropia, hyperopia, lacrimal drainage abnormalities, microcornea, microphthalmia, myopia, optic disk coloboma, ptosis (Fig. 2.4), nystagmus, pronounced convex arched eyebrows, strabismus, telecanthus (Fig. 2.4)

*Inheritance*: AD, 50% de novo

*Known genes or gene locus*: FOXL2

### Branchiootorenal Syndrome[19,69,70]

OMIM: #113650, #610896

*Description*: Branchiootorenal syndrome is a developmental defect of the second branchial arch caused

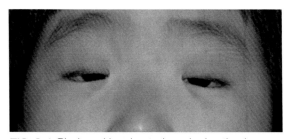

FIG. 2.4 Blepharophimosis, ptosis, and epicanthus inversus syndrome. Note the characteristic blepharophimosis, bilateral ptosis, epicanthus inversus, and telecanthus. (Courtesy Sa HS, MD, Lee JH, MD, Woo KI, MD, Kim YD, MD. A new method of medial epicanthoplasty for patients with Blepharophimosis-Ptosis-Epicanthus Inversus Syndrome. *Ophthalmology*. November 1, 2012;119(11):2402–2407. © 2012.)

by mutations in *EYA1* at 8q13.3 or *SIX5* at 19q13.32. It is characterized by branchial cysts and fistulas, hearing loss and structural ear deformities, and renal hypoplasia.

*Epidemiology*: prevalence of 1/40,000

*Eye findings*: eyes absent, iris atrophy, lacrimal duct aplasia

*Inheritance*: AD, 10% de novo

*Known genes or gene locus*: EYA1 (branchiootorenal syndrome 1), SIX5 (branchiootorenal syndrome 2)

### Cantu Syndrome[71-73]

OMIM: #239850

*Description*: Cantu syndrome involves a mutation of *ABCC9* at 12p12.1. The condition is characterized by congenital hypertrichosis, osteochondrodysplasia, cardiomegaly, and macrosomia, as well as delayed motor and speech development, and learning disabilities. Distinctive facial features include macrocephaly, coarse facies, broad nasal bridge, long philtrum, gingival hyperplasia, thick lips, epicanthal folds, and long curly eyelashes.

*Epidemiology*: unknown; fewer than 50 cases reported

*Eye findings*: epicanthal folds, long eyelashes

*Inheritance*: AD

*Known genes or gene locus*: ABCC9

### Char Syndrome[74-76]

OMIM: #169100

*Description*: Char syndrome is a rare developmental disorder characterized by patent ductus arteriosus, digital abnormalities, and dysmorphic faces. Digital abnormalities include fifth finger clinodactyly and distal interphalangeal joint symphalangism, facial abnormalities include broad forehead, prominent low-set ears, short philtrum, broad nasal bridge, thick lips, triangular mouth, ptosis, hypertelorism, and downslanting palpebral fissures.

*Epidemiology*: unknown

*Eye findings*: downslanting palpebral fissures, hypertelorism, ptosis, strabismus, thick, flared eyebrows

*Inheritance*: AD

*Known genes or gene locus*: TFAP2B

### Cherubism[77-81]

OMIM: #118400

*Description*: Cherubism is characterized by swelling and painless cystlike masses of the mandible and maxilla, beginning in the first few years of life until puberty. This fibrous dysplasia can progress to other parts of the head including the eyes, leading to a series of ocular changes in some patients.

*Epidemiology*: unknown; about 250 cases reported

*Eye findings*: diminished visual field and acuity, globe displacement, lesions in orbital floor, lower eyelid retraction, optic neuropathy, proptosis, scarring of macula, striae of macula, upward turned eyes

*Inheritance*: AD

*Known genes or gene locus*: SH3BP2

## Cohen Syndrome[82-84]

*OMIM*: #216550

*Description*: Cohen syndrome is a developmental abnormality characterized by hypotonia, intellectually disability, delayed milestones, microcephaly, neutropenia, joint laxity, characteristic facial features, overly friendly behavior, and truncal obesity. Characteristic facial features include downslanting palpebral fissures, high-arched eyelids, thick eyebrows, short philtrum, micrognathia, prominent nasal bridge, prominent upper incisors, and open mouth appearance.

*Epidemiology*: unknown; more common in Finnish populations

*Eye findings*: almond-shaped eyes, bull's eye maculopathy, cataract, chorioretinal dystrophy, coloboma of lids and retina, downslanting palpebral fissures, exophthalmos, high-arched eyelids, iris atrophy, microcornea, microphthalmia, myopia, nyctalopia, optic atrophy, oval pupil, ptosis, retinal dystrophy, slow pupillary response, spherophakia, strabismus

*Inheritance*: AR

*Known genes or gene locus*: VPS13B

## Congenital Microcoria[3,85,86]

*OMIM*: #15660

*Description*: Congenital microcoria is caused by mutation at 13q32 and is characterized by pupils less than 2 mm in diameter bilaterally. Defects are localized to the iris, including hypoplastic dilator muscles and underdeveloped iris features, and can result in elevated goniodysgenesis and glaucoma.

*Epidemiology*: unknown

*Eye findings*: astigmatism, elevated intraocular pressure, goniodysgenesis, glaucoma, hypoplasia of iris dilator muscle, iris transillumination defects, microcoria, myopia, photophobia, poorly developed collarettes and crypts, poorly reactive pupils, thickened juxtacanalicular tissue, translucent peripheral iris

*Inheritance*: AD

*Known genes or gene locus*: 13q32, includes TGDS and GPR180

## Cornelia De Lange Syndrome[20,87]

*OMIM*: #122470, #300590, #610759, #614701, #300882

*Description*: Cornelia de Lange syndrome is a heterogenous multisystem developmental disorder characterized by distinctive facial features, microcephaly, hearing loss, intellectually disability, delayed development, upper extremity skeletal deformities, GERD, and hirsutism. Characteristic facial features include low-set ears, short nose, anteverted nares, long smooth philtrum, narrow palpebral fissures, long eyelashes, arched eyebrows, synophrys, ptosis, and hooded eyelids.

*Epidemiology*: incidence of 1/10,000

*Eye findings*: arched eyebrows (Fig. 2.5), blepharitis, cataract, deep-set eyes, downslanting palpebral fissures, glaucoma, hooding of eyelids, hypertelorism, long eyelashes (Fig. 2.5), myopia, nasolacrimal duct obstruction, nystagmus, ptosis, synophrys (Fig. 2.5), telecanthus

*Inheritance*: AD (Type 1, 3, 4), X-linked (Type 2, 5), majority de novo

*Known genes or gene locus*: NIPBL (type 1), SMC1A (type 2), SMC3 (type 3), RAD21 (type 4), HDAC8 (type 5)

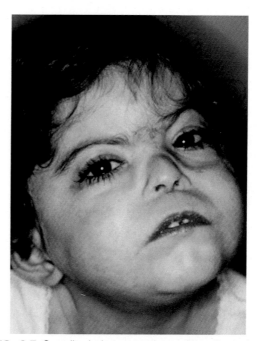

FIG. 2.5 Cornelia de Lange syndrome. Note the arched eyebrows, prominent long eyelashes, and synophrys. (Courtesy Graham JM, Burkardt DDC, Rimoin DL. *Abnormal Body Size and Proportion, Emery and Rimoin's Principles and Practice of Medical Genetics*; January 1, 2013:1–25. © 2013.)

## Crigler-Najjar/Gilbert Syndrome[21,88,89]

*OMIM*: #218800, #606785, #143500

*Description*: Crigler-Najjar and Gilbert syndrome are unconjugated hyperbilirubinemias caused by mutation of *UGT1A1* at 2q37.1. Type II Crigler-Najjar syndrome is sensitive to phenobarbital treatment, whereas type I is not and is more severe.

*Epidemiology*: crigler-Najjar syndrome is rare with incidence about 1/1,000,000; Gilbert syndrome involves 5%–10% of Western European populations

*Eye findings*: jaundice

*Inheritance*: Crigler-Najjar–AD; Gilbert–AR and AD

*Known genes or gene locus*: UGT1A1

## Cutis Laxa, Debre Type[90,91]

*OMIM*: #219200

*Description*: Cutis laxa debre type is a member of a series of rare connective tissue disorders caused by mutation of *ATP6V0A2* at 12q24.31 resulting in abnormal protein glycosylation. It is characterized by cutis laxa, developmental delay and abnormalities, wide fontanelles, hypotonia, ataxia, spasticity, and seizures.

*Epidemiology*: unknown

*Eye findings*: downslanting palpebral fissures, myopia, reverse-V eyebrows, strabismus, telecanthus

*Inheritance*: AR

*Known genes or gene locus*: ATP6V0A2

## Dopamine β-Hydroxylase Deficiency[92–94]

*OMIM*: #223360

*Description*: Dopamine β-hydroxylase deficiency is a rare mutation of *DBH* at 9q34.2, leading to absent norepinephrine and epinephrine and autonomic nervous system changes. This deficiency is characterized by orthostatic hypotension, hypoglycemia, hypotension, syncope, seizures, retrograde ejaculation, nasal congestion, and ptosis.

*Epidemiology*: unknown

*Eye findings*: blepharoptosis, delayed eye opening as a neonate, ptosis

*Inheritance*: AR

*Known genes or gene locus*: DBH

## Dubowitz Syndrome[95–97]

*OMIM*: %223370

*Description*: Dubowitz syndrome is a rare developmental syndrome of an unknown genetic change characterized by intellectual disability, growth retardation, microcephaly, short stature, genital abnormalities, eczema, and characteristic facial features. Facial features include small triangular face, broad and flat nose, sloping forehead, ptosis, and short palpebral fissures.

*Epidemiology*: unknown

*Eye findings*: aniscoria, astigmatism, blue sclera, blepharophimosis, epicanthal folds, esotropia, hyperopia, iris coloboma, iris hypoplasia, megalocornea, microphthalmia, optic nerve cupping, ptosis, short palpebral fissures, sparse lateral eyebrows, strabismus, telecanthus

*Inheritance*: AR (possibly AD)

*Known genes or gene locus*: Unknown

## Dyskeratosis Congenita[98–102]

*OMIM*: #127550, #613989, #613987, #613990, #615190, #268130, #616553, #224230, #613988, #616353, #616553, #305000

*Description*: Dyskeratosis congenita is a progressive bone marrow disorder caused by defective telomerase maintenance. It is characterized by the triad of dystrophic nails, abnormal skin pigmentation, and oral hairy leukoplakia. A series of other systemic abnormalities can also occur, including enteropathy, cardiomyopathy, cirrhosis, intellectual disability, skeletal abnormalities, and many others.

*Epidemiology*: prevalence of 1/1,000,000

*Eye findings*: cataract, conjunctival leukoplakia, epiphora (excessive watering), obstruction of lacrimal ducts, optic atrophy, retinopathy, sparse eyelashes, strabismus

*Inheritance*: AD, AR, X-linked, often de novo

*Known genes or gene locus*: TERC (AD 1), TERT (AD 1, AR 4), TINF2 (AD 3, AD 5), RTEL1 (AD 4, AR 5), ACD (AD 6, AR 7), NOLA3 (AR 1), NOLA2 (AR 2), WRAP53 (AR 3), PARN (AR 6), DKC1 (X-linked), CTC1

## Ectrodactyly-Ectodermal Dysplasia-Clefting Syndrome[103–107]

*OMIM*: %129900, #604292.

*Description*: Ectrodactyly-ectodermal dysplasia-clefting (EEC) syndrome is a rare developmental disorder most commonly caused by a mutation of either *TP63* at 3q28 or an unknown gene linked to 7q11.2-q21.3, characterized by ectrodactyly and syndactyly, cleft lip, and ectodermal dysplasia.

*Epidemiology*: unknown

*Eye findings*: blepharitis, blepharophimosis, corneal clouding, corneal perforation, corneal scarring, dacryocystitis, entropion with trichiasis, glaucoma, lacrimal duct abnormalities, limbal stem cell deficiency, pannus, photophobia, sparse eyelashes and eyebrows

*Inheritance*: AD

*Known genes or gene locus*: 7q11.2-q21.3 (EEC1), *TP63* (EEC3)

*Special note*: May have considerable phenotypic and genotypic overlap with ADULT syndrome, Hays-Wells syndrome, and Limb-Mammary syndrome.

## Frontofacionasal Dysplasia[108,109]

*OMIM*: %229400

*Description*: Frontofacionasal dysplasia is a rare developmental disorder characterized by midface hypoplasia, telecanthus, ocular malformations, S-shaped palpebral fissures, and cranium bifidum.

*Epidemiology*: unknown

*Eye findings*: ankyloblepharon, blepharophimosis, cataract, hypertelorism, incomplete eye closure, lower lid lagophthalmos, microcornea, microphthalmia, ptosis, S-shaped palpebral fissures, telecanthus, upper eyelid and iris coloboma

*Inheritance*: AR

*Known genes or gene locus*: Unknown

## Gillespie Syndrome[110–112]

*OMIM*: #206700

*Description*: Gillespie syndrome is a rare neurologic disorder caused by mutation of *ITPR1* at 3p26.1 and characterized by aniridia, iris hypoplasia, scalloped iris edges, hypotonia, progressive cerebellar hypoplasia, ataxia, and intellectual disability.

*Epidemiology*: unknown

*Eye findings*: aniridia, fixed dilated pupils, iris hypoplasia, nystagmus, photophobia, scalloped pupillary margins of iris, visual impairment

*Inheritance*: AR, AD

*Known genes or gene locus*: *ITPR1*

## Griscelli Syndrome Type 3[113,114]

*OMIM*: #609227

*Description*: Griscelli syndrome type 3, a rare melanocyte transport disorder caused by mutations in *MLPH* at 2q37.3 or in *MYO5A* at 15q21 is characterized by hypopigmentation and gray-silver hair without immunologic or neurologic symptoms.

*Epidemiology*: unknown

*Eye findings*: silver-gray eyelashes and eyebrows

*Inheritance*: AR

*Known genes or gene locus*: *MLPH*, *MYO5A*

## Hays-Wells Syndrome[115,116]

*OMIM*: #106260

*Description*: Hays-Wells syndrome, also known as ankyloblepharon-ectodermal defects-cleft lip/palate, is a rare ectodermal dysplasia caused by mutation of *TP63* at 3q28. This syndrome is characterized by recurring skin erosions, hypodontia, malformed nails, hearing loss, cleft palate/lip, and ankyloblepharon.

*Epidemiology*: unknown

*Eye findings*: ankyloblepharon filiforme adnatum, blepharitis, conjunctivitis, lacrimal duct atresia, sparse eyelashes

*Inheritance*: AD

*Known genes or gene locus*: *TP63*

*Special note*: May have considerable phenotypic and genotypic overlap with ADULT syndrome, EEC syndrome, and Limb-Mammary syndrome. Mutations in *TP63* can cause seven different autosomal dominant syndromes with variable phenotypes, an example of allelic heterogeneity.

## Hereditary Hemorrhagic Telangiectasia (Osler-Rendu-Weber Disease)[22,117–120]

*OMIM*: #187300, #600376, %601101, %610655, #615506 #175050

*Description*: Hereditary hemorrhagic telangiectasia is a vascular dysplasia characterized by telangiectases, epistaxis, and visceral legions. It may involve brain, liver, lungs, and skin. Juvenile hereditary hemorrhagic telangiectasia is also characterized by gastrointestinal polyps.

*Epidemiology*: incidence of 1/5000

*Eye findings*: branch retinal artery occlusion, choroidal hemorrhage, conjunctival telangiectases, hematic epiphora, retinal vascular abnormalities, visceral angiodysplasia

*Inheritance*: AD

*Known genes or gene locus*: *ENG* (Type 1), *ACVRL1* (Type 2), *HHT3* (Type 3), *HHT4* (Type 4), *GDF2* (Type 5)

## Hermansky-Pudlak Syndrome[121–123]

*OMIM*: #203300, #608233, #614072, #614073, #614074, #614075, #614076, #614077, #614171, #617050

*Description*: Hermansky-Pudlak syndrome is a disorder characterized by OCA, ceroid deposition, and platelet deficiency caused by a series of different mutations affecting lysosomal trafficking. Other manifestations include issues with coagulation, granulomatous colitis, pulmonary fibrosis, kidney failure, neutropenia, and increased risk of skin cancers.

*Epidemiology*: prevalence of 1/500,000–1,000,000 worldwide; 1/1800 in Puerto Rico

*Eye findings*: diminished visual acuity, esotropia, foveal hypoplasia, hypermetropic astigmatism, hypopigmented retina, iris heterochromia, iris transillumination, ocular melanocytosis, OCA, nystagmus, photophobia, reduced iris pigment

*Inheritance*: AR
*Known genes or gene locus*: *HPS1* (HSP1), *AP3B1* (HSP2), *HPS3* (HSP), *HPS4* (HSP4), *HPS5* (HSP5), *HPS6* (HSP6), *DTNBP1* (HSP7), *BLOC1S3* (HSP8), *BLOC1S6* (HSP9), *AP3D1* (HSP10)

## Ichthyosis Lamellar[124–128]

OMIM: #242300, #242100, #606545, #601277, #242500, #604777, #612281, #615022, #613943, #615023, #615024, #602400, #617320, #617574, #617571, 146750

*Description*: Ichthyosis lamellar is a series of skin disorders caused by a variety of mutations, characterized by abnormal keratinization. Manifestations include collodion membrane at birth, erythroderma, keratoderma, scaly skin, alopecia, hypohidrosis, joint deformities, eclabium (turning outward of the lip), and ectropion.

*Epidemiology*: incidence of 1/300,000–500,000

*Eye findings*: cicatricial lagophthalmos, ectropion leading to corneal damage, eyelash retraction madarosis

*Inheritance*: AR (recessive type 1–14), AD (no genes identified)

*Known genes or gene locus*: *TGM1* (Type 1), *ALOX12B* (Type 2), *ALOXE3* (Type 3), *ABCA12* (Type 4A, 4B), *CYP4F22* (Type 5), *NIPAL4* (Type 6), *ARCI7* (Type 7), *LIPN* (Type 8), *CERS3* (Type 9), *PNPLA1* (Type 10), *ST14* (Type 11), *CASP14* (Type 12), *SDR9C7* (Type 13), *SULT2B1* (Type 14)

## Juberg-Marsidi Syndrome[129–131]

OMIM: #309580

*Description*: Juberg-Marsidi syndrome belongs to a group of X-Linked intellectual disability syndromes caused by mutation of *ATRX* at Xq21.1. This syndrome is characterized by severe intellectual disability, impaired growth, hypotonic facies, hearing deficits, and hypogonadism. Facial dysmorphism characterized by flat and broad nasal bridge, midface hypoplasia, small low-set ears, macrostomia, prominent upper incisors, epicanthal folds, ptosis, exotropia, and upslanting palpebral fissures.

*Epidemiology*: unknown

*Eye findings*: epicanthal folds, exotropia, hypertelorism, optic atrophy, ptosis, upslanting palpebral fissures

*Inheritance*: XLR

*Known genes or gene locus*: *ATRX*

## Kabuki Syndrome[23,132,133]

OMIM: #147920, #300867

*Description*: Kabuki syndrome is a multisystem cognitive impairment syndrome characterized by intellectual disability, growth deficiency, hypotonia, seizures, microcephaly, skeletal abnormalities, fetal finger pads, frequent otitis media, cardiovascular abnormalities, and characteristic facies. Facial features include prominent nose, large ears, high-arched palate, long palpebral fissures, ptosis, thick eyelashes, and arched eyebrows.

*Epidemiology*: prevalence of 1/32,000

*Eye findings*: arched and sparse eyebrows, blue sclera, cataract, eversion of lower eyelid, long thick eyelashes, long palpebral fissures, Marcus Gunn phenomenon, megalocornea, microcornea, nystagmus, optic nerve hypoplasia, Peter's anomaly, ptosis, retinal and ocular coloboma strabismus

*Inheritance*: AD (Kabuki syndrome 1), XLD (Kabuki syndrome 2)

*Known genes or gene locus*: *KMT2D* (Kabuki syndrome 1), *KDM6A* (Kabuki syndrome 2)

## Kaufman Oculocerebrofacial Syndrome[134,135]

OMIM: #244450

*Description*: Kaufman oculocerebrofacial syndrome is a rare developmental disorder caused by mutation of *UBE3B* at 12q24.11, characterized by intellectual disability, microcephaly, distinctive facial features, growth deficiency, and hypotonia. Facial features include flat philtrum, micrognathia, high palate, anteverted nares, broad eyebrows, telecanthus, blepharophimosis, ptosis, and epicanthal folds.

*Epidemiology*: unknown

*Eye findings*: blepharophimosis, coloboma, entropion, epicanthal folds, hyperopia, microcornea, microphthalmia, myopia, nasolacrimal duct stenosis, nystagmus, optic nerve hypoplasia, pale optic disc sparse and broad eyebrows, ptosis, strabismus, telecanthus, upslanting palpebral fissures

*Inheritance*: AR

*Known genes or gene locus*: *UBE3B*

## Lacrimo-Auriculo-Dento-Digital Syndrome[136–141]

OMIM: #149730

*Description*: Lacrimo-auriculo-dento-digital syndrome is a rare multiple congenital abnormality disorder caused by mutation of fibroblast growth factor genes. It is characterized by lacrimal duct abnormalities, low-set cup-shaped ears and hearing loss, underdeveloped salivary glands, and teeth and finger abnormalities.

*Epidemiology*: unknown

*Eye findings*: alacrima, corneal ulcerations and perforation, dacryocystitis, diffuse ophthalmoplegia, downslanting palpebral fissures, epiblepharon, epiphora, hypesthesia, hypertelorism, keratoconjunctivitis sicca, lacrimal duct and puncta hypoplasia, lacrimal duct obstruction, limbal stem cell deficiency, ptosis, recurrent conjunctivitis, telecanthus

*Inheritance*: AD

*Known genes or gene locus*: FGFR3, FGF10, FGFR2

## LEOPARD Syndrome[142–144]

*OMIM*: #151100, #611554, #613707

*Description*: LEOPARD syndrome is a rare multisystem disorder characterized by multiple lentigines, electrocardiographic conduction abnormalities, ocular hypertelorism, pulmonic stenosis, abnormal genitalia, retardation of growth, and sensorineural deafness. The syndrome is caused by dysregulated RAS-MAPK trafficking, most frequently a mutation of *PTPN11* at 12q24.13.

*Epidemiology*: unknown; about 200 cases reported

*Eye findings*: epicanthal folds, hypertelorism, ptosis, strabismus

*Inheritance*: AD

*Known genes or gene locus*: PTPN11 (LEOPARD syndrome 1), RAF1 (LEOPARD syndrome 2), BRAF (LEOPARD syndrome 3), MAP2K1

## Limb-Mammary Syndrome[107,145]

*OMIM*: #603543

*Description*: Limb-Mammary syndrome is a rare developmental disorder caused by mutation of *TP63* at 3q28 characterized by nipple and mammary gland hypoplasia, ectrodactyly, hypodontia, hypohidrosis, clef palate, and lacrimal duct atresia.

*Epidemiology*: unknown

*Eye findings*: lacrimal duct atresia

*Inheritance*: AD

*Known genes or gene locus*: TP63

*Special note*: May have considerable phenotypic and genotypic overlap with ADULT syndrome, EEC syndrome, and Hays-Wells syndrome.

## Lymphedema-Distichiasis Syndrome[10,11]

*OMIM*: #153400

*Description*: Lymphedema-distichiasis syndrome is a rare disorder caused by the mutation of *FOXC2* at 16q24.1 and characterized by lymphedema, distichiasis, cardiac defects, varicose veins, cleft palate, spinal extradural cysts, photophobia, and ptosis.

*Epidemiology*: unknown

*Eye findings*: astigmatism, conjunctivitis, corneal irritation, distichiasis, ptosis, photophobia, stye

*Inheritance*: AD

*Known genes or gene locus*: FOXC2

## Melnick-Needles Syndrome[146,147]

*OMIM*: #309350

*Description*: Melnick-Needles syndrome is caused by mutations in the *FLNA* gene. Phenotypic characteristics include curvature of the spine, joint dislocations, and unusually long fingers and toes. Abnormalities with bone structure exist including bowed limbs, underdeveloped, irregular ribs, and absent bones.

*Epidemiology*: unknown; fewer than 100 reported cases

*Eye findings*: exophthalmos, proptosis

*Inheritance*: XLD

*Known genes or gene locus*: FLNA

## Menkes Disease[148,149]

*OMIM*: #309400

*Description*: Menkes disease, a disorder of copper transport, is characterized by features including sparse, kinky hair, failure to thrive, and deterioration of the nervous system. Additional features include weak muscle tone, sagging facial features, seizures, developmental delay, intellectual disability, and early death.

*Epidemiology*: incidence of 1/100,000–1/250,000

*Eye findings*: retinal degeneration

*Inheritance*: XLR

*Known genes or gene locus*: ATP7A

## Mental Retardation, X-Linked, With Cerebellar Hypoplasia and Distinctive Facial Appearance[150,151]

*OMIM*: #300486

*Description*: Features of this disease include hypotonia with motor delay, marked strabismus, early-onset complex partial seizures, and moderate to severe intellectual disability.

*Epidemiology*: unknown

*Eye findings*: deep-set eyes, hypotelorism, nystagmus, strabismus

*Inheritance*: XLR

*Known genes or gene locus*: OPHN15

## Mevalonic Aciduria[152,153]

*OMIM*: #610377

*Description*: Mevalonic aciduria is a genetic disorder affecting cholesterol and isoprenoid biosynthesis that causes short stature, psychomotor retardation, progressive cerebellar ataxia, febrile crises, hepatosplenomegaly, lymphadenopathy, arthralgia, and skin rashes. Affected individuals have mevalonic aciduria and low to normal cholesterol levels, as well as elevated creatine kinase levels. It is allelic to hyper-IgD syndrome.

*Epidemiology*: prevalence of <1/1,000,000

*Eye findings*: attenuation of retinal vessel, blue sclerae, central cataracts, downslanting palpebral fissures, moderate atrophy of optic disc, nuclear cataract, nystagmus, retinal dystrophy, undetectable rod and cone responses on electroretinography

*Inheritance*: AR

*Known genes or gene locus*: MVK

### Methylmalonic Aciduria and Homocystinuria, CblF [154,155]

OMIM: #277380

*Description*: This disease is characterized by megaloblastic anemia, lethargy, failure to thrive, developmental delay, intellectual deficit, and seizures. This is a disorder of cobalamin metabolism that affects biosynthesis of both adenosylcobalamin (AdoCbl) and methylcobalamin (MeCbl) resulting in absent methylmalonyl-CoA mutase and methionine synthase activities, accounting for the presence of methylmalonic aciduria and homocystinuria.

*Epidemiology*: prevalence of <1/1,000,000

*Eye findings*: epicanthal folds, nystagmus, retinopathy

*Inheritance*: AR

*Known genes or gene locus*: LMBRD1

### Miller Syndrome [156–158]

OMIM: #263750

*Description*: Miller syndrome features facial abnormalities including underdeveloped cheek bones, a small lower jaw, cleft lip and/or palate, abnormalities of the eyes, absent fifth (pinky) fingers and toes. Additional skeletal abnormalities include abnormal bones in the forearms and lower legs.

*Epidemiology*: prevalence of 1/1,000,000

*Eye findings*: downslanting palpebral fissures, ectropion, eyelid coloboma

*Inheritance*: AR

*Known genes or gene locus*: DHODH

### Moyamoya Disease, Syndromic [159–161]

OMIM: #300845

*Description*: Patients with Moyamoya disease have short stature, hypergonadotropic hypogonadism, and facial dysmorphism. Other variable features include dilated cardiomyopathy, premature graying of the hair, and early-onset cataracts.

*Epidemiology*: incidence of 1/1,000,000

*Eye findings*: cataracts, deep-set eyes, hypertelorism, ptosis

*Inheritance*: XLR

*Known genes or gene locus*: Deletion of Xq28

### Mucopolysaccharidosis Type IIIA (Sanfilippo Syndrome A) [162–164]

OMIM: #252900

*Description*: This lysosomal storage disease involves neurologic symptoms such as progressive dementia, aggressive behavior, hyperactivity, seizures, deafness, loss of vision, and insomnia. Dysostosis multiplex is also commonly seen, although there is variable presence of macrocephaly and coarse facial features. This condition is associated with accumulation of heparan sulfate. The MPS III disorders are examples of locus heterogeneity. The syndrome involves a deficiency of the enzyme heparan N-sulfatase.

*Epidemiology*: incidence of 1–9/100,000

*Eye findings*: clear corneas, synophrys

*Inheritance*: AR

*Known genes or gene locus*: SGSH

### Mucopolysaccharidosis Type IIIB (Sanfilippo Syndrome B) [165–167]

OMIM: #252920

*Description*: This lysosomal storage disease that results in accumulation of heparan sulfate, features progressive neurodegeneration, behavioral problems, mild skeletal changes, and reduced life span. Macrocephaly and coarse facial features may also be present. The syndrome involves a deficiency of the enzyme alpha-N-acetylglucosaminidase.

*Epidemiology*: incidence of <1/1,000,000

*Eye findings*: clear corneas, synophrys

*Inheritance*: AR

*Known genes or gene locus*: NAGLU

### Mucopolysaccharidosis Type IIIC (Sanfilippo Syndrome C) [168,169]

OMIM: #252930

*Description*: This lysosomal storage disease that results in accumulation of heparan sulfate features severe neurologic symptoms, including progressive dementia, aggressive behavior, hyperactivity, seizures, deafness, and loss of vision. Macrocephaly and coarse facial features may also be present. The syndrome involves a deficiency of the enzyme acetyl CoA:alpha-glucosaminide acetyltransferase.

*Epidemiology*: incidence of <1/1,000,000

*Eye findings*: clear corneas, pigmentary retinopathy, synophrys

*Inheritance*: AR

*Known genes or gene locus*: HGSNAT

### Mucopolysaccharidosis Type IIID (Sanfilippo Syndrome D) [170,171]

OMIM: #252940

*Description*: This lysosomal storage disease that result in accumulation of heparin sulfate features severe neurologic symptoms, including progressive dementia, aggressive behavior, hyperactivity, seizures, deafness, loss of vision. Macrocephaly and coarse facial features may also be present. The syndrome involves a deficiency of the enzyme N-acetylglucosamine 6-sulfatase.

*Epidemiology*: incidence of <1/1,000,000

*Eye findings*: clear corneas, synophrys

*Inheritance*: AR

*Known genes or gene locus*: GNS

## Nager Acrofacial Dysostosis[172–174]

*OMIM*: #154400

*Description*: Nager acrofacial dysotosis features facial abnormalities including downslanted palpebral fissures, midface retrusion, and micrognathia. Limb skeletal anomalies found with the disorder include small or absent thumbs, triphalangeal thumbs, radial hypoplasia or aplasia, radioulnar synostosis, phocomelia of the upper limbs, and occasionally lower-limb defects.

*Epidemiology*: unknown

*Eye findings*: downslanting palpebral fissures, lower lid coloboma, partial-total absence of lower eyelashes

*Inheritance*: AD

*Known genes or gene locus*: SF3B4

## Native American Myopathy[175,176]

*OMIM*: #255995

*Description*: Native American myopathy features weakness, arthrogryposis, kyphoscoliosis, short stature, cleft palate, ptosis, and susceptibility to malignant hyperthermia.

*Epidemiology*: prevalence of 1/5000 within the Native American Lumbee population in North Carolina, USA

*Eye findings*: ptosis, short and downslanting palpebral fissures, telecanthus

*Inheritance*: AR

*Known genes or gene locus*: STAC3

## Neonatal Progeroid Syndrome[177,178]

*OMIM*: %264090

*Description*: Neonatal progeroid syndrome is characterized by a noticeably aged appearance at birth, intrauterine growth restriction, feeding difficulties, distinctive craniofacial features, hypotonia, developmental delay, and intellectual disability.

*Epidemiology*: prevalence of <1/1,000,000

*Eye findings*: blue sclerae, entropion, hypertelorism, nystagmus, sparse eyelashes, upward slanting palpebral fissures

*Inheritance*: AR

*Known genes or gene locus*: Unknown

## Neurofibromatosis-Noonan Syndrome[179,180]

*OMIM*: #601321

*Description*: Neurofibromatosis-Noonan syndrome is a disorder characterized by abnormal facial features, short stature, hypertelorism, cardiac anomalies, neurologic anomalies, deafness, motor delay, and bleeding disorders.

*Epidemiology*: unknown

*Eye findings*: downslanting palpebral fissures, epicanthal folds, hypertelorism, Lisch nodules, ptosis

*Inheritance*: AD

*Known genes or gene locus*: NF1

## Noonan Syndrome[24,181,182]

*OMIM*: #163950

*Description*: Noonan syndrome contains features including distinctive facial appearance, short stature, a broad or webbed neck, congenital heart defects, bleeding problems, skeletal malformations, and developmental delay.

*Epidemiology*: prevalence of 6/10,000–9/10,000

*Eye findings*: downslanting palpebral fissures (Fig. 2.6), epicanthal folds, hypertelorism (Fig. 2.6), myopia, ptosis

*Inheritance*: AD

*Known genes or gene locus*: PTPN11, KRAS, SOS1, SOS2, BRAF, RAF1, NRAS, RIT1, LZTR1

## Ocular Albinism[15,183]

*OMIM*: #300500

*Description*: Ocular albinism phenotypic features include nystagmus, impaired vision, iris hypopigmentation with translucency, albinotic fundus, macular hypoplasia; individuals generally have normally pigmented skin and hair. Female carriers may have a punctate iris translucency with mottling of the fundus. Individuals of black or Asian heritage may have brown irides without translucency and a variable hypopigmentation of the fundus.

*Epidemiology*: prevalence of 1/50,000

*Eye findings*: decreased iris pigment, foveal hypoplasia nystagmus, strabismus, translucent iris (Fig. 2.7)

*Inheritance*: X-linked

*Known genes or gene locus*: GPR143

## Oculoauriculofrontonasal Syndrome[184–186]

*OMIM*: #601452

*Description*: The oculoauriculofrontonasal syndrome phenotypic features originate from anomalies of the embryological first and second branchial arches. Clinical features include microtia/skin tags, epibulbar dermoids, cleft lip/palate, mandibular hypoplasia, and facial asymmetry; malformations are due to the anomalous development of the frontonasal eminence and maxillary processes.

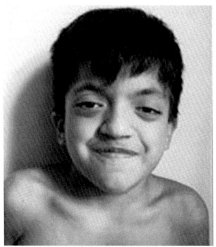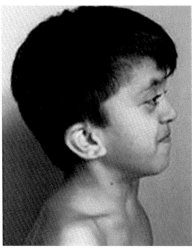

FIG. 2.6 Noonan syndrome. Note the downslanting palpebral fissures and hypertelorism (left photo) with low-set and posteriorly rotated ears (right photo). (Courtesy Koch A, DDS, MD, Eisig S, DDS. Syndromes with unusual Facies. *Atlas Oral Maxillofac Surg Clin N Am*. September 1, 2014;22(2):205–210. © 2014; From Tartaglia M, Gelb BD, Zenker M. Noonan syndrome and clinically related disorders. *Best Pract Res Clin Endocrinol Metab*. 2011;25(1):161–79; with permission.)

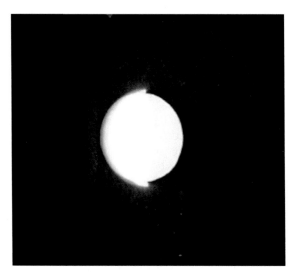

FIG. 2.7 Diffuse iris transillumination defects by retroillumination on slit-lamp examination. (Courtesy Kubal A, MD, Dagnelie G, PhD, Goldberg M, MD. Ocular albinism with absent foveal pits but without nystagmus, photophobia, or severely reduced vision. *Journal AAPOS*. December 1, 2009;13(6):610–612. © 2009.)

*Epidemiology*: prevalence: < 1/1,000,000
*Eye findings*: downslanted palpebral fissures, hypertelorism, ocular dermoids
*Inheritance*: Unknown
*Known genes or gene locus*: Unknown

## Oculocerebral Syndrome With Hypopigmentation[187,188]

*OMIM*: #257800

*Description*: Oculocerebral hypopigmentation syndrome is a rare congenital syndrome characterized by cutaneous and ocular hypopigmentation, ocular anomalies, growth deficiency, intellectual deficit and progressive neurologic anomalies such as spastic tetraplegia, hyperreflexia, and/or athetoid movements.

*Epidemiology*: unknown

*Eye findings*: blue sclerae, corneal and lens opacity, nystagmus, ocular hypopigmentation, spastic ectropium

*Inheritance*: AR

*Known genes or gene locus*: 3q27.1q29

## Oculocutaneous Albinism[16,108,189,190,251]

*OMIM*: #20310

*Description*: Oculocutaneous albinism affects pigmentation of the skin, hair, and eyes. Affected individuals typically have very fair skin and white- or light-colored hair.

*Epidemiology*: prevalence of 1/20,000

*Eye findings*: decreased iris pigment, foveal hypoplasia nystagmus, strabismus, translucent iris

*Inheritance*: AR

*Known genes or gene gocus*: TYR, OCA2, TYRP1, SLC45A2, MC1R, SLC24A5, C10orf11

## Oculopharyngeal Muscular Dystrophy[191,192]

OMIM: #164300

*Description*: Oculopharyngeal muscular dystrophy is an adult-onset genetic disorder characterized by slowly progressing muscle disease affecting the muscles of the upper eyelids and the throat. Patients experience eyelid drooping, arm and leg weakness, and difficulty in swallowing due to their muscle weakness. This condition is caused by (GCG)n repeat expansion from the normal 6 repeats to pathologic 8−13 repeats, with severity depending upon the number of polyalanine repeats present as well as concomitant presence of a (GCG)7 polymorphism. Rarely, homozygosity for a (GCG)7 polymorphism results in recessive disease.

*Epidemiology*: prevalence of 1/100,000−9/100,000; more common in individuals of French-Canadian, Bukhara Jewish, and French populations

*Eye findings*: extraocular movements may be mildly decreased, ptosis

*Inheritance*: AD, AR (rare)

*Known genes or gene locus: PABPN1*

## Oral-Facial-Digital Syndrome[193,194]

OMIM: #311200

*Description*: Oral-facial-digital syndrome is a genetic condition that affects the development of the oral cavity, facial features, and digits. The condition can also be associated with polycystic kidney disease.

*Epidemiology*: prevalence of 1/50,000−1/250,000

*Eye findings*: downslanting palpebral fissures, epicanthus, hypertelorism, nystagmus, strabismus, telecanthus

*Inheritance*: AR, XLD

*Known genes or gene locus: OFD1*

## Osteogenesis Imperfecta[25,195,196]

OMIM: #166200

*Description*: Osteogenesis imperfecta is a genetic disorder in which bone development is severely affected which causes them to break easily. Other distinctive features include weak muscles, brittle teeth, a curved spine, dental problems, and hearing loss.

*Epidemiology*: prevalence of 6/100,000−7/100,000

*Eye findings*: blue or gray sclera

*Inheritance*: AD (most common), AR, sporadic

*Known genes or gene locus: COL1A1, COL1A2, CRTAP, LEPRE1*

## Phenylketonuria[197−199]

OMIM: #261600

*Description*: Phenylketonuria or PKU, a genetic metabolic disorder caused by deficiency of phenylalanine hydroxylase. Clinical features may include eczema, light skin, intellectual disability, seizures, delayed development, musty odor, behavioral problems, and psychiatric disorders. The disorder is included on the Recommended Uniform Screening Panel (RUSP) for newborn screening, and outcome is generally good with strict adherence to specific lifetime diet modifications. Deficient enzyme activity results in both elevated phenylalanine and its derivatives, as well as decreased levels of tyrosine which is necessary for generation of melanin and neurotransmitters.

*Epidemiology*: incidence of 1/10,000−15,000

*Eye findings*: possible cataracts and blue eyes in untreated

*Inheritance*: AR

*Known genes or gene locus: PAH*

## Piebaldism[200,201]

OMIM: #172800

*Description*: Piebaldism is an extremely rare autosomal dominant trait characterized by the congenital absence of melanocytes in affected areas of the skin and hair, white forelock of hair. Other dermatologic anomalies may include irregularly shaped white patches on the face, trunk, and extremities.

*Epidemiology*: unknown

*Eye findings*: heterochromia iridis

*Inheritance*: AD

*Known genes or gene locus: KIT, SNAI2*

## Popliteal Pterygium Syndrome[202−204]

OMIM: #119500

*Description*: Popliteal pterygium syndrome is a genetic disease characterized by abnormal development of the face, skin, and genitals. Phenotypic expression of this disease includes cleft lip, with or without cleft palate, contractures of the lower extremities with skin webbing at the back of the knee, abnormal external genitalia, syndactyly of fingers and/or toes, and a pyramidal skin fold over the hallux nail.

*Epidemiology*: incidence of 1/300,000

*Eye findings*: congenital ankyloblepharon filiforme

*Inheritance*: AD

*Known genes or gene locus: IRF6*

## Prieto Syndrome[205,206]

OMIM: %309610

*Description*: Prieto syndrome is a genetic disorder characterized by intellectual disability, facial dysmorphism, patella luxation, clinodactyly, subcortical cerebral atrophy, and abnormal teeth growth.

*Epidemiology*: unknown

*Eye findings*: epicanthal folds, hypertelorism, nystagmus, ptosis, strabismus

*Inheritance*: XLR

*Known genes or gene locus: Xp11-q21*

## Proud Syndrome[207,208]

*OMIM*: #300004

*Description*: Proud syndrome is a genetic and developmental disorder characterized by agenesis of the corpus callosum, intellectual disability, spasticity, seizures, microcephaly, limb contractures, scoliosis, tapered fingers with hyperconvex nails, abnormal facial features including large eyes, prominent supraorbital ridges, synophrys, optic atrophy, broad alveolar ridges. Renal and urologic anomalies include renal dysplasia, cryptorchidism, and hypospadias.

*Epidemiology*: unknown

*Eye findings*: nystagmus, optic atrophy, strabismus, synophrys

*Inheritance*: X-linked

*Known genes or gene locus*: ARX

## Roberts Syndrome[209,210]

*OMIM*: #268300

*Description*: Roberts syndrome is a rare autosomal recessive disorder characterized by pre- and postnatal growth deficiency, microcephaly, encephalocele, bilateral cleft lip and palate, and mesomelic symmetric upper and lower limb reduction. Prominent craniofacial features include cleft lip, cleft palate, and micrognathia, ear abnormalities, hypertelorism, downslanting palpebral fissures, and small nostrils.

*Epidemiology*: unknown; 150 reported cases

*Eye findings*: bluish sclerae, cataracts, corneal clouding, downslanting palpebral fissures, exophthalmos, hypertelorism, lid coloboma, microphthalmia

*Inheritance*: AR

*Known genes or gene locus*: ESCO2

## Russell-Silver Syndrome[211–213]

*OMIM*: #180860

*Description*: Russell-Silver syndrome is characterized by severe intrauterine growth retardation, poor postnatal growth, failure to thrive, abnormal craniofacial features including triangular shaped face and a broad forehead, and body asymmetry.

*Epidemiology*: incidence of 1/30,000–100,000

*Eye findings*: blue sclera

*Inheritance*: AD, AR, sporadic (most cases); epigenetic hypomethylation of the H19/IGF2-imprinting control region; maternal uniparental disomy of chromosome 7

*Known genes or gene locus*: H19, IGF2

## Schwartz Jampel Syndrome[214–216]

*OMIM*: #255800

*Description*: Schwartz Jampel syndrome is a rare autosomal recessive disorder characterized by permanent myotonia and abnormal skeletal development and dysplasia which results in reduced stature, kyphoscoliosis, bowing of the diaphyses, and irregular epiphyses.

*Epidemiology*: prevalence of <1/1,000,000

*Eye findings*: cataract, blepharophimosis, long eyelashes in irregular rows, microcornea, myopia. narrow palpebral fissures, ptosis

*Inheritance*: AR

*Known genes or gene locus*: HSPG2

## Shashi X-Linked Mental Retardation Syndrome (Mental Retardation, X-Linked, Syndromic 11)[217,218]

*OMIM*: #300238

*Description*: This genetic disease is characterized by moderate intellectual deficiency, obesity, macroorchidism, and characteristic facial features.

*Epidemiology*: unknown

*Eye findings*: narrow palpebral fissures, periorbital fullness, prominent supraorbital ridges

*Inheritance*: XLR

*Known genes or gene locus*: RBMX

## SHORT Syndrome[219,220]

*OMIM*: #269880

*Description*: A rare, multisystem disease characterized by short stature; anomalies of the anterior chamber of the eye; craniofacial features such as triangular facies, lack of facial fat, and hypoplastic nasal alae with overhanging columella, partial lipodystrophy, hernias, hyperextensibility, and poor dentition.

*Epidemiology*: prevalence of <1/1,000,000

*Eye findings*: cataracts, deep-set eyes glaucoma, megalocornea, myopia, Rieger anomaly, telecanthus

*Inheritance*: AD

*Known genes or gene locus*: PIK3R1

## Simpson-Golabi-Behmel Syndrome[221–223]

*OMIM*: #312870, #300209

*Description*: Simpson-Golabi-Behmel syndrome is characterized by distinctive facial features including widely spaced eyes, large mouth and tongue, a broad nose with an upturned tip, and abnormalities of the palate.

*Epidemiology*: unknown
*Eye findings*: downslanting palpebral fissures, epicanthal folds, hypertelorism
*Inheritance*: XLR
*Known genes or gene locus*: GPC3, OFD1

## Sotos Syndrome[224–226]
OMIM: #117550
*Description*: Sotos syndrome is a genetic disease with a general overgrowth along with developmental delay, intellectual disability advanced bone age, and abnormal craniofacial morphology including macrodolichocephaly with frontal bossing, frontoparietal sparseness of hair, apparent hypertelorism, downslanting palpebral fissures, and facial flushing.
*Epidemiology*: incidence of 1/10,000–1/14,000
*Eye findings*: downslanting palpebral fissures, hyperopia, nystagmus, strabismus
*Inheritance*: AD
*Known genes or gene locus*: NSD1

## Tangier Disease[227,228]
OMIM: #205400
*Description*: Tangier disease is an autosomal recessive disorder characterized by markedly reduced levels of plasma high-density lipoproteins resulting in tissue accumulation of cholesterol esters. Clinical features include very large, yellow-orange tonsils, enlarged liver, spleen and lymph nodes, and hypocholesterolemia.
*Epidemiology*: unknown
*Eye findings*: cicatricial ectropion, corneal opacities, decreased corneal sensation due to peripheral neuropathy, exposure keratopathy, incomplete eyelid closure
*Inheritance*: AR
*Known genes or gene locus*: ABCA1

## Tarp Syndrome[229,230]
OMIM: #311900
*Description*: Tarp syndrome features talipes equinovarus, atrial septal defect, robin sequence, and persistent left superior vena cava and generally affects males.
*Epidemiology*: unknown
*Eye findings*: hypertelorism, optic atrophy, short palpebral fissures, underdeveloped supraorbital ridges
*Inheritance*: XLR
*Known genes or gene locus*: RBM10

## Tietz Syndrome[231–233]
OMIM: #103500
*Description*: Tietz syndrome, also called Tietz albinism-deafness syndrome (TADS), is a genetic disease that is characterized by congenital bilateral sensorineural hearing loss and generalized albino-like hypopigmentation of skin, eyes, and hair.
*Epidemiology*: prevalence of <1/1,000,000
*Eye findings*: blue eyes, hypopigmented fundi, no heterochromia iridis, white eyebrows, white eyelashes
*Inheritance*: AD
*Known genes or gene locus*: MITF

## Triple A Syndrome[234–236]
OMIM: #231550
*Description*: Triple A syndrome is an autosomal recessive disorder characterized by adrenocorticotropic hormone–resistant adrenal failure, achalasia of the esophageal cardia, and alacrima. Neurologic impairment involving the central, peripheral, and autonomic nervous system occurs. Other features of this disorder include palmoplantar hyperkeratosis, short stature, facial dysmorphy, and osteoporosis.
*Epidemiology*: unknown
*Eye findings*: alacrima, anisocoria due to autonomic dysfunction, optic atrophy
*Inheritance*: AR
*Known genes or gene locus*: AAAS

## Tucker Syndrome[237,250]
OMIM: 193240
*Description*: Tucker syndrome features bilateral ptosis of the eyelids and bilateral recurrent laryngeal nerve paralysis.
*Epidemiology*: unknown
*Eye findings*: bilateral ptosis
*Inheritance*: AD
*Known genes or gene locus*: Unknown

## Waardenburg Syndrome[238–241]
OMIM: #193500
*Description*: Waardenburg syndrome is a genetic condition characterized by hearing loss and varied pigmentation of the eyes, hair, and skin. A distinctive white forelock (hair just above the forehead) or early graying of scalp hair may be noted.
*Epidemiology*: incidence of 1/40,000
*Eye findings*: blepharophimosis, blue irides, heterochromia iridis (Fig. 2.8), hypertelorism, synophrys, hypertelorism, dystopia canthorum (W index > 1.95 as a major criteria for Waardenburg syndrome type I)
*Inheritance*: AD, AR
*Known genes or gene locus*: EDN3, EDNRB, MITF, PAX3, SNAI2, SOX10

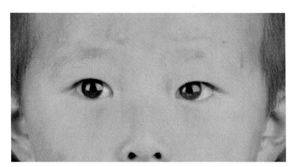

FIG. 2.8 Waardenburg syndrome. Note the iris hetero-chromia and dystopia canthorum. (Courtesy Ma J, Zhang TS, Lin K, Sun H, Jiang HC, Yang YL, Low F, Gao YQ, Ruan B. Waardenburg syndrome type II in a Chinese patient caused by a novel nonsense mutation in the SOX10 gene. *Int J Pediatr Otorhinolaryngol.* June 1, 2016;85:56−61. © 2016.)

*Special note*: To calculate W index in millimeters, see below; abnormal is W > 1.95.

a = inner canthal distance, in millimeters
b = interpupillary distance, in millimeters
c = outer canthal distance, in millimeters
$$X = (2a − (0.2119c + 3.909))/c$$
$$Y = (2a − (0.2479\, b + 3.909))/b$$
$$W = X + Y + a/b$$

### WAGR Syndrome[14,242,243]

*OMIM*: #194072

*Description*: WAGR syndrome is a rare genetic syndrome in which affected children are predisposed to develop *W*ilms tumor, *A*niridia (absence of the colored part of the eye, the iris), *G*enitourinary anomalies, and intellectual disability (formerly called mental *R*etardation).

*Epidemiology*: prevalence of 1/500,000−1/1,000,000
*Eye findings*: aniridia
*Inheritance*: AD, sporadic
*Known genes or gene locus*: PAX6, WT1, BDNF

### Watson Syndrome[244,245]

*OMIM*: #193520

*Description*: Watson syndrome is an autosomal dominant disorder characterized by pulmonic stenosis, cafe-au-lait macules, decreased intellectual ability, and short stature. Most affected individuals have relative macrocephaly and Lisch nodules, and about one-third of those affected reportedly have neurofibromas. This condition may be a variant of neurofibromatosis.

*Epidemiology*: unknown

*Eye findings*: lisch nodules
*Inheritance*: AD
*Known genes or gene locus*: NF1

### X-Linked Hypohidrotic Ectodermal Dysplasia[246−249]

*OMIM*: #305100

*Description*: This genetic disease is characterized by sparse hair, abnormal or missing teeth and inability to sweat, dryness of the skin, eyes, airways, and mucous membranes.

*Epidemiology*: prevalence of 1/1,000,000−9/1,000,000
*Eye findings*: absent meibomian glands, absent tears, periorbital hyperpigmentation, periorbital wrinkles, scant or absent eyelashes, scant or absent eyebrows
*Inheritance*: XLR
*Known genes or gene locus*: EDA

## REFERENCES

1. Lee K, Couser NL. Genetic testing for eye diseases: a comprehensive guide and review of ocular genetic manifestations from anterior segment malformation to retinal dystrophy. *Curr Genet Med Rep.* 2016;4:41−48.
2. Bobilev AM, et al. Assessment of PAX6 alleles in 66 families with aniridia. *Clin Genet.* 2016;89(6):669−677.
3. Ramirez-Miranda A, et al. Ultrabiomicroscopic-histopathologic correlations in individuals with autosomal dominant congenital microcoria: three-generation family report. *Case Rep Ophthalmol.* 2011; 2(2):160−165.
4. Rüfer F, Schröder A, Erb C. White-to-white corneal diameter: normal values in healthy humans obtained with the Orbscan II topography system. *Cornea.* 2005;24(3):259−261.
5. Gordon-Shaag A, et al. The genetic and environmental factors for keratoconus. *Biomed Res Int.* 2015;2015:795738.
6. Khan AO. Genetic diseases of the eye. In: Traboulsi EI, ed. *Chapter 7, Cornea Plana.* 2nd ed. Oxford University Press; 2012.
7. Herwig MC, et al. Anterior segment developmental anomalies in a 33-week-old fetus with MIDAS syndrome. *Pediatr Dev Pathol.* 2014;17(6):491−495.
8. Weiss AH, et al. Simple microphthalmos. *Arch Ophthalmol.* 1989;107(11):1625−1630.
9. Kallish S, et al. Ablepharon−macrostomia syndrome−extension of the phenotype. *Am J Med Genet.* 2011; 155(12):3060−3062.
10. Brice G, et al. Analysis of the phenotypic abnormalities in lymphoedema-distichiasis syndrome in 74 patients with FOXC2 mutations or linkage to 16q24. *J Med Genet.* 2002;39(7):478−483.
11. Fang J, et al. Mutations in FOXC2 (MFH-1), a forkhead family transcription factor, are responsible for the

hereditary lymphedema-distichiasis syndrome. *Am J Hum Genet.* 2000;67(6):1382–1388.

12. Hingorani M, Hanson I, van Heyningen V. Aniridia. *Eur J Hum Genet.* 2012;20(10):1011–1017.

13. Bobilev AM, et al. Assessment of PAX6 alleles in 66 families with aniridia. *Clin Genet.* 2015.

14. Tezcan B, Rich P, Bhide A. Prenatal diagnosis of WAGR syndrome. *Case Rep Obstet Gynecol.* 2015;2015:928585.

15. Lang GE, Rott HD, Pfeiffer RA. X-linked ocular albinism. *Ophthalm Genet.* 1990;11:265–271.

16. Montoliu L, et al. Increasing the complexity: new genes and new types of albinism. *Pigment Cell Melanoma Res.* 2014;27(1):11–18.

17. Weksberg R, Shuman C, Beckwith JB. Beckwith-wiedemann syndrome. *Eur J Hum Genet.* 2010;18:8–14.

18. Graziadio C, et al. Blepharophimosis-ptosis-epicanthus inversus syndrome. *Pediatr Int.* 2011;53(3):390–392.

19. Frazer FC, et al. Frequency of the branchio-oto-renal (BOR) syndrome in children with profound hearing loss. *Am J Med Genet.* 1980;7(3):341–349.

20. Boyle MI, et al. Cornelia de Lange syndrome. *Clin Genet.* 2015;88(1):1–12.

21. Fretzayas A, et al. Eponym: Gilbert syndrome. *Eur J Pediatr.* 2012;71(1):11–15.

22. Dupuis-Girod S, Bailly S, Plauchu H. Hereditary hemorrhagic telangiectasia: from molecular biology to patient care. *J Thromb Haemost.* 2010;8(7):1447–1456.

23. Adam MP, Hudgins L. Kabuki syndrome: a review. *Clin Genet.* 2005;67(3):209–219.

24. Van Der Burgt I. Noonan syndrome. *Orphanet J Rare Dis.* 2007;2.

25. Forlino A, Marini JC. Osteogenesis imperfecta. *Lancet.* 2016;387:1657–1671.

26. Marchegiani S, et al. Recurrent mutations in the basic domain of TWIST2 cause Ablepharon macrostomia and Barber-Say syndromes. *Am J Hum Genet.* 2015;97: 99–110.

27. Maria DM, et al. Barber–say syndrome and Ablepharon–macrostomia syndrome: an overview. *Am J Med Genet.* 2016;170(8):1989–2001.

28. Stevens CA, Sargent LA. Ablepharon-macrostomia syndrome. *Am J Med Genet.* 2001;107(1):30–37.

29. Propping P, Zerres K. ADULT syndrome: an autosomal-dominant disorder with pigment anomalies, ectrodactyly, nail dysplasia, and hypodontia. *Am J Hum Genet.* 1993;45(5):642–648.

30. Resiler TT, Patton MA, Meagher PP. Further phenotypic and genetic variation in ADULT syndrome. *Am J Med Genet.* 2006;140(22):2495–2500.

31. Slavotinek AM, et al. Acro-dermato-ungual-lacrimal-tooth (ADULT) syndrome: report of a child with phenotypic overlap with ulnar-mammary syndrome and a new mutation in TP63. *Am J Med Genet.* 2005;138(2): 146–149.

32. van Zelst-Stams WA, van Steensel MA. A novel TP63 mutation in family with ADULT syndrome presenting with eczema and hypothelia. *Am J Med Genet.* 2009;149(7): 1558–1560.

33. Hingorani M, et al. Ocular abnormalities in Alagille syndrome. *Ophthalmology.* 1999;106(2):330–337.

34. Ho NC, et al. Severe hypodontia and oral xanthomas in Alagille syndrome. *Am J Med Genet.* 2000;93(3): 250–252.

35. Kanath BM, et al. Facial features in Alagille syndrome: specific or cholestasis facies? *Am J Med Genet.* 2002; 112(2):163–170.

36. Felbor U, et al. Ocular ochronosis in alkaptonuria patients carrying mutations in the homogentisate 1,2-dioxygenase gene. *Br J Ophthalmol.* 1999;83(6): 680–683.

37. Linder M, Bertelmann T. On the ocular findings in ochronosis: a systematic review of literature. *BMC Ophthalmol.* 2014;14(12).

38. Milch RA. Studies of Alcaptonuria: inheritance of 47 cases in eight highly inter-related Dominican Kindreds. *Am J Hum Genet.* 1960;12(1):76–85.

39. Vilboux T, et al. Mutation spectrum of homogentisic acid oxidase (HGD) in alkaptonuria. *Hum Mutat.* 2009; 30(12):1611–1619.

40. Ihnatko R, et al. Congenital aniridia and the ocular surface. *Ocul Surf.* 2016;14(2):196–206.

41. Cheong S, et al. Mutations in CPAMD8 cause a unique form of autosomal-recessive anterior segment dysgenesis. *Cell.* 2016;99(6):1338–1352.

42. Choi A, et al. Novel mutations in PXDN cause microphthalmia and anterior segment dysgenesis. *Eur J Hum Genet.* 2015;23(3):337–341.

43. Nischal KK. Genetics of congenital corneal opacification–impact on diagnosis and treatment. *Cornea.* 2015;10(34 suppl):S24–S34.

44. Smith JE, Traboulsi EE. Genetic diseases of the eye. In: Traboulsi EI, ed. *Chapter 7, Malformations of the Anterior Segment of the Eye.* 2nd ed. Oxford University Press; 2012.

45. Sowden JC. Molecular and developmental mechanisms of anterior segment dysgenesis. *Eye (Lond).* 2007;21(1): 1310–1318.

46. Alward WL. Axenfeld-Rieger syndrome in the age of molecular genetics. *Am J Ophthalmol.* 2000;130(1):107–115.

47. Lines MA, Kozlowski K, Walter MA. Molecular genetics of Axenfeld-Rieger malformations. *Hum Mol Genet.* 2002; 11(10):1177–1184.

48. Waldron JM, et al. Axenfeld–Rieger Syndrome (ARS): a review and case report. *Spec Care Dentist.* 2010;30(5): 218–222.

49. Donato ND, et al. Severe forms of Baraitser–Winter syndrome are caused by ACTB mutations rather than ACTG1 mutations. *Eur J Hum Genet.* 2014;22(2):179–183.

50. Rivière JB, et al. De novo mutations in the actin genes ACTB and ACTG1 cause Baraitser-Winter syndrome. *Nat Genet.* 2012;44(4):440–444.

51. Verloes A, et al. Baraitser–Winter cerebrofrontofacial syndrome: delineation of the spectrum in 42 cases. *Eur J Hum Genet.* 2015;23(3):292–301.

52. David A, et al. Macrostomia, ectropion, atrophic skin, hypertrichosis: another observation. *Am J Med Genet.* 1991;39(1):112–115.

53. Tenea D, Jacyk WK. Barber–say syndrome. *Pediatr Dermatol.* 2006;23(2):183–184.

54. Clarke SL, et al. Barth syndrome. *Orphanet J Rare Dis.* 2013;8(23).

55. Schlame M, Ren M. Barth syndrome, a human disorder of cardiolipin metabolism. *FEBS Lett.* 2006;580(23): 5450–5455.

56. De Jong PT, et al. Medullated nerve fibers: a sign of multiple basal cell Nevi (Gorlin's) syndrome. *Arch Ophthalmol.* 1985;103(12):1833–1836.

57. Farndon PA, et al. Location of gene for Gorlin syndrome. *Lancet.* 1992;339(8793):581–582.

58. Lam C, Ou JC, Billingsley EM. "PTCH"-ing it together: a basal cell nevus syndrome review. *Dermatol Surg.* 2013; 39(11):1557–1572.

59. Pino LC, et al. Basal cell nevus syndrome: clinical and molecular review and case report. *Int J Dermatol.* 2016; 55(4):367–375.

60. Kidd A, et al. A Scottish family with Bazex-Dupre-Christol syndrome: follicular atrophoderma, congenital hypotrichosis, and basal cell carcinoma. *J Med Genet.* 1996; 33(6):493–497.

61. Rodrigues Jr IA, et al. Bazex syndrome. *An Bras Dermatol.* 2013;88(6 suppl 1):209–211.

62. Torrelo A, et al. Bazex–dupre–christol syndrome. *Pediatr Dermatol.* 2006;23(3):286–290.

63. Winter SC, et al. Prenatal diagnosis of the Beckwith-Wiedemann syndrome. *Am J Med Genet.* 1986;24(1): 137–141.

64. Kanazawa N, et al. Early-onset sarcoidosis and CARD15 mutations with constitutive nuclear factor-κB activation: common genetic etiology with Blau syndrome. *Blood.* 2005;105(3):1195–1197.

65. Latkany PA, et al. Multifocal choroiditis in patients with familial juvenile systemic granulomatosis. *Am J Ophthalmol.* 2002;134(6):897–904.

66. Martin T, et al. Blau syndrome. *QJM.* 2011;104(11): 997–998.

67. Corrêa FJ, et al. A new FOXL2 gene mutation in a woman with premature ovarian failure and sporadic blepharophimosis-ptosis-epicanthus inversus syndrome. *Fertil Steril.* 2010;93(3):1006.e3–e6.

68. Shah BM, et al. Novel occurrence of axenfeld: Rieger syndrome in a patient with blepharophimosis ptosis epicanthus inversus syndrome. *Indian J Ophthalmol.* 2014;62(3): 358–360.

69. Kochhar A, et al. Branchio-oto-renal syndrome. *Am J Med Genet.* 2007;143(14):1671–1678.

70. Morisada N, Kandai N, Iijima K. Branchio-oto-renal syndrome: comprehensive review based on nationwide surveillance in Japan. *Pediatr Int.* 2014;56(3):309–314.

71. Robertson SP, et al. Congenital hypertrichosis, osteochondrodysplasia, and cardiomegaly: Cantú syndrome. *Am J Med Genet.* 1999;85(4):395–402.

72. Scurr I, et al. Cantú syndrome: report of nine new cases and expansion of the clinical phenotype. *Am J Med Genet.* 2011;155(3):508–518.

73. van Bon BWM, et al. Cantú syndrome is caused by mutations in ABCC9. *Am J Hum Genet.* 2012;90(6):1094–1101.

74. Mani A, et al. Syndromic patent ductus arteriosus: evidence for haploinsufficient TFAP2B mutations and identification of a linked sleep disorder. *PNAS.* 2004;102(8): 2975–2979.

75. Satoda M, et al. Mutations in TFAP2B cause Char syndrome, a familial form of patent ductus arteriosus. *Nat Genet.* 2000;25(1):42–46.

76. Sweeney E, et al. Char syndrome: a new family and review of the literature emphasizing the presence of symphalangism and the variable phenotype. *Clin Dysmoprhol.* 2000;9(3):177–182.

77. Ahmadi AJ, Pirinjian GE, Sires BS. Optic neuropathy and macular chorioretinal folds caused by orbital cherubism. *Arch Ophthalmol.* 2003;121(4):570–573.

78. Kömerik N, Taş B, Önal L. *Cherub Head Neck Pathol.* 2014; 8(2):164–167.

79. Patel JR. Cherubism: report of three cases. *ASDC J Dent Child.* 1987;54(4):289–290.

80. Silva EC, et al. Cherubism: clinicoradiographic features, treatment, and long-term follow-up of 8 cases. *J Oral Maxillofac Surg.* 2007;65(3):517–522.

81. Stiller M, et al. Craniosynostosis in cherubism. *Am J Med Genet.* 2000;95(4):325–331.

82. Hurmerinta K, et al. Craniofacial features in Cohen syndrome: an anthropometric and cephalometric analysis of 14 patients. *Clin Genet.* 2002;62(2):157–164.

83. Norio R. Finnish disease heritage I: characteristics, causes, background. *Hum Genet.* 2003;112(5–6):441–456.

84. Taban M, et al. Cohen syndrome: report of nine cases and review of the literature, with emphasis on ophthalmic features. *J AAPOS.* 2007;11(5):431–437.

85. Rouillac C, et al. Mapping of a congenital microcoria locus to 13q31-q32. *Am J Hum Genet.* 1998;62(5): 1117–1122.

86. Toulemont PJ, et al. Association of congenital microcoria with myopia and glaucoma: a study of 23 patients with congenital microcoria. *Ophthalmology.* 1995;102(2): 193–198.

87. Minor A, et al. Two novel RAD21 mutations in patients with mild Cornelia de Lange syndrome-like presentation and report of the first familial case. *Gene.* 2014;537(2): 279–284.

88. Bosma PJ. Inherited disorders of bilirubin metabolism. *J Hepatol.* 2003;38(1):107–117.

89. Sneitz N, et al. Crigler-najjar syndrome in The Netherlands: identification of four novel UGT1A1 alleles, genotype–phenotype correlation, and functional analysis of 10 missense mutants. *Hum Mutat.* 2010;31(1): 52–59.

90. Van Maldergem L, et al. Cobblestone-like brain dysgenesis and altered glycosylation in congenital cutis laxa, Debré type. *Neurology*. 2008;71(20):1602−1608.

91. Van Maldergem L, et al. Facial anomalies in congenital cutis laxa with retarded growth and skeletal dysplasia. *Am J Med Genet*. 1989;32(2):265.

92. Kim CH, et al. Mutations in the dopamine β-hydroxylase gene are associated with human norepinephrine deficiency. *Am J Med Genet*. 2002;108(2):140−147.

93. Senard JM, Rouet P. Dopamine beta-hydroxylase deficiency. *Orphanet J Rare Dis*. 2006;2006(7):1.

94. Timmers HJ, et al. Congenital dopamine-β-hydroxylase deficiency in humans. *Ann NY Acad Sci*. 2004;1018(1):520−523.

95. Kuster W, Majewski F. The Dubowitz syndrome. *Eur J Pediatr*. 1986;144(6):574−578.

96. Tsukahara M, Optiz JM. Dubowitz syndrome, review of 141 cases including 36 previously unreported patients. *Am J Med Genet*. 1996;63(1):277−289.

97. Yesilkaya E, et al. Dubowitz syndrome: a cholesterol metabolism disorder? *Genet Couns*. 2008;19(3):287−290.

98. Barbaro PM, Ziegler DS, Reddel RR. The wide-ranging clinical implications of the short telomere syndromes. *Inter Med J*. 2016;46(4):393−403.

99. Bessler M, Wilson DB, Mason PJ. Dyskeratosis congenita. *FEBS Lett*. 2010;584(17):3831−3838.

100. Keller RB, et al. CTC1 Mutations in a patient with dyskeratosis congenita. *Pediatr Blood Cancer*. 2012;59(2):311−314.

101. Scully C, Langdon J, Evans J. Marathon of eponyms: 26 Zinsser-Engman-Cole syndrome (Dyskeratosis congenita). *Oral Dis*. 2012;18(5):522−523.

102. Tsilou ET, et al. Ocular and orbital manifestations of the inherited bone marrow failure syndromes: Fanconi anemia and dyskeratosis congenita. *Ophthalmology*. 2010;117(3):615−622.

103. Di Iorio E, et al. Limbal stem cell deficiency and ocular phenotype in ectrodactyly-ectodermal dysplasia-clefting syndrome caused by p63 mutations. *Ophthalmology*. 2012;119(1):74−83.

104. Gün I, Kizilaslan C, Atalay MA. Familial ectrodactyly−ectodermal dysplasia−clefting syndrome. *Int J Gynaecol Obstet*. 2012;119(1):86−87.

105. McNab AA, Potts MJ, Welham RA. The EEC syndrome and its ocular manifestations. *Br J Ophthalmol*. 1989;73(4):261−264.

106. Rosenberg JB, Butrus S, Bazemore MG. Ectrodactyly-ectodermal dysplasia-clefting syndrome causing blindness in a child. *J AAPOS*. 2011;15(1):80−82.

107. van Bokhoven H, et al. p63 Gene mutations in EEC syndrome, limb-mammary syndrome, and isolated split hand-split foot malformation suggest a genotype-phenotype correlation. *Am J Hum Genet*. 2001;69(3):481−492.

108. Gollop TR. Fronto-Facio-nasal dysostosis—a new autosomal recessive syndrome. *Am J Med Genet*. 1981;10(4):409−412.

109. Suthers G, David D, Clark B. Fronto-facio-nasal dysplasia. *Clin Dysmorphol*. 1997;6(3):245−249.

110. Carvalho DR, et al. Additional features of Gillespie syndrome in two Brazilian siblings with a novel ITPR1 homozygous pathogenic variant. *Eur J Med Genet*. 2017.

111. Gerber H, et al. Recessive and dominant de novo ITPR1 mutations cause Gillespie syndrome. *Am J Hum Genet*. 2016;98(5):971−980.

112. Mariën P, et al. Cerebellar cognitive affective syndrome without global mental retardation in two relatives with Gillespie syndrome. *Cortex*. 2008;44(1):54−67.

113. Ménasché G, et al. Griscelli syndrome restricted to hypopigmentation results from a melanophilin defect (GS3) or a MYO5A F-exon deletion (GS1). *J Clin Investig*. 2003;112(3):450−456.

114. Sanal O, et al. Griscelli disease: genotype−phenotype correlation in an array of clinical heterogeneity. *J Clin Immunol*. 2002;22(4):237−243.

115. Hay RJ, Wells RS. The syndrome of ankyloblepharon, ectodermal defects and cleft lip and palate: an autosomal dominant condition. *Br J Dermatol*. 1976;94(3):277−289.

116. Hida T, et al. Ankyloblepharon-ectodermal defects-cleft lip/palate syndrome: a case with a novel p63 mutation associated with abnormal keratohyalin granules. *Eur J Dermatol*. 2014;24(4):495−497.

117. Bayrak-Toydemir P, et al. A fourth locus for hereditary hemorrhagic telangiectasia maps to chromosome 7. *Am J Genet A*. 2006;140(20):2155−2162.

118. Cole S, et al. A new locus for hereditary haemorrhagic telangiectasia (HHT3) maps to chromosome 5. *J Med Genet*. 2005;42(7):577−582.

119. Rinalids M, et al. Ocular manifestations in hereditary hemorrhagic telangiectasia (Rendu-Osler-Weber disease): a case-series. *Ophthalm Genet*. 2011;32(1):12−17.

120. Wooderchak-Donahue WL, et al. BMP9 mutations cause a vascular-anomaly syndrome with phenotypic overlap with hereditary hemorrhagic telangiectasia. *Am J Hum Genet*. 2013;93(3):530−537.

121. Ammann S, et al. Mutations in AP3D1 associated with immunodeficiency and seizures define a new type of Hermansky-Pudlak syndrome. *Blood*. 2016;127(8):997−1006.

122. Haneef SA, Doss GP. Advances in protein chemistry and structural biology. In: Donev R, ed. *Chapter 8, Personalized Pharmacoperones for Lysosomal Storage Disorder: Approach for Next-Generation Treatment*. Vol. 102. Academic Press; 2016.

123. Kinnear PE, Tuddenham EG. Albinism with haemorrhagic diathesis: Hermansky-Pudlak syndrome. *Br J Ophthalmol*. 1985;69(12):904−908.

124. Cruz AA, et al. Eyelid abnormalities in lamellar ichthyoses. *Ophthalmology*. 2000;107(10):1895−1898.

125. Heinz L, et al. Mutations in SULT2B1 cause autosomal-recessive congenital ichthyosis in humans. *Am J Hum Genet*. 2017;100(6):926–939.

126. Lefèvre C, et al. Mutations in a new cytochrome P450 gene in lamellar ichthyosis type 3. *Hum Mol Genet*. 2006;15(5):767–776.

127. Melnik B, et al. Autosomal dominant lamellar ichthyosis exhibits an abnormal scale lipid pattern. *Clin Genet*. 1989;35(2):152–156.

128. Rodríguez-Pazos L, et al. Autosomal recessive congenital ichthyosis. *Actas Dermosifiliogr*. 2013;104(4):270–284.

129. Saugier-Veber P, et al. Lumping Juberg-Marsidi syndrome and X-linked alpha-thalassemia/mental retardation syndrome? *Am J Hum Genet*. 1995;55(3):300–301.

130. Saugier-Veber P, et al. The Juberg-Marsidi syndrome maps to the proximal long arm of the X chromosome (Xq12-q21). *Am J Hum Genet*. 1993;52(6):1040–1045.

131. Tsukahara M, et al. Juberg-Marsidi syndrome: report of an additional case. *Am J Hum Genet*. 1995;58(4):353–355.

132. Kobayashi O, Sakuragawa N. Inheritance in Kabuki make-up (Niikawa-Kuroki) syndrome. *Am J Med Genet*. 1996;61(1):92–93.

133. Miyake N, et al. MLL2 and KDM6A mutations in patients with Kabuki syndrome. *Am J Med Genet*. 2013;161(9):2234–2243.

134. Kaufman RL, et al. An oculocerebrofacial syndrome. *Birth Defects Orig Artic Ser*. 1971;7(1):135–138.

135. Yilmanz R, et al. Kaufman oculocerebrofacial syndrome: novel UBE3B mutations and clinical features in four unrelated patients. *Am J Med Genet*. 2018;176(1):187–193.

136. Bamforth JS, Kaurah P. Lacrimo-auriculo-dento-digital syndrome: evidence for lower limb involvement and severe congenital renal anomalies. *Am J Med Genet*. 1992;43(6):932–937.

137. Cortes M, et al. Limbal stem cell deficiency associated with LADD syndrome. *Arch Ophthalmol*. 2005;123(5):691–694.

138. Lim LT, et al. Lacrimal-auricular-dental-digital (LADD) syndrome with diffuse ophthalmoplegia—a new finding. *Semin Ophthalmol*. 2012;27(3–4):59–60.

139. Mundos S, Horn D. Lacrimo-Auriculo-Dento-digital (LADD) syndrome. In: *Limb Malformations*. 1st ed. Berlin, Heidelberg: Springer; 2014.

140. Rohmann E, et al. Mutations in different components of FGF signaling in LADD syndrome. *Nat Genet*. 2006;38(4):414–417.

141. Wiedemann HR, Drescher J. LADD syndrome: report of new cases and review of the clinical spectrum. *Eur J Pediatr*. 1986;144(6):579–582.

142. Lehmann LH, et al. A patient with LEOPARD syndrome and PTPN11 mutation. *Circulation*. 2009;119(9):1328–1329.

143. Sarkozy A, Digilio MC, Dallapiccola B. Leopard syndrome. *Oprhanet J Rare Dis*. 2008;3(13).

144. Sarkozy A, et al. Germline BRAF mutations in Noonan, LEOPARD, and cardiofaciocutaneous syndromes: molecular diversity and associated phenotypic spectrum. *Hum Mutat*. 2009;30(4):695–702.

145. van Bokhoven H, et al. Limb mammary syndrome: a new genetic disorder with mammary hypoplasia, ectrodactyly, and other Hand/Foot anomalies maps to human chromosome 3q27. *Am J Hum Genet*. 1996;64(2):538–546.

146. Krajewska-walasek M, Kozlowski K. Melnick-Needles syndrome. *Australas Radiol*. 1994;38:146–147.

147. Robertson SP. Otopalatodigital syndrome spectrum disorders: otopalatodigital syndrome types 1 and 2, frontometaphyseal dysplasia and Melnick-Needles syndrome. *Eur J Hum Genet*. 2007;15:3–9.

148. Kodama H, Murata Y. Molecular genetics and pathophysiology of Menkes disease. *Pediatr Int*. 1999;41:430–435.

149. Tumer Z, Moller LB. Menkes disease. *Eur J Hum Genet*. 2010;18:511–518.

150. Bergmann C, et al. Oligophrenin 1 (OPHN1) gene mutation causes syndromic X-linked mental retardation with epilepsy, rostral ventricular enlargement and cerebellar hypoplasia. *Brain*. 2003;126:1537–1544.

151. des Portes V, et al. Specific clinical and brain MRI features in mentally retarded patients with mutations in the Oligophrenin-1 gene. *Am J Med Genet A*. 2004;124A:364–371.

152. Bretón Martínez JR, Cánovas Martínez A, Casaña Pérez S, Escribá Alepuz J, Giménez Vázquez F. Mevalonic aciduria: report of two cases. *J Inherit Metab Dis*. 2007;30:829.

153. Kožich V, et al. Mevalonic aciduria. *J Inherit Metab Dis*. 1991;14:265–266.

154. Frattini D, Fusco C, Ucchino V, Tavazzi B, Della Giustina E. Early onset methylmalonic aciduria and homocystinuria cblC type with demyelinating neuropathy. *Pediatr Neurol*. 2010;43:135–138.

155. Wang X, Sun W, Yang Y, Jia J, Li C. A clinical and gene analysis of late-onset combined methylmalonic aciduria and homocystinuria, cblC type, in China. *J Neurol Sci*. 2012;318:155–159.

156. Miller M, Fineman R, Smith DW. Postaxial acrofacial dysostosis syndrome. *J Pediatr*. 1979;95:970–975.

157. Pereira SCS, Rocha CMG, Guion-Almeida ML, Richieri-Costa A. Postaxial acrofacial dysostosis: report on two patients. *Am J Med Genet*. 1992;44:274–279.

158. Vigneron J, Stricker M, Vert P, Rousselot JM, Levy M. Postaxial acrofacial dysostosis (Miller) syndrome: a new case. *J Med Genet*. 1991;28:636–638.

159. Hervé D, et al. A hereditary moyamoya syndrome with multisystemic manifestations. *Neurology*. 2010;75:259–264.

160. Kuroda S, Houkin K. Moyamoya disease: current concepts and future perspectives. *Lancet Neurol*. 2008;7:1056–1066.

161. Pollak L. Moyamoya disease and moyamoya syndrome. *N Engl J Med*. 2009;361:98.

162. Meyer A, et al. Scoring evaluation of the natural course of mucopolysaccharidosis type IIIA (Sanfilippo syndrome type A). *Pediatrics.* 2007;120:e1255−e1261.

163. Valstar MJ, et al. Mucopolysaccharidosis type IIIA: clinical spectrum and genotype-phenotype correlations. *Ann Neurol.* 2010;68:876−887.

164. White KK, Karol LA, White DR, Hale S. Musculoskeletal manifestations of sanfilippo syndrome (mucopolysaccharidosis type III). *J Pediatr Orthop.* 2011;31:594−598.

165. Shapiro E, et al. The neurobehavioral phenotype in mucopolysaccharidosis Type IIIB: an exploratory study. *Mol Genet Metab Rep.* 2016;6:41−47.

166. Valstar MJ, et al. Mucopolysaccharidosis type IIIB may predominantly present with an attenuated clinical phenotype. *J Inherit Metab Dis.* 2010;33:759−767.

167. Yogalingam G, Weber B, Meehan J, Rogers J, Hopwood JJ. Mucopolysaccharidosis type IIIB: characterisation and expression of wild-type and mutant recombinant alpha-N-acetylglucosaminidase and relationship with Sanfilippo phenotype in an attenuated patient. *Biochim Biophys Acta Mol Basis Dis.* 2000;1502:415−425.

168. Huh HJ, et al. The first Korean case of mucopolysaccharidosis IIIC (sanfilippo syndrome type C) confirmed by biochemical and molecular investigation. *Ann Lab Med.* 2013;33(1):75−79.

169. Ruijter GJG, et al. Clinical and genetic spectrum of Sanfilippo type C (MPS IIIC) disease in The Netherlands. *Mol Genet Metab.* 2008;93:104−111.

170. Mok A, Cao H, Hegele RA. Genomic basis of mucopolysaccharidosis type IIID (MIM 252940) revealed by sequencing of GNS encoding N-acetylglucosamine-6-sulfatase. *Genomics.* 2003;81:1−5.

171. Valstar MJ, et al. Mucopolysaccharidosis type IIID: 12 new patients and 15 novel mutations. *Hum Mutat.* 2010;31.

172. Chemke J, Mogilner BM, Ben-Itzhak I, Zurkowski L, Ophir D. Autosomal recessive inheritance of Nager acrofacial dysostosis. *J Med Genet.* 1988;25:230−232.

173. Herrmann BW, Karzon R, Molter DW. Otologic and audiologic features of Nager acrofacial dysostosis. *Int J Pediatr Otorhinolaryngol.* 2005;69:1053−1059.

174. Kavadia S, Kaklamanos EG, Antoniades K, Lafazanis V, Tramma D. Nager syndrome (preaxial acrofacial dysostosis): a case report. *Oral Surg Oral Med Oral Pathol Oral Radiol Endod.* 2004;97:732−738.

175. Stamm DS, et al. Native American myopathy: congenital myopathy with cleft palate, skeletal anomalies, and susceptibility to malignant hyperthermia. *Am J Med Genet Part A.* 2008;146:1832−1841.

176. Stamm DS, et al. Novel congenital myopathy locus identified in Native American Indians at 12q13.13-14.1. *Neurology.* 2008;71:1764−1769.

177. Hou JW. Natural course of neonatal progeroid syndrome. *Pediatr Neonatol.* 2009;50:102−109.

178. Jacquinet A, et al. Neonatal progeroid variant of Marfan syndrome with congenital lipodystrophy results from mutations at the 3′ end of FBN1 gene. *Eur J Med Genet.* 2014;57:230−234.

179. Buehning L, Curry CJ. Neurofibromatosis-noonan syndrome. *Pediatr Dermatol.* 1995;12:267−271.

180. Reig I, et al. Neurofibromatosis-Noonan syndrome: case report and clinicopathogenic review of the Neurofibromatosis-Noonan syndrome and RAS-MAPK pathway. *Dermatol Online J.* 2011;17:4.

181. Nishi E, et al. A novel heterozygous MAP2K1 mutation in a patient with Noonan syndrome with multiple lentigines. *Am J Med Genet.* 2015;167(2):407−411.

182. Roberts AE, Allanson JE, Tartaglia M, Gelb BD. Noonan syndrome. *Lancet.* 2013;381:333−342.

183. Lewen RM. Ocular albinism. *Arch Ophthalmol.* 1988;106:120−121.

184. Butler MG, Regier EJ, Begleiter ML, Ishmael HA. Oculoauriculofrontonasal syndrome (OAFNS) in a nine-month-old male. *Am J Med Genet.* 2002;107:169−173.

185. Gabbett MT, et al. Characterizing the oculoauriculofrontonasal syndrome. *Clin Dysmorphol.* 2008;17:79−85.

186. Tunc T, et al. Oculoauriculofrontonasal dysplasia syndrome with additional clinical features. *Cleft Palate Craniofacial J.* 2017;54:749−753.

187. Chabchoub E, et al. Oculocerebral hypopigmentation syndrome maps to chromosome 3q27.1q29. *Dermatology.* 2012;223:306−310.

188. Ozkan H, Unsal E, Köse G. Oculocerebral hypopigmentation syndrome (Cross syndrome). *Turk J Pediatr.* 1991;33:247−252.

189. Grønskov K, Ek J, Brondum-Nielsen K. Oculocutaneous albinism. *Orphanet J Rare Dis.* 2007;2.

190. Okulicz JF, Shah RS, Schwartz RA, Janniger CK. Oculocutaneous albinism. *J Eur Acad Dermatol Venereol.* 2003;17:251−256.

191. Fischmann A. Oculopharyngeal muscular dystrophy. *Neuromuscul Imag.* 2013:305−311.

192. Luigetti M, et al. Oculopharyngeal muscular dystrophy: clinical and neurophysiological features. *Clin Neurophysiol.* 2015;126:2406−2408.

193. Olney AH, Kolodziej P, Bradley Schaefer G, Buehler BA. Oral-facial-digital syndrome type I. *Ear Nose Throat J.* 1997;76:778.

194. Sukarova-Angelovska E, Angelkova N, Palcevska-Kocevska S, Kocova M. The many faces of oral-facial-digital syndrome. *Balk J Med Genet.* 2012;15:37−44.

195. Huber MA, Clare M, Vanisha P, Rouin A, Martin G. Osteogenesis imperfecta. *Curr Orthop.* 2007;21:236−241.

196. Rauch F, Glorieux FH. Osteogenesis imperfecta. *Lancet.* 2004;363:1377−1385.

197. Blau N, Van Spronsen FJ, Levy HL. Phenylketonuria. *Lancet.* 2010;376:1417−1427.

198. Cleary MA. Phenylketonuria. *Paediatr Child Health.* 2015;25:108−112.

199. Cleary MA. Phenylketonuria. *Paediatr Child Health.* 2011;21:61−64.

200. Agarwal S, Ojha A. Piebaldism: a brief report and review of the literature. *Indian Dermatol Online J.* 2012;3:144−147.
201. Oiso N, Fukai K, Kawada A, Suzuki T. Piebaldism. *J Dermatol.* 2013;40:330−335.
202. Devadas S, Belvadi GB, Premlatha R, Ramya S. Popliteal pterygium syndrome. *Perinatology.* 2012;13:32−33.
203. Qasim M, Shaukat M. Popliteal pterygium syndrome: a rare entity. *APSP J Case Rep.* 2012;3:5.
204. Ratbi I, et al. Clinical and molecular findings in a Moroccan patient with popliteal pterygium syndrome: a case report. *J Med Case Rep.* 2014;8.
205. Raymond FL. X linked mental retardation: a clinical guide. *J Med Genet.* 2006;43:193−200.
206. Ropers H-H, Hamel BCJ. X-linked mental retardation. *Nat Rev Genet.* 2005;6:46−57.
207. Bonneau D, et al. X-linked lissencephaly with absent corpus callosum and ambiguous genitalia (XLAG): clinical, magnetic resonance imaging, and neuropathological findings. *Ann Neurol.* 2002;51:340−349.
208. Hartmann H, et al. Agenesis of the corpus callosum, abnormal genitalia and intractable epilepsy due to a novel familial mutation in the aristaless-related homeobox gene. *Neuropediatrics.* 2004;35:157−160.
209. Abbas R, et al. A child with Roberts syndrome. *J Coll Physicians Surg Pakistan.* 2011;21:431−433.
210. da Silva EO, Bezerra LHGE. The Roberts syndrome. *Hum Genet.* 1982;61:372−374.
211. Eggermann T. Russell-Silver syndrome. *Am J Med Genet Part C Semin Med Genet.* 2010;154:355−364.
212. Plotts CA, Livermore CL. Russell-silver syndrome and nonverbal learning disability: a case study. *Appl Neuropsychol.* 2007;14:124−134.
213. Wee SA. Russell-Silver syndrome. *Dermatol Online J.* 2007;13:16.
214. Arya R, et al. Schwartz Jampel syndrome in children. *J Clin Neurosci.* 2013;20:313−317.
215. Ferrannini E, Perniola T, Krajewska G, Serlenga L, Trizio M. Schwartz-Jampel syndrome with autosomal-dominant inheritance. *Eur Neurol.* 1982;21:137−146.
216. Mathur N, Ghosh PS. Schwartz-jampel syndrome. *Pediatr Neurol.* 2017;68:77−78.
217. Frints SGM, Froyen G, Marynen P, Fryns JP. X-linked mental retardation: vanishing boundaries between non-specific (MRX) and syndromic (MRXS) forms. *Clin Genet.* 2002;62:423−432.
218. Kleefstra T, Hamel BCJ. X-linked mental retardation: further lumping, splitting and emerging phenotypes. *Clin Genet.* 2005;67:451−467.
219. Innes AM, Dyment DA. SHORT syndrome. In: *GeneReviews®.* 1993.
220. Koenig R, Brendel L, Fuchs S. Short syndrome. *Clin Dysmorphol.* 2003;12:45−49.
221. Neri G, Gurrieri F, Zanni G, Lin A. Clinical and molecular aspects of the Simpson-Golabi-Behmel syndrome. *Am J Med Genet.* 1998;79:279−283.
222. Tenorio J, et al. Simpson-Golabi-Behmel syndrome types I and II. *Orphanet J Rare Dis.* 2014;9:138.
223. Young EL, Wishnow R, Nigro MA. Expanding the clinical picture of simpson-golabi-behmel syndrome. *Pediatr Neurol.* 2006;34:139−142.
224. Baujat G, Cormier-Daire V. Sotos syndrome. *Orphanet J Rare Dis.* 2007;2.
225. Juneja A, Sultan A. Sotos syndrome. *J Indian Soc Pedod Prev Dent.* 2011;29:S48−S51.
226. Kurotaki N, Matsumoto N. Sotos syndrome. In: *Genomic Disorders: The Genomic Basis of Disease.* 2006:237−246.
227. Haas LF, Austad WI, Bergin JD. Tangier disease. *Brain.* 1974;97:351−354.
228. Puntoni M, Sbrana F, Bigazzi F, Sampietro T. Tangier disease: epidemiology, pathophysiology, and management. *Am J Cardiovasc Drugs.* 2012;12:303−311.
229. Gripp KW, et al. Long-term survival in TARP syndrome and confirmation of RBM10 as the disease-causing gene. *Am J Med Genet Part A.* 2011;155:2516−2520.
230. Johnston JJ, et al. Expansion of the TARP syndrome phenotype associated with de novo mutations and mosaicism. *Am J Med Genet Part A.* 2014;164:120−128.
231. Amiel J, Watkin PM, Tassabehji M, Read AP, Winter RM. Mutation of the MITF gene in albinism-deafness syndrome (Tietz syndrome). *Clin Dysmorphol.* 1998;7:17−20.
232. Izumi T, et al. Tietz syndrome: unique phenotype specific to mutations of MITF nuclear localization signal. *Clin Genet.* 2008;74:93−95.
233. Smith SD, Kelley PM, Kenyon JB, Hoover D. Tietz syndrome (hypopigmentation/deafness) caused by mutation of MITF. *J Med Genet.* 2000;37:446−448.
234. Brooks BP, et al. Triple-A syndrome with prominent ophthalmic features and a novel mutation in the AAAS gene: a case report. *BMC Ophthalmol.* 2004;4:1−7.
235. Prpic I, Huebner A, Persic M, Handschug K, Pavletic M. Triple A syndrome: genotype-phenotype assessment. *Clin Genet.* 2003;63:415−417.
236. Sarathi V, Shah NS. Triple-a syndrome. *Adv Exp Med Biol.* 2010;685:1−8.
237. Parmeggiani A, Posar A, Leonardi M, Rossi PG. Neurological impairment in congenital bilateral ptosis with ophthalmoplegia. *Brain Dev.* 1992;14:107−109.
238. Ekinci S, Ciftci AO, Senocak ME, Büyükpamukçu N. Waardenburg syndrome associated with bilateral renal anomaly. *J Pediatr Surg.* 2005;40:879−881.
239. Read AP, Newton VE. Waardenburg syndrome. *J Med Genet.* 1997;34:656−665.
240. Milunsky JM. Waardenburg syndrome type I. In: Adam MP, Ardinger HH, Pagon RA, et al., eds. *GeneReviews® [Internet].* Seattle, WA: University of Washington, Seattle; 2001, 1993−2018. [Updated 2017 May 4].
241. Farrer LA, Grundfast KM, Amos J, et al. Waardenburg syndrome (WS) type I is caused by defects at multiple loci, one of which is near ALPP on chromosome 2: first report of the WS Consortium. *Am J Hum Genet.* 1992;50:902−913.

242. Fischbach BV, Trout KL, Lewis J, Luis CA, Sika M. WAGR syndrome: a clinical review of 54 cases. *Pediatrics.* 2005; 116:984−988.

243. Prasher VP, Ali M, Nasritdinova N, Routhu S, Thalitaya MD. Longevity in WAGR syndrome. *Int J Dev Disabil.* 2012;58:20−23.

244. Allanson JE, et al. Watson syndrome: is it a subtype of type 1 neurofibromatosis? *J Med Genet.* 1991;28: 752−756.

245. Watson GH. Pulmonary stenosis, café-au-lait spots, and dull intelligence. *Arch Dis Child.* 1967;42:303−307.

246. Kere J, et al. X-linked anhidrotic (hypohidrotic) ectodermal dysplasia is caused by mutation in a novel transmembrane protein. *Nat Genet.* 1996;13: 409−416.

247. Lexner MO, et al. Anthropometric and cephalometric measurements in X-linked hypohidrotic ectodermal dysplasia. *Orthod Craniofacial Res.* 2007;10:203−215.

248. Nakata M, Koshiba H, Eto K, Nance WE. A genetic study of anodontia in X-linked hypohidrotic ectodermal dysplasia. *Am J Hum Genet.* 1980;32:908−919.

249. Nortjé CJ, Farman AG, Thomas CJ, Watermeyer GJJ. X-linked hypohidrotic ectodermal dysplasia-An unusual prosthetic problem. *J Prosthet Dent.* 1978;40:137−142.

250. Tucker HM. Congenital bilateral recurrent nerve paralysis and ptosis: a new syndrome? *Laryngoscope.* 1983;93: 1405−1407.

251. Goldberg RA, Lally DR, Heier JS. Oculocutaneous albinism. *JAMA Ophthalmol.* 2015;133:e143518.

# CHAPTER 3

# Genetic Abnormalities With Anophthalmia, Microphthalmia, and Colobomas

NIKISHA Q. RICHARDS • ADAM E. PFLUGRATH • CHETNA PANDE • NATARIO L. COUSER

Anophthalmia, microphthalmia, and colobomas represent dysgenesis of ocular development. Anophthalmia and microphthalmia are severe eye malformations, with an incidence of 0.4−2.4 per 100,000 and 10.0−10.8 per 100,000 infants, respectively.[1] Colobomas have a prevalence of 4.9 per 100,000[2]; these range from a minor eye anomaly affecting the cosmetic appearance of the iris or eyelid, to an optic nerve or chorioretinal coloboma that may significantly impair vision. Ocular development begins early in gestation with molecular patterning involving a complex network of signaling molecules and transcription factors. The earliest physical evidence of ocular development occurs by gestational day 22 with the thickening of surface ectoderm and the concurrent formation of optic pits in the neural ectoderm. By gestational day 25, the optic pits become the optic vesicles with connections to the developing forebrain. By gestational day 28, the optic vesicles encounter the surface ectoderm and invaginate to form the bilayered optic cups. Mesodermal and neural crest cells migrate into the space between the cup and the surface ectoderm. By the fifth week of gestation, the optic fissures begin to fuse and close, thus providing a framework for complete development of ocular structures. Failure of the optic fissures to close results in a "typical" uveal coloboma, often present in the inferior-nasal location due to the location of the fetal fissure; these may involve the iris, ciliary body, optic nerve, and/or choroid structures. Atypical colobomas, which may represent an anterior hyaloid system remnant, generally involve other ocular anatomical locations and often have less

posterior segment involvement. Eyelid colobomas result as a failure of the mesodermal lid folds to fuse. Disruptions in patterning or formation, or the regression of early ocular structures can result in anophthalmia or microphthalmia.

Anophthalmia, microphthalmia, and coloboma may occur as separate entities along a phenotypic spectrum, occurring with a combined prevalence of 19 per 100,000 live births.[3] Additionally, anophthalmia, microphthalmia, and coloboma can be found in a variety of systemic syndromes.[4] Many of the syndromes highlighted in this chapter display genetic heterogeneity, i.e., Fraser syndrome, Micro syndrome, and muscular dystrophy-dystroglycanopathy, type A (MDDGA). While other syndromes listed display pleiotropy, i.e., COACH syndrome, Joubert syndrome, and Meckel syndrome. The phenotypic and genetic heterogeneity, severity, and rare nature of many of these conditions highlights the importance of the role of genetic counseling for individuals and families affected, and provides incentive to investigate the genetic aspects of this group of disorders further.

## GENETIC DISORDERS
### Cerebral-Cerebellar-Coloboma Syndrome[5,6]
OMIM: 300864.

*Description*: Cerebral-Cerebellar-Coloboma syndrome is associated with hydrocephalus, macrocephaly, low-set ears, aberrant origin of the right subclavian artery, hyperpnea, and periodic apnea, 13 ribs, and a multitude of central nervous system deficits such as cerebellar agenesis or hypoplasia, agenesis of the corpus callosum, misshapen posterior fossa, seizures, and delayed psychomotor development. The syndrome is considered a distinct phenotype from Joubert syndrome, due to the X-linked inheritance and the absence of the molar tooth sign on neuroimaging.

*Epidemiology*: unknown; one family reported.

*Eye Findings*: chorioretinal coloboma.

*Inheritance*: XLR.

*Known Genes or Gene Locus*: unknown.

### Cerebrooculofacioskeletal Syndrome[7,8]

*OMIM*: #214150.

*Description*: Cerebrooculofacioskeletal syndrome (COFS1), also known as COFS syndrome and Pena-Shokeir syndrome Type II, is associated with failure to thrive, microcephaly, micrognathia, sensorineural hearing loss, prominent nasal root, overhanging upper lip, arthrogryposis, hirsutism, cerebellar hypoplasia, infantile spasms, and hypotonia. There is significant developmental delay, profound intellectual disability, photosensitivity, and often death in childhood. Shares clinical manifestations with Cockayne syndrome.

*Epidemiology*: unknown.

*Eye Findings*: cataracts, blepharophimosis, microphthalmia, nystagmus, and deep-set eyes.

*Inheritance*: AR.

*Known Genes or Gene Locus*: *ERCC6* (COFS1), *ERCC5* (COFS3), and *ERCC1* (COFS4).

### Cerebrooculonasal Syndrome[9,10]

*OMIM*: %605627.

*Description*: Cerebrooculonasal syndrome is associated with anophthalmia, proboscis-like nares, central nervous system abnormalities, and intellectual disability.

*Epidemiology*: unknown.

*Eye Findings*: anophthalmia, sparse eyebrows and eyelashes, epicanthal folds, and hypertelorism.

*Inheritance*: AD.

*Known Genes or Gene Locus*: *PTCH*.

### CHARGE Syndrome[11,12]

*OMIM*: #214800.

*Description*: CHARGE syndrome, also known as Hall-Hittner syndrome, is characterized by the presence of ocular coloboma, heart anomalies, choanal atresia, retarded growth and development, genital hypoplasia, ear anomalies, and deafness. Other features associated with CHARGE syndrome include esophageal malformations, cleft palate, cranial nerve dysfunction, limb abnormalities, renal anomalies, and thymic hypoplasia.

*Epidemiology*: incidence of 1/12,000.

*Eye Findings*: anophthalmia; coloboma in iris, optic nerve, or retina (Fig. 3.1); epicanthus; hypertelorism; microphthalmia; ptosis, downslanting palpebral fissures; and telecanthus.

*Inheritance*: AD.

*Known Genes or Gene Locus*: *CHD7* and *SEMA3E*.

### CHIME Syndrome[13,14]

*OMIM*: #280000.

*Description*: CHIME syndrome, also known as zunich neuroectodermal syndrome and glycosylphosphatidylinositol biosynthesis defect 5 (GPIBD5), is characterized by ocular coloboma, congenital heart disease, ichthyosiform dermatosis, mental retardation, ear defects/conductive hearing loss, and epilepsy.

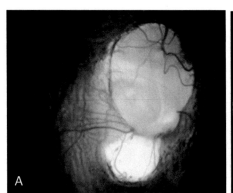 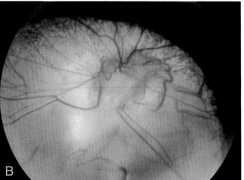

FIG. 3.1 Optic disc and choroidal colobomas in the right eye **(A)** and left eye **(B)**. (Courtesy Yang HK, Choi BY. CHARGE syndrome with oculomotor nerve palsy. *J AAPOS*. December 1, 2015;19(6): 555–557. © 2015.)

*Epidemiology*: unknown.

*Eye Findings*: coloboma, epicanthal folds, and hypertelorism.

*Inheritance*: AR.

*Known Genes or Gene Locus*: PIGL.

## Chondrodysplasia With Platyspondyly, Distinctive Brachydactyly, Hydrocephaly, and Microphthalmia[15,16]

*OMIM*: #300863.

*Description*: Chondrodysplasia with platyspondyly, distinctive brachydactyly, hydrocephaly, and microphthalmia is an X-linked disorder associated with intrauterine growth restriction, hydrocephaly with frontal bossing, small low-set ears, a short and flat nose with microphthalmia, and other distinctive bony features. Radiographs show platyspondyly with osseous abnormalities, including metaphyseal cupping of metacarpals, metatarsals, and phalanges. Affected females display body asymmetry and intellectual disability.

*Epidemiology*: unknown.

*Eye Findings*: microphthalmia.

*Inheritance*: XLD.

*Known Genes or Gene Locus*: HDAC6.

## COACH Syndrome[17–19]

*OMIM*: #216360.

*Description*: COACH syndrome, also known as Joubert syndrome with cerebellar vermis hypo/aplasia, oligophrenia, congenital ataxia, ocular coloboma and hepatic fibrosis, is associated with intellectual disability and ataxia secondary to cerebellar hypo/aplasia. Renal and ocular coloboma findings are variable.

*Epidemiology*: unknown.

*Eye Findings*: hypertelorism, nystagmus, ocular coloboma, and oculomotor apraxia.

*Inheritance*: AR.

*Known Genes or Gene Locus*: CC2D2A, TMEM67, and RPGRIP1L.

## Congenital Disorder of Glycosylation, Type Iq[20–22]

*OMIM*: #612379.

*Description*: Congenital disorder of glycosylation, Type Iq (CDG1Q), also known as coloboma, ccular with ichthyosis, brain malformations and endocrine abnormalities, is associated with ocular colobomas, ichthyosis, intellectual disability, and midline brain malformations with associated endocrine abnormalities.

*Epidemiology*: unknown.

*Eye Findings*: hypertelorism, nystagmus, ocular coloboma, optic nerve hypoplasia, and variable vision loss.

*Inheritance*: AR.

*Known Genes or Gene Locus*: SRD5A3.

## Corpus Callosum, Agenesis of, With Mental Retardation, Ocular Coloboma, and Micrognathia[23]

*OMIM*: #300472.

*Description*: Agenesis of corpus callosum with mental retardation, ocular coloboma, and micrognathia, also known as syndromic X-linked mental retardation 28 (MRXS28) and Graham-Cox syndrome, is characterized by agenesis of the corpus callosum, intellectual disability, retrognathia, and ocular coloboma.

*Epidemiology*: unknown.

*Eye Findings*: coloboma, downslanting palpebral fissures, and visual impairment.

*Inheritance*: XLR.

*Known Genes or Gene Locus*: IGBP1.

## Delleman Syndrome (Oculocerebrocutaneous Syndrome)[24–26]

*OMIM*: 164180.

*Description*: Delleman syndrome, also known as oculocerebrocutaneous syndrome or orbital cyst with cerebral and focal dermal malformations, is characterized by orbital cysts and microphthalmia/anophthalmia, central nervous system cysts, hydrocephalus, agenesis of the corpus callosum, large tectum, absence of cerebellar vermis, lipomatous skin tags, and focal dermal aplasia or hypoplasia. Children who survive have psychomotor retardation and epilepsy.

*Epidemiology*: unknown.

*Eye Findings*: anophthalmia, eyelid and iris coloboma, dermoids, microphthalmia, nystagmus, orbital cyst, and opacified cornea.

*Inheritance*: possible AD.

*Known Genes or Gene Locus*: unknown.

## Duane-Radial Ray Syndrome[27–29]

*OMIM*: #607323.

*Description*: Duane-Radial Ray syndrome, also called Okihiro syndrome or acro-renal-ocular syndrome, is associated with radial ray defects, renal anomalies, iris and optic nerve colobomas, microphthalmia, Duane anomaly, and deafness. Cognitive abilities and growth are normal.

*Epidemiology*: unknown.

*Eye Findings*: cataracts, Duane anomaly (limitations in abduction, globe retraction, and palpebral fissure narrowing on adduction), epicanthal folds, hypertelorism, iris/retinal coloboma, microphthalmia, optic disc hypoplasia, and strabismus.

*Inheritance*: AD.

*Known genes or gene locus*: SALL4.

## Focal Dermal Hypoplasia[30–32]

*OMIM*: #305600.

*Description*: Focal dermal hypoplasia, also known as Goltz syndrome or Goltz-Gorlin syndrome, is a multisystem disorder characterized by linear areas of skin atrophy with variable pigmentation, fat herniation, skeletal anomalies, papillomas, digital abnormalities (syndactyly, polydactyly, camptodactyly, ectrodactyly, and absence), nail and tooth abnormalities, ocular anomalies, and sparse hair. Cognitive abilities are typically intact for the majority of affected individuals. Ninety percent of cases are female.

*Epidemiology*: unknown.

*Eye Findings*: aniridia, anophthalmia, coloboma, ectopia lentis, microcornea, microphthalmia, nystagmus, optic atrophy, papillomas of conjunctiva and eyelid, strabismus, lacrimal drainage system abnormalities, and cysts.

*Inheritance*: XLD.

*Known Genes or Gene Locus*: PORCN.

## Fraser Syndrome[33–36]

*OMIM*: #219000, #617666, #617667.

*Description*: Fraser syndrome, also known as cryptophthalmos with other malformations and cryptophthalmos-syndactyly syndrome, is characterized by cryptophthalmos, syndactyly, and laryngeal and genitourinary system abnormalities. Intellectual disability is uncommon.

*Epidemiology*: prevalence of 0.2/100,000−0.43/100,000.

*Eye Findings*: blindness, coloboma of the upper eyelid, cryptophthalmos (Fig. 3.2), hypertelorism, lacrimal drainage system malformations, microphthalmia, and supernumerary eyebrows.

*Inheritance*: AR.

*Known Genes or Gene Locus*: FRAS1 (Fraser syndrome 1), FREM2 (Fraser syndrome 2), and GRIP1 (Fraser syndrome 3).

## Goldberg-Shprintzen Megacolon Syndrome[37–39]

*OMIM*: #609460.

*Description*: Goldberg-Shprintzen syndrome is characterized by dysmorphic facial features, microcephaly, and intellectual disability. It is associated

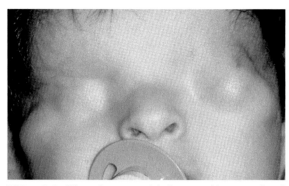

FIG. 3.2 Bilateral cryptophthalmos with associated orbitopalpebral cysts extending to the lateral orbital rims. (Courtesy Mocan MC, Ozgen, B, Irkec, M. Bilateral orbitopalpebral cysts in a case of cryptophthalmos associated with Fraser syndrome. *J AAPOS*. April 1, 2008;12(2):210−211. © 2008.)

with Hirschsprung disease and gyral abnormalities of the brain.

*Epidemiology*: unknown.

*Eye Findings*: blue sclerae, corneal ulcers, curled eyelashes, downslanting palpebral fissures, high-arched and dense eyebrows, iris coloboma, megalocornea, optic disc pallor, ptosis, synophrys, and telecanthus.

*Inheritance*: AR.

*Known Genes or Gene Locus*: KIAA1279.

## Meckel Syndrome[40–42]

*OMIM*: #249000.

*Description*: Meckel syndrome, also known as Meckel-Gruber syndrome, dysencephalia splanchnocystica and Gruber syndrome, is characterized by the triad of occipital encephalocele, postaxial polydactyly, and polycystic kidneys. Death typically occurs in utero or shortly after birth.

*Epidemiology*: incidence varies by region, estimated to occur worldwide in 1/3500−1/149,000; increased frequency reported in Finland, Belgium, and amongst Gujarati Indians.

*Eye Findings*: hypertelorism, hypotelorism, microphthalmia, ocular colobomas, and optic nerve hypoplasia.

*Inheritance*: AR.

*Known Genes or Gene Locus*: MKS1 (Meckel syndrome 1), TMEM216 (Meckel syndrome 2), TMEM67 (Meckel syndrome 3), CEP290 (Meckel syndrome 4), RPGRIP1L (Meckel syndrome 5), CC2D2A (Meckel syndrome 6), NPHP3 (Meckel syndrome 7), TCTN2 (Meckel syndrome 8), B9D1 (Meckel syndrome 9), B9D2 (Meckel syndrome 10), TMEM231 (Meckel syndrome 11),

*KIF14* (Meckel syndrome 12), and *TMEM107* (Meckel syndrome 13).

## Micro Syndrome[43,44]

*OMIM*: #600118.

*Description*: Micro syndrome, also known as Warburg Micro syndrome, is characterized by ocular abnormalities, corpus callosum hypoplasia, microcephaly, spastic diplegia, severe intellectual disability, and hypogonadism.

*Epidemiology*: unknown.

*Eye Findings*: congenital cataracts, deep-set eyes, microcornea, microphakia, microphthalmia, nystagmus, optic atrophy, and ptosis.

*Inheritance*: AR.

*Known Genes or Gene Locus*: *RAB3GAP1* (Micro syndrome 1), *RAB3GAP2* (Micro syndrome 2), *RAB18* (Micro syndrome 3), and *TBC1D20* (Micro syndrome 4).

## Microcephaly Microcornea Syndrome Seemanova Type[45]

*OMIM*: −.

*Description*: Microcephaly microcornea syndrome Seemanova type, also known as Seemanova-Lesny syndrome, is characterized by microcephaly, microphthalmia, congenital cataracts, hypogenitalism, delayed growth, and intellectual disability. The syndrome represents a rare X-linked intellectual disability disorder.

*Epidemiology*: unknown; three reported cases.

*Eye Findings*: congenital cataracts, epicanthal folds, hypertelorism, microcornea, microphthalmia, and upslanting palpebral fissures.

*Inheritance*: X-linked.

*Known Genes or Gene Locus*: unknown.

## Microphthalmia, Isolated[46−48]

*OMIM*: %251600.

*Description*: Group of inherited conditions with isolated microphthalmia.

*Epidemiology*: unknown.

*Eye Findings*: microphthalmia, high hyperopia, and glaucoma.

*Inheritance*: AR, AD.

*Known Genes or Gene Locus*: *CHX10*, *RAX*, *GDF6*, *MFRP*, *PRSS56*, *GDF3*, and *ALDH1A3*.

## Microtia Eye Coloboma and Imperforation of the Nasolacrimal Duct[49,50]

*OMIM*: #611863.

*Description*: The microtia, eye coloboma, and imperforation of the nasolacrimal duct disorder is characterized by the presence of microtia and an imperforated

nasolacrimal duct; ocular coloboma findings were variable. It is a rare disorder, described in a single, but large family.

*Epidemiology*: unknown.

*Eye Findings*: chorioretinal and iris coloboma, and imperforate nasolacrimal duct.

*Inheritance*: AD.

*Known Genes or Gene Locus*: 4p16-p15.

## Muscular Dystrophy-Dystroglycanopathy, Type A[51,52]

*OMIM*: #236670.

*Description*: Muscular dystrophy-dystroglycanopathy (congenital with brain and eye anomalies), also known as HARD syndrome, Walker-Warburg syndrome, muscle-eye-brain disease, cerebro-oculo-muscular syndrome, is characterized by lissencephaly, hydrocephalus, cerebellar malformations, ocular abnormalities, and congenital muscular dystrophy. Growth and intellectual disability are common. The majority of cases are lethal within first few months of life.

*Epidemiology*: prevalence of 1.2/100,000.

*Eye Findings*: cataracts, colobomas, deep-set eyes, glaucoma, persistent hyperplastic primary vitreous, iris malformations/hypoplasia, microcornea, microphthalmia (Fig. 3.3), myopia, optic nerve hypoplasia, Peter anomaly, retinal detachment, and retinal dysplasia.

*Inheritance*: AR.

*Known Genes or Gene Locus*: *POMT1* (MDDGA1), *POMT2* (MDDGA2), *POMGNT1* (MDDGA3), *FKTN*

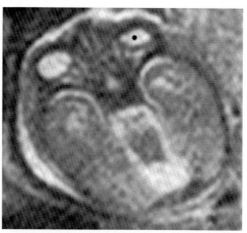

FIG. 3.3 Walker-Warburg syndrome. Fetal imaging (axial view) through the orbits shows left microphthalmia. (Courtesy Shekdar K, Feygin T. Fetal Neuroimaging, Neuroimaging Clinics of North America. August 1, 2011;21(3):677−703. © 2011.)

(MDDGA4), *FKRP* (MDDGA5), *LARGE* (MDDGA6), *ISPD* (MDDGA7), *GTDC2* (MDDGA8), *DAG1* (MDDGA9), *TMEM5* (MDDGA10), *B3GALNT2* (MDDGA11), *SGK196* (MDDGA12), B3GNT1 (MDDGA13), and *GMPPB* (MDDGA14).

## Nanophthalmos[53,54]

*OMIM*: %600165.

*Description*: Nanophthalmos is characterized by an inherited short axial length of the eyes; typically bilateral and symmetrical.

*Epidemiology*: unknown.

*Eye Findings*: small eye, high hyperopia, high incidence of angle closure glaucoma, and choroidal detachment.

*Inheritance*: AD.

*Known Genes or Gene Locus*: *MFRP* and *TMEM98*.

## Oculodentodigital Dysplasia[55,56]

*OMIM*: #164200.

*Description*: Oculodentodigital dysplasia, also known as oculodentoosseous dysplasia or ODD syndrome, is characterized by microphthalmia, dental anomalies, and syndactyly of the fourth and fifth digits. Neurologic symptoms are frequent and include spasticity, nystagmus, hearing loss, and bladder and bowel dysfunction. Cognitive impairment occurs in some patients.

*Epidemiology*: unknown.

*Eye Findings*: cataract, ciliary body cysts, epicanthal folds, glaucoma, hypotelorism, iris anomalies and iridocorneal angle dysgenesis, microcornea, microphthalmia, nystagmus, optic nerve and retinal dysplasia, and short palpebral fissures.

*Inheritance*: AD (majority), AR.

*Known Genes or Gene Locus*: *GJA1*.

## Osteoporosis-Pseudoglioma Syndrome[57,58]

*OMIM*: #259770.

*Description*: Osteoporosis-pseudoglioma syndrome, also known as ocular form of osteogenesis imperfecta, is characterized by osteoporosis associated with ocular abnormalities and visual impairment. Affected individuals are prone to fractures. Cognitive development is typically normal.

*Epidemiology*: unknown.

*Eye Findings*: absent anterior chamber, blindness, cataracts, corneal opacities, glaucoma, iris atrophy, leukocoria, microphthalmia, phthisis bulbi, pseudoglioma, and persistent hyperplasia of primary vitreous.

*Inheritance*: AR.

*Known Genes or Gene Locus*: *LRP5*.

## Papillorenal Syndrome[59–61]

*OMIM*: #120330.

*Description*: Papillorenal syndrome, also known as renal coloboma syndrome, optic nerve coloboma with renal disease, or congenital anomalies of the kidney and urinary tract (CAKUT) with or without ocular abnormalities, is characterized by ocular malformations and renal hypodysplasia. Cognitive and growth development is normal.

*Epidemiology*: unknown.

*Eye Findings*: microcornea, microphthalmia, "morning glory" optic disc anomaly, nystagmus, optic disc and retinal coloboma, optic nerve cysts, retinal detachment, retinal dysplasia, and staphyloma.

*Inheritance*: AD.

*Known Genes or Gene Locus*: *PAX2*.

## PHACE Association[62–64]

*OMIM*: 606519.

*Description*: PHACE association, also known as PHACE(S) syndrome, Pascual-Castroviejo type II syndrome, is a neurocutaneous syndrome characterized by posterior fossa brain malformations, facial hemangiomas, arterial anomalies, cardiac anomalies, and eye anomalies. PHACE syndrome is more common in females than males (9:1).

*Epidemiology*: unknown.

*Eye Findings*: facial and choroidal hemangioma, congenital cataracts, congenital glaucoma, congenital third and fourth nerve palsies, cryptophthalmos, exophthalmos, Horner syndrome, iris coloboma, iris heterochromia, iris hypoplasia, iris vessel hypertrophy, microphthalmia, Mittendorf dots, "morning-glory" optic disc anomaly, optic nerve hypoplasia and atrophy, peripapillary staphyloma, persistent fetal vasculature, posterior embryotoxon, proptosis, ptosis, retinal coloboma, retinal vascular abnormalities, sclerocornea, and strabismus.

*Inheritance*: sporadic.

*Known Genes or Gene Locus*: unknown; potential locus of 7q33.

## Renpenning Syndrome (Mental Retardation, X-Linked, Renpenning Type)[65,66]

*OMIM*: #309500.

*Description*: Renpenning syndrome, also known as Sutherland-Haan X-linked mental retardation syndrome, Golabi-Ito-Hall syndrome or syndromic X-linked mental retardation (MRXS3, MRXS8, and MRXS55) is an X-linked disorder characterized by intellectual disability, microcephaly, long and narrow face, short stature, and variable ocular abnormalities. Females typically show little or no phenotypic expression.

*Epidemiology*: unknown.

*Eye Findings*: cataracts, colobomas, epicanthus, hypermetropia, microphthalmia, long eyelashes, sparse eyebrows, strabismus, and upslanting palpebral fissures.

*Inheritance*: XLR.

*Known Genes or Gene Locus*: PQBP1.

## Syndromic Microphthalmia 1 (Lenz Microphthalmia Syndrome)[67,68]

*OMIM*: #309800.

*Description*: Syndromic microphthalmia 1, also known as Lenz microphthalmia syndrome or Lenz dysplasia, is characterized by anophthalmia or microphthalmia, and skeletal and genitourinary defects. Intellectual disability, behavioral abnormalities, and seizures are seen in most cases.

*Epidemiology*: unknown.

*Eye Findings*: anophthalmia, colobomas, microcornea, microphthalmia, and ptosis.

*Inheritance*: X-linked.

*Known Genes or Gene Locus*: NAA10.

## Syndromic Microphthalmia 2 (Oculofaciocardiodental Syndrome)[69,70]

*OMIM*: #300166.

*Description*: Syndromic microphthalmia 2, also known as oculofaciocardiodental syndrome and formerly known as ANOP2 and MAA, is characterized by ocular anomalies, facial anomalies, cardiac anomalies, and dental anomalies. The syndrome is lethal in males. Patients often have delayed motor development and mild intellectual disability.

*Epidemiology*: unknown.

*Eye Findings*: anophthalmia, blepharophimosis, congenital cataract, cryptophthalmia, glaucoma, iris synechiae, microcornea, microphthalmia, persistent hyperplasia of primary vitreous, ptosis, retinal detachment, strabismus, and thick eyebrows.

*Inheritance*: XLD.

*Known Genes or Gene Locus*: BCOR.

## Syndromic Microphthalmia 3 (Microphthalmia and Esophageal Atresia Syndrome)[71–73]

*OMIM*: #206900.

*Description*: Syndromic microphthalmia 3, also known as microphthalmia (or anophthalmia)-esophageal atresia syndrome, anophthalmia-esophageal-genital syndrome and SOX2 anophthalmia syndrome, is characterized by severe ocular anomalies, esophageal atresia, brain abnormalities, and hypogonadotropic hypogonadism.

Neurocognitive delays and sensorineural hearing loss is common.

*Epidemiology*: unknown.

*Eye Findings*: anophthalmia, aphakia, coloboma, hypotelorism, microphthalmia, optic nerve hypoplasia, sclerocornea, short/small palpebral fissure, and sparse eyebrows.

*Inheritance*: AD.

*Known Genes or Gene Locus*: SOX2.

## Syndromic Microphthalmia 4[74]

*OMIM*: %301590.

*Description*: Syndromic microphthalmia 4, also known as microphthalmia with ankyloblepharon and intellectual disability, is characterized by clinical anophthalmia, ankyloblepharon, and underdevelopment of bony orbits. Subjects lacked other features found in Lenz microphthalmia syndrome.

*Epidemiology*: unknown.

*Eye Findings*: ankyloblepharon and anophthalmia.

*Inheritance*: XLR.

*Known Genes or Gene Locus*: Xq27-q28.

## Syndromic Microphthalmia 5[75,76]

*OMIM*: #610125.

*Description*: Syndromic microphthalmia 5, also known as early-onset retinal dystrophy with or without pituitary dysfunction, is characterized by unilateral or bilateral microphthalmia or clinical anophthalmia with variable additional ocular features, hypotonia, central nervous system malformations, pituitary dysfunction, developmental delay, and seizures.

*Epidemiology*: unknown.

*Eye Findings*: anophthalmia, cataracts, colobomas, microcornea, microphthalmia, optic nerve hypoplasia, and retinal dystrophy.

*Inheritance*: AD.

*Known Genes or Gene Locus*: OTX2.

## Syndromic Microphthalmia 6[77–80]

*OMIM*: #607932.

*Description*: Syndromic microphthalmia 6, also known as microphthalmia with brain and digital anomalies, is characterized by anophthalmia or microphthalmia, pituitary hypoplasia, facial asymmetry, ear and digital abnormalities. Intellectual disability and developmental delay is common.

*Epidemiology*: unknown.

*Eye Findings*: anophthalmia, cataracts, colobomas, congenital aphakia, cryptophthalmos, glaucoma, microcornea, microphthalmia, overdeveloped eyebrows, Peters anomaly, and retinal dystrophy.

*Inheritance*: AD.

*Known Genes or Gene Locus*: BMP4.

## Syndromic Microphthalmia 7 (MIDAS Syndrome)[81,82]

*OMIM*: #309801.

*Description*: Syndromic microphthalmia 7, also known as MIDAS (microphthalmia, dermal aplasia and sclerocornea) syndrome, microphthalmia with linear skin defects, or linear skin defects with multiple congenital anomalies, is characterized by microphthalmia and linear aplastic skin defects of the face and neck. There is no fatty tissue herniation associated with the aplastic skin defects in MIDAS syndrome. MIDAS syndrome is lethal in utero for males.

*Epidemiology*: unknown.

*Eye Findings*: cataracts, colobomas, microphthalmia, pigmentary retinopathy, and sclerocornea.

*Inheritance*: XLD.

*Known Genes or Gene Locus*: HCCS.

## Syndromic Microphthalmia 8[83–86]

*OMIM*: %601349.

*Description*: Syndromic microphthalmia 8, also known as microcephaly-microphthalmia-ectrodactyly of lower limbs-prognathism syndrome, is characterized by intellectual disability, microcephaly, microphthalmia, ectrodactyly, and prognathism.

*Epidemiology*: unknown.

*Eye Findings*: lateral deficiency of eyebrows, microcornea, microphthalmia, and short palpebral fissures.

*Inheritance*: AD (most commonly), sporadic cases have been reported.

*Known Genes or Gene Locus*: 6q21.

## Syndromic Microphthalmia 9 (Matthew-Wood Syndrome)[87–90]

*OMIM*: #601186.

*Description*: Syndromic microphthalmia 9, also known as Matthew-Wood syndrome, Spear syndrome, pulmonary hypoplasia-diaphragmatic hernia-anophthalmia-cardiac defect (PDAC) or pulmonary agenesis, microphthalmia and diaphragmatic defect, is characterized by clinical anophthalmia or microphthalmia and pulmonary hypoplasia or aplasia. Severity of phenotypic presentation varies and can include multiple organ system defects, hypoplasia, or agenesis. The condition is typically lethal.

*Epidemiology*: unknown.

Eye Findings: anophthalmia, blepharophimosis, broad eyebrows, colobomas, microphthalmia, optic nerve hypoplasia, and retinal dysplasia.

*Inheritance*: AR.

*Known Genes or Gene Locus*: STRA6.

## Syndromic Microphthalmia 10[91]

*OMIM*: %611222.

*Description*: Syndromic microphthalmia 10, also known as microphthalmia and brain atrophy syndrome, is characterized by microphthalmia, microcephaly, and intellectual disability. Psychomotor development is normal in the first few months of life; however, it rapidly declines within the first year of life. Magnetic resonance imaging studies of the brain are notable for diffuse degenerative and atrophic changes.

*Epidemiology*: unknown.

*Eye Findings*: blindness and microphthalmia.

*Inheritance*: AR.

*Known Genes or Gene Locus*: unknown.

## Syndromic Microphthalmia 11[92]

*OMIM*: #614402.

*Description*: Syndromic microphthalmia 11 is characterized by microphthalmia, agenesis of the corpus callosum, cleft lip and palate. Cognitive abilities and growth are delayed.

*Epidemiology*: unknown.

*Eye Findings*: microphthalmia and optic nerve hypoplasia.

*Inheritance*: AR.

*Known Genes or Gene Locus*: VAX1.

## Syndromic Microphthalmia 12[88,89,93]

*OMIM*: #615524.

*Description*: Syndromic microphthalmia 12, also known as microphthalmia with or without pulmonary hypoplasia, diaphragmatic hernia and/or cardiac defects, is characterized by anophthalmia/microphthalmia and diaphragmatic hernia with variable degrees of pulmonary hypoplasia and/or cardiac defects resembling syndromic microphthalmia 9 (Matthew-Wood or PDAC syndrome) but lacking STRA6 mutation. Cognitive and developmental delay is prominent.

*Epidemiology*: unknown.

*Eye Findings*: anophthalmia, microphthalmia, and short palpebral fissures.

*Inheritance*: AD, AR.

*Known Genes or Gene Locus*: RARB.

## Syndromic Microphthalmia 13[94,95]

*OMIM*: #300915.

*Description*: Syndromic microphthalmia 13, also known as Maine microphthalmos or colobomatous microphthalmia with microcephaly, short stature, and psychomotor retardation, is characterized by microphthalmia, microcephaly, short stature, and intellectual disability.

*Epidemiology*: unknown.

*Eye Findings*: coloboma, esotropia, microcornea, microphthalmia, pendular nystagmus, and ptosis.

*Inheritance*: X-linked.

*Known Genes or Gene Locus*: HMGB3.

## Syndromic Microphthalmia 14[96–98]

*OMIM*: #615877.

*Description*: Syndromic microphthalmia 14, also known as microphthalmia/coloboma and skeletal dysplasia syndrome, is characterized by anophthalmia/microphthalmia, and coloboma with or without skeletal dysplasia. Intellectual disability and joint contractures are common.

*Epidemiology*: unknown.

*Eye Findings*: anophthalmia, cataracts, colobomas, corectopia, epicanthal folds, microcornea, microphthalmia, nystagmus, sclerocornea, and strabismus.

*Inheritance*: AR, AD (most).

*Known Genes or Gene Locus*: MAB21L2.

## Temtamy Syndrome[99–101]

*OMIM*: #218340.

*Description*: Temtamy syndrome (mental retardation with or without craniofacial dysmorphism, ocular coloboma, or abnormal corpus callosum), is characterized by microphthalmia, coloboma, and profound global developmental delay with seizures and abnormalities of the corpus callosum.

*Epidemiology*: unknown.

*Eye Findings*: arched eyebrows, coloboma, dislocated lens, downslanting palpebral fissures, hypertelorism, microcornea, microphthalmia, myopia, and optic disc atrophy.

*Inheritance*: AR.

*Known Genes or Gene Locus*: C12orf57.

## REFERENCES

1. Dharmasena A, Keenan T, Goldacre R, Hall N, Goldacre MJ. Trends over time in the incidence of congenital anophthalmia, microphthalmia and orbital malformation in England: database study. *Br J Ophthalmol*. 2017;101(6):735–739.
2. Bermejo E, Martínez-Frías ML. Congenital eye malformations: clinical-epidemiological analysis of 1,124,654 consecutive births in Spain. *Am J Med Genet*. 1998; 75(5):497–504.
3. Morrison D, Fitzpatrick D. National study of microphthalmia, anophthalmia, and coloboma (MAC) in Scotland: investigation of genetic aetiology. *J Med Genet*. 2002;39:16–22.
4. Lee K, Couser NL. Genetic testing for eye diseases: a comprehensive guide and review of ocular genetic manifestations from anterior segment malformation to retinal dystrophy. *Curr Genet Med Rep*. 2016;4: 41–48.
5. Kroes YH, Nievelstein R. Cerebral, cerebellar, and colobomatous anomalies in three related males: sex-linked inheritance in a newly recognized syndrome with features overlapping with Joubert syndrome. *Am J Medical Genetics*. 2005:297–301.
6. Laugel V, Dalloz C. Cerebro-oculo-facio-skeletal syndrome: three additional cases with CSB mutations, new diagnostic criteria and an approach to investigation. *J Med Genet*. 2008:564–571.
7. Meira BL. Manitoba aboriginal kindred with original cerebro-oculo-facio-skeletal syndrome has a mutation in the Cockayne syndrome Group B (CSB) gene. *Am J Hum Genet*. 2000:1221–1228.
8. Yew Weng Y, Giordano NC. Understanding photodermatoses associated with defective DNA repair: photosensitive syndromes without associated cancer predisposition. *J Am Acad Dermatol*. 2016:873–882.
9. Guion-Almeida Leine M, Zechi-Ceide Maria R. Cerebro-oculo-nasal syndrome: 13 new Brazilian cases. *Am J Med Genet*. 2007;143(24):3252–3266.
10. Kokitsu-Nakata NM. Cerebro-oculo-nasal syndrome: report of a case with a severe phenotype. *Am J Med Genet A*. 2009;149(3):519–520.
11. Charge syndrome. In: Chen H, ed. *Atlas of Genetic Diagnosis and Counseling*. 2nd ed. New York, NY: Springer; 2012:323–330.
12. Verloes A. Updated diagnostic criteria for CHARGE syndrome: a proposal. *Am J Med Genet*. 2005;133A: 306–308.
13. Ng B, Hackmann K. Mutations in the glycosylphosphatidlinositol gene PIGL cause CHIME syndrome. *Am J Hum Genet*. 2012;90:685–688.
14. Shashi V, Zunich J. Neuroectodermal (CHIME) syndrome: an additional case with long term follow up of all reported cases. *J Med Genet*. 1995;32:465–469.
15. Chassaing N. X-linked dominant chondrodysplasia with platyspondyly, distinctive brachydacyly, hydrocephaly and microphthalmia. *Am J Med Genet*. 2005;136A:307–312.
16. Simon D. A mutation in the 3′-UTR of the HDAC6 gene abolishing the post-transcriptional regulation mediated by hsa-miR-433 is linked to a new form of dominant X-link chondrodysplasia. *Hum Mol Genet*. 2010;19(10): 2015–2027.
17. Brancati F. MKS3/TMEM67 mutations are a major cause of COACH syndrome, a Joubert syndrome related disorder with liver involvement. *Hum Mutat*. 2009;30: E432–E442.

18. Doherty D. Mutations in 3 genes (MKS3, CC2D2A and RPGRIP1L) cause COACH syndrome (Joubert syndrome with congenital hepatic fibrosis). *J Med Genet.* 2010;47: 8−21.

19. Verloes A, Lambotte C. Further delineation of a syndrome of cerebellar vermis hypo/aplasia, oligophrenia, congenital ataxia, coloboma, and hepatic fibrosis. *Am J Med Genet.* 1989;32:227−232.

20. Al-Gazali LA. New autosomal recessive syndrome of ocular colobomas, ichthyosis, brain malformations and endocrine abnormalities in an Inbred Emirati family. *Am J Med Genet Part A.* 2008;146A:813−819.

21. Cantagrel V. SRD5A3 is required for converting polyprenol to dolichol and is mutated in a congenital glycosylation disorder. *Cell.* 2010;142:203−217.

22. Morava EA. Novel cerebello-ocular syndrome with abnormal glycosylation due to abnormalities in dilichol metabolism. *Brain.* 2010;133:3210−3220.

23. Graham MJ. A new X-linked syndrome with agenesis of the corpus callosum, mental retardation, coloboma, micrognathia, and a mutation in the alpha 4 gene at Xq13. *Am J Med Genet Part A.* 2003;123A:37−44.

24. McCandless S, Robin N. Severe oculocerebrocutaneous (Delleman) syndrome: overlap with Goldenhar anomaly. *Am J Med Genet A.* 1998;78:282−285.

25. Moog U, de Die-Smulders C. Oculocerebrocutaneous syndrome: report of three additional cases and aetiological considerations. *Clin Genet.* 1997;52:219−225.

26. Moog U, Jones MC. Oculocerebrocutaneous syndrome: the brain malformation defines a phenotype. *J Med Genet.* 2005;42:913−921.

27. Al-Baradie R. Duane radial ray syndrome (Okihiro syndrome) maps to 20q13 and results from mutations in SALL4, a new member of the SAL family. *Am J Hum Genet.* 2002;71:1195−1199.

28. Hayes A. The Okihiro syndrome of Duane anomaly, radial ray abnormalities, and deafness. *Am J Med Genet.* 1985;22:273−280.

29. Kohlhase J, Chitayat D. SALL4 mutations in Okihiro syndrome (Duane-radial ray syndrome), acro-renal-ocular syndrome and related disorders. *Hum Mutat.* 2005;26: 176−183.

30. Deidrick KK. Cognitive and psychological functioning in focal dermal hypoplasia. *Am J Med Genet C.* 2016;172C: 34−40.

31. Gisseman DJ, Herce HH. Ophthalmic manifestations of focal dermal hypoplasia (Goltz syndrome): a case series of 18 patients. *Am J Med Genet Part C.* 2016; 172C:59−63.

32. Sanchez-Valle A, Sutton RV. Focal dermal hypoplasia. In: *Harper's Textbook of Pediatric Dermatology.* 3rd ed. Oxford, UK: Wiley-Blackwell; 2011:133.1−133.9.

33. Fraser syndrome. In: Chen H, ed. *Atlas of Genetic Diagnosis and Counseline.* 2nd ed. New York, NY: Springer; 2012: 875−882.

34. Barisic I. Fraser syndrome: epidemiological study in a European population. *Am J Med Genet Part A.* 2013; 161A:1012−1018.

35. van Haelst MM. Fraser syndrome: a clinical study of 59 cases and evaluation of diagnostic criteria. *Am J Med Genet Part A.* 2007;143A:3194−3203.

36. Vogel JM. Mutations in GRIP1 cause Fraser syndrome. *J Med Genet.* 2012;49:303−306.

37. Brooks SA. Homozygous nonsense mutations in KIAA1279 are associated with malformations of the central and enteric nervous system. *Am J Hum Genet.* 2005; 77:120−126.

38. Hurst AJ. Unknown syndrome: hirschsprung's disease, microcephaly, and iris coloboma: a new syndrome of defective neuronal migration. *J Med Genet.* 1988;25: 494−497.

39. Yomo A. Goldberg−Shprintzen syndrome: Hirschsprung disease, hypotonia, and ptosis in sibs. *Am J Med Genet Part A.* 1991;41:188−191.

40. Meckel-gruber syndrome. In: Chen H, ed. *Atlas of Genetic Diagnosis and Counseling.* 2nd ed. New York, NY: Springer; 2012:1335−1340.

41. Morgan N. A novel locus for Meckel-Gruber syndrome, MKS3, maps to chromosome 8q24. *Hum Genet.* 2002; 111:456−461.

42. Salonen R, Paavola P. Meckel syndrome. *J Med Genet.* 1998;35:497−501.

43. Aligianis AI. Mutations of the catalytic subunit of RAB3-GAP cause Warburg Micro syndrome. *Nat Genet.* 2005; 37:221−224.

44. Picker-Minh S. Large homozygous RAB3GAP1 gene microdeletion causes Warburg micro syndrome 1. *Orphanet J Rare Dis.* 2014;9:113.

45. Seemanova E, Lesny I. X-linked microcephaly, microphthalmia, microcornea, congenital cataract, hypogenitalism, mental deficiency, growth retardation, spasticity: possible new syndrome. *Am J Med Genet.* 1996;66:179−183.

46. Warburg M. Classification of microphthalmos and coloboma. *J Med Genet.* 1993;30:664−669.

47. Bessant DAR, Anwar K, Khaliq S, et al. Phenotype of autosomal recessive congenital microphthalmia mapping to chromosome 14q32. *Br J Ophthal.* 1999;83: 919−922 [PubMed: 10413693, images, related citations].

48. Bessant DAR, Khaliq S, Hameed A, et al. A locus for autosomal recessive congenital microphthalmia maps to chromosome 14q32. *Am J Hum Genet.* 1998;62: 1113−1116.

49. Alasti F, Van Camp G. Genetics of microtia and associated syndromes. *J Med Genet.* 2009;46:361−369.

50. Balikova I. Autosomal-dominant microtia linked to five tandem copies of a copy-number-variable region at chromosome 4p16. *Am J Hum Genet.* 2008;82:181−187.

51. Dobyns BW. Diagnostic criteria for Walker-Warburg syndrome. *Am J Med Genet.* 1989;32:195−210.

52. Vajsar J, Schachter H. Walker-Warburg syndrome. *Orphanet Journal Rare Diseases.* 2006;1:29.

53. Fuchs J, Holm K, Vilhelmsen K, Rosenberg T, Scherfig E, Fledelius HC. Hereditary high hypermetropia in the Faroe Islands. *Ophthal Genet.* 2005;26:9−15 [PubMed: 15823920, related citations].

54. Othman MI, Sullivan SA, Skuta GL, et al. Autosomal dominant nanophthalmos (NNO1) with high hyperopia and angle-closure glaucoma maps to chromosome 11. *Am J Hum Genet*. 1998;63:1411−1418.

55. Gabriel LAR, Sachdeva R. Oculodentodigital dysplasia-new ocular findings and a novel connexin 43 mutation. *Arch Ophthalmol*. 2011;129:781−784.

56. Judisch Frank G. Oculodentodigital dysplasia: four new reports and a literature review. *Arch Ophthalmol*. 1979; 97:878−884.

57. Frontali M. Osteoporosis-pseudoglioma syndrome: report of three affected sibs and an overview. *Am J Med Genet*. 1985;22:35−47.

58. Steinmann B, Royce P. Osteoporosis-pseudoglioma syndrome. In: *Connective Tissue and its Heritable Disorders*. 2nd ed. Hoboken, NJ, USA: John Wiley & Sons; 2003: 1119−1121.

59. Amiel J. PAX2 mutations in renal-coloboma syndrome: mutational hotspot and germline mosaicism. *Eur J Hum Genet*. 2000;8:820−826.

60. Schimmenti AL. Renal coloboma syndrome. *Eur J Hum Genet*. 2011;19:1207−1212.

61. Schimmenti AL, Cunliffe H. Further delineation of renal-coloboma syndrome in patients with extreme variability of phenotype and identical PAX2 mutations. *Am J Hum Genet*. 1997;60:869−878.

62. Assari R. PHACE(S) syndrome: report of a case with new ocular and systemic manifestations. *J Curr Ophthalmol*. 2017;29:136−138.

63. Metry D. Consensus statement on diagnostic criteria for PHACE syndrome. *Pediatrics*. 2009;124:1447−1456.

64. Mitchell S, Siegel D. Candidate locus analysis for PHACE syndrome. *Am J Med Genet A*. 2012;158A:1363−1367.

65. Kalscheuer MV. Mutations in the polyglutamine binding protein 1 gene cause X-linked mental retardation. *Nat Genet*. 2003;35:313−315.

66. Stevenson RE. Renpenning syndrome comes into focus. *Am J Med Genet A*. 2005;134:415−421.

67. Esmailpour T. A splice donor mutation in NAA10 results in the dysregulation of the retinoic acid signaling pathway and causes Lenz microphthalmia syndrome. *J Med Genet*. 2014;51:185−196.

68. Forrester S. Manifestations in four males with and an obligate carrier of the Lenz microphthalmia syndrome. *Am J Med Genet*. 2001;98:92−100.

69. Gorlin JR. Oculo-facio-cardio-dental (OFCD) syndrome. *Am J Med Genet*. 1996;63:290−292.

70. Hilton E. BCOR analysis in patients with OFCD and Lenz microphthalmia syndromes, mental retardation with ocular anomalies, and cardiac laterality defects. *Eur J Hum Genet*. 2009;17:1325−1335.

71. Fantes J. Mutations in SOX2 cause anophthalmia. *Nat Genet*. 2003;33:462−463.

72. Numakura C. Supernumerary impacted teeth in a patient with SOX2 anophthalmia syndrome. *Am J Med Genet Part A*. 2010;152A:2355−2359.

73. Ragge N. SOX2 anophthalmia syndrome. *Am J Med Genet Part A*. 2005;135:1−7.

74. Graham CA. X-linked clinical anophthalmos. Localization of the gene to Xq27-Xq28. *Ophthalmic Paediatr Genet*. 1991;12:43−48.

75. Ragge N. Heterozygous mutations of OTX2 cause severe ocular malformations. *Am J Hum Genet*. 2005;76: 1008−1022.

76. Tajima T. OTX2 loss of function mutation causes anophthalmia and combined pituitary hormone deficiency with a small anterior and ectopic posterior pituitary. *J Clin Endocrinol Metab*. 2009;94:314−319.

77. Ahmad EM. 14q(22) deletion in a familial case of anophthalmia with polydactyly. *Am J Med Genet Part A*. 2003; 120A:117−122.

78. Bakrania P. Mutations in BMP4 cause eye, brain, and digit developmental anomalies: overlap between the BMP4 and hedgehog signaling pathways. *Am J Hum Genet*. 2008;82:304−319.

79. Bennett PC. Deletion 14q (q22q23) associated with anophthalmia, absent pituitary and other abnormalities. *J Med Genet*. 1991;28:280−281.

80. Nolen L. Deletion at 14q22-23 indicates a contiguous gene syndrome comprising anophthalmia, pituitary hypoplasia, and ear anomalies. *Am J Med Genet Part A*. 2006;140A:1711−1718.

81. Al-Gazali L. Two 46,XX,t(X;Y) females with linear skin defects and congenital microphthalmia: a new syndrome at Xp22.3. *J Med Genet*. 1990;27:59−63.

82. Wimplinger I. Mutations of the mitochondrial holocytochrome c-type synthase in X-linked dominant microphthalmia with linear skin defects syndrome. *Am J Hum Genet*. 2006;79:878−889.

83. Kumar AR. Absence of mutations in NR2E1 and SNX3 in five patients with MMEP (microcephaly, microphthalmia, ectrodactyly, and prognathism) and related phenotypes. *BMC Med Genet*. 2007;8:48.

84. Suthers G, Morris L. A second case of microcephaly, microphthalmia, ectrodactyly (split-foot) and prognathism (MMEP). *Clin Dysmorphol*. 1996;5:77−79.

85. Vervoort SV. Sorting nexin 3 (SNX3) is disrupted in a patient with a translocation t(6;13)(q21;q12) and microcephaly, microphthalmia, ectrodactyly, prognathism (MMEP) phenotype. *J Med Genet*. 2002;39: 893−899.

86. Viljoen DL, Smart RL. Split-foot anomaly, microphthalmia, cleft-lip and cleft-palate, and mental retardation associated with a chromosome 6;13 translocation. *Clin Dysmorphol*. 1993;2:274−277.

87. Casey J. First implication of STRA6 mutations in isolated anophthalmia, microphthalmia and coloboma: a new dimension to the STRA6 phenotype. *Hum Mutat*. 2011; 32:1417−1426.

88. Chassaing N. Mutation analysis of the STRA6 gene in isolated and non-isolated anophthalmia/microphthalmia. *Clin Genet*. 2013;83:244−250.

89. Chitayat D. The PDAC syndrome (pulmonary hypoplasia/agenesis, diaphragmatic hernia/eventration, anophthalmia/microphthalmia, and cardiac defect) (Spear syndrome, Matthew-Wood syndrome): report of eight cases including a living child and further evidence for autosomal recessive inheritance. *Am J Med Genet A*. 2007;143A:1268−1281.

90. Pasutto F. Mutations in STRA6 cause a broad spectrum of malformations including anophthalmia, congenital heart defects, diaphragmatic hernia, alveolar capillary dysplasia, lung hypoplasia and mental retardation. *Am J Hum Genet*. 2007;80:550−560.

91. Kanavin JO. Microphthalmia and brain atrophy: a novel neurodegenerative disease. *Ann Neurol*. 2006;59:719−723.

92. Slavotinek MA. VAX1 mutation associated with microphthalmia, corpus callosum agenesis, and orofacial clefting: the first description of a VAX1 phenotype in humans. *Hum Mutat*. 2012;33:364−368.

93. Srour M. Recessive and dominant mutations in retinoic acid receptor beta in cases with microphthalmia and diaphragmatic hernia. *Am J Hum Genet*. 2013;93:765−772.

94. Goldberg FM, McKusick AV. X-linked colobomatous microphthalmos and other congenital anomalies: a disorder resembling Lenz's dysmorphogenetic syndrome. *Am J Ophthal*. 1971;71:1128−1133.

95. Scott FA. Identification of an HMGB3 frameshift mutation in a family with an X-linked colobomatous microphthalmia syndrome using whole-genome and X-exome sequencing. *JAMA Ophthal*. 2014;132:1215−1220.

96. Deml B. Mutations in MAB21L2 result in ocular coloboma, microcornea and cataracts. *PLoS Genet*. 2015;11: e1005002.

97. Horn D. A novel oculo-skeletal syndrome with intellectual disability caused by a particular MAB21L2 mutation. *Eur J Med Genet*. 2015;58:387−391.

98. Rainger J. Monoallelic and biallelic mutations in MAB21L2 cause a spectrum of major eye malformations. *Am J Hum Genet*. 2014;94:915−923.

99. Akizu N. Whole-exome sequencing identifies mutated c12orf57 in recessive corpus callosum hypoplasia. *Am J Hum Genet*. 2013;92:392−400.

100. Li J. Agenesis of the corpus callosum, optic coloboma, intractable seizures, craniofacial and skeletal dysmorphisms: an autosomal recessive disorder similar to Temtamy syndrome. *Am J Med Genet Part A*. 2007;143A:1900−1905.

101. Zahrani F. Mutations in C12orf57 cause a syndromic form of colobomatous microphthalmia. *Am J Hum Genet*. 2013;92:387 (gon).

## FURTHER READING

1. Brooks B, Traboulsi E. Anophthalma, colobomatous, microphthalmia, and optic fissure closure defects. In: Traboulsi EI, ed. *Genetic Diseases of the Eye*. 2nd ed. New York: Oxford University Press; 2012.

2. Gentile M. COACH syndrome: report of two brothers with congenital hepatic fibrosis, cerebellar vermis hypoplasia, oligophrenia, ataxia and mental retardation. *Am J Med Genet*. 1996;64:514−520.

3. Gonzalez-Rodriguez J. Mutational screening of CHX10, GDF6, OTX2, RAX and SOX2 genes in 50 unrelated microphthalmia-anophthalmia-coloboma (MAC) spectrum cases. *Br J Ophthalmol*. 2010;94:1100−1104.

4. Schneider A. Novel SOX2 mutations and genotype-phenotype correlation in anophthalmia and microphthalmia. *Am J Med Genet Part A*. 2009;149A:2706−2715.

5. Williamson KA, Fitzpatrick DR. The genetic architecture of microphthalmia, anophthalmia and coloboma. *Eur J Med Genet*. 2014;57(8):369−380.

# CHAPTER 4

# Craniofacial Syndromes and Conditions

JENNIFER RHODES • ELEANOR LOVE • HIND AL SAIF • NATARIO L. COUSER

The craniofacial syndromes and conditions include synostotic and nonsynostotic disorders. Craniosynostosis is a malformation that involves the early closure of one or more sutures of the skull. This malformation can be an isolated finding, or it may occur as part of a syndrome. Craniosynostosis is a feature in nearly 200 known syndromes. The particular suture involved and dysmorphic features present along with the identification of the gene affected help characterize each specific disorder. The prognosis may vary considerably, indeed neurodevelopmental outcomes range from unaffected to severely delayed. Mutations within the *FGFR1*, *FGFR2*, and *FGFR3* genes have been identified to cause many of the craniosynostotic syndromes.[1] Crouzon syndrome, Apert syndrome, Pfeiffer syndrome types 1, 2, and 3, Jackson-Weiss syndrome, Beare-Stevenson syndrome, and FGFR2-related isolated coronal synostosis involve *FGFR2* gene mutations.[1,2] A small percentage of patients with Pfeiffer syndrome type 1 will have mutations in *FGFR1* responsible for the phenotype.[2] Crouzon syndrome with acanthosis nigricans and Muenke syndrome are both caused by mutations in the *FGFR3* gene.[3] A craniosynostosis malformation may be suspected in as early as the prenatal period from signs of increased biparietal dimensions or ventriculomegaly during an ultrasound evaluation. While theoretically prenatal ultrasound identification of an abnormal head shape leading to a specific diagnosis is possible, it is rare. Noninvasive pregnancy testing may assist in screening the previously mentioned conditions early in pregnancy. Most of these genetic disorders have an autosomal dominant (AD) pattern of inheritance; if a familial mutation is known, preimplantation genetic diagnosis testing may be considered.[4] Genetic testing methodology for these conditions may include a sequence analysis or deletion and duplication analyses involving polymerase chain reaction techniques, multiplex ligation-dependent probe amplification, and an analysis by a chromosomal microarray.[5]

Craniofacial conditions that are nonsynostotic include Treacher Collins syndrome, Pierre Robin sequence, and craniofacial microsomia. Treacher Collins syndrome, also called mandibulofacial dysostosis, is an AD condition with variable expressivity that is characterized by underdevelopment of the facial bones. Additional features include coloboma, downslanting palpebral fissures, ear underdevelopment, conductive hearing loss, and micrognathia. Pierre Robin sequence refers to a combination of micrognathia, glossoptosis, and cleft palate. These combinations of anomalies can be in isolation or can be observed in numerous syndromes, such as Stickler syndrome. Hemifacial microsomia is a condition in which the lower portion of one-half of the face, including the ipsilateral external and middle ear, is underdeveloped resulting in facial asymmetry. Goldenhar syndrome, also called facioauriculovertebral sequence, is characterized by bilateral hemifacial microsomia, cervical spine abnormalities, and the presence of epibulbar and limbal dermoids.

## GENETIC DISORDERS
### Antley-Bixler Syndrome[6–9]
OMIM: #207410.

*Description*: Antley-Bixler syndrome (ABS) is characterized by radiohumeral synostosis present from the perinatal period and is associated with mid-face hypolasia, choanal stenosis or atresia, and multiple joint contractures. Genital anomalies and disordered steroidogenesis may be present.

*Epidemiology*: unknown; 50 reported cases.

*Eye Findings*: hypertelorism, downslanting palpebral fissures, proptosis, and strabismus.

*Inheritance*: primarily AR; minority of cases are de novo.

*Known Genes or Gene Locus*: FGFR2.

## Apert Syndrome[8,10−12]

*OMIM*: #101200.

*Description*: Apert syndrome is associated with craniosynostosis, syndactyly, and hypoplasia of the midface. Intellectual disability or normal intelligence may be present.

*Epidemiology*: incidence of 1/65,000−1/160,000.

*Eye Findings*: hypertelorism (Fig. 4.1), downslanting palpebral fissures (Fig. 4.1), proptosis (Fig. 4.1), and shallow orbits.

*Inheritance*: AD, although majority of cases are de novo.

*Known Genes or Gene Locus*: FGFR2.

## Baller-Gerold Syndrome[8,13−15]

*OMIM*: #218600.

*Description*: The primary features of Baller-Gerold syndrome are craniosynstosis and radial aplasia. Spinal and pelvic skeletal abnormalities and small stature are commonly seen.

*Epidemiology*: estimated prevalence of fewer than 1/1,000,000.

*Eye Findings*: hypertelorism and proptosis.

*Inheritance*: AR.

*Known Genes or Gene Locus*: RECQL4.

## Beare-Stevenson Syndrome[16−18]

*OMIM*: #123790.

*Description*: Beare-Stevenson cutis gyrata syndrome is characterized by craniosynostosis, mid-facial hypoplasia, cutis gyrata, and acanthosis nigricans. Other signs and symptoms include choanal atresia, ear defects, and a prominent umbilical stump.

*Epidemiology*: unknown; fewer than 20 cases have been reported worldwide.

*Eye Findings*: hypertelorism, downslanting palpebral fissures, and proptosis.

*Inheritance*: AD, although all cases observed to date have been de novo.

*Known Genes or Gene Locus*: FGFR2.

## Carpenter Syndrome[8,19−21]

*OMIM*: #201000.

*Description*: The primary features of Carpenter syndrome are acrocephaly with craniofacial asymmetry and brachydactyly, syndactyly, or polydactyly of the

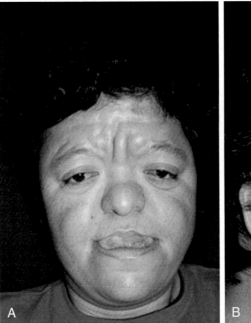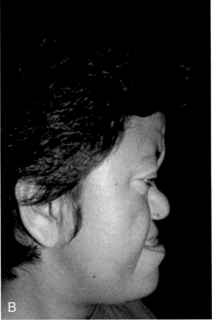

FIG. 4.1 Front view showing hypertelorism, downslanting palpebral fissures **(A)**, and ocular proptosis, bulbous tip of the nose, and hypoplastic middle face seen on lateral view **(B)**. (Courtesy Costa, FWG, Rodrigues RR, Batista ACB; Ribeiro, T.R., Pereira KMA. Multiple radiopaque mandibular esions in a patient with Apert syndrome. *J Endod*. December 1, 2012;38(12):1639−1643. © 2012.)

hands and feet. Other clinical features include obesity, congenital heart defects, umbilical hernia, and cryptorchidism. Intellectual disability ranging from mild to profound is common among people with Carpenter syndrome; however, some individuals have normal intelligence.

*Epidemiology*: incidence of 1/1,000,000.

*Eye Findings*: corneal abnormalities such as microcornea, improper development and/or clouding; downslanting palpebral fissures; epicanthal folds; hypoplastic supraorbital ridges; and optic atrophy.

*Inheritance*: AR.

*Known Genes or Gene Locus*: RAB23.

## Craniometaphyseal Dysplasia[22,23]

*OMIM*: #123000.

*Description*: The cardinal features of craniometaphyseal dysplasia are hyperstosis and sclerosis of the craniofacial bones, macrocephaly, metaphyseal dysplasia, and sensorineural deafness.

*Epidemiology*: unknown.

*Eye Findings*: blindness, hypertelorism, and proptosis.

*Inheritance*: AD or AR.

*Known Genes or Gene Locus*: ANKH, GJA1.

## Craniosynostosis—Adelaide and Philadelphia Types[8,24,25]

*OMIM*: #185900 (Philadelphia type), %600593 (Adelaide type).

*Description*: Craniosynostosis—Adelaide and Philadelphia types are characterized by sagittal craniosynostosis causing facial asymmetry, broad forehead, brachyturricephaly. Syndactyly of the hands and feet are also associated.

*Epidemiology*: unknown.

*Eye Findings*: hypertelorism and proptosis.

*Inheritance*: AD.

*Known Genes or Gene Locus*: FGFR3 (Adelaide), 2q34-q36 (Philadelphia).

## Craniosynostosis—Boston Type[8,26]

*OMIM*: #604757.

*Description*: Features of Boston-type craniosynostosis include forehead retrusion, frontal bossing, brachyturricephaly, and the Kleeblattschädel deformity (cloverleaf skull). Intelligence is typically normal; some affected individuals may experience seizures.

*Epidemiology*: unknown.

*Eye Findings*: hyperopia, hypotelorism, and myopia.

*Inheritance*: AD.

*Known Genes or Gene Locus*: MSX2.

## Craniosynostosis Mental Retardation Syndrome of Lin and Gettig[8,27,28]

*OMIM*: 218649.

*Description*: This condition, craniosynostosis mental retardation syndrome of Lin and Gettig, is characterized by craniosynostosis, severe intellectual disability, agenesis of the corpus callosum, camptodactyly, hypogonadism, and distinctive facial features. Only three cases have been reported.

*Epidemiology*: unknown.

*Eye Findings*: blepharophimosis, downslanting/upslanting palpebral fissures, epicanthal folds, hypertelorism, hypotelorism, neural palpebral fissures, ptosis, and strabismus.

*Inheritance*: AR.

*Known Genes or Gene Locus*: unknown (possibly due to mutation in KAT6B gene).

## Craniotelencephalic Dysplasia[29–31]

*OMIM*: 218670.

*Description*: Craniotelencephalic dysplasia is a very rare condition characterized by craniosynostosis, psychomotor delay, seizures, and numerous brain abnormalities that include arhinencephaly, lissencephaly, septo-optic dysplasia, and agenesis of the corpus callosum.

*Epidemiology*: unknown.

*Eye Findings*: hypotelorism, microphthalmia, and optic nerve hypoplasia.

*Inheritance*: AR.

*Known Genes or Gene Locus*: unknown.

## Crouzon Syndrome[8,18,32,33]

*OMIM*: #123500.

*Description*: Craniosynostosis in Crouzon syndrome causes alterations of the facial structure due to abnormal growth of the facial bones. Common features include exophthalmos, vision problems caused by shallow orbits, strabismus, a beaked nose, and an underdeveloped upper jaw. Individuals with Crouzon syndrome are usually of normal intelligence.

*Epidemiology*: incidence of 1.6/100,000.

*Eye Findings*: amblyopia, exophthalmos, exposure conjunctivitis/keratitis, hypertelorism, iris coloboma, optic atrophy, poor vision, proptosis, ptosis shallow orbits, and strabismus.

*Inheritance*: AD.
*Known Genes or Gene Locus*: FGFR2.

## Crouzon Syndrome With Acanthosis Nigricans (Crouzonodermoskeletal Syndrome)[18,34−36]

*OMIM*: #612247.

*Description*: Individuals with this condition, Crouzon Syndrome with Acanthosis Nigricans (Crouzonodermoskeletal Syndrome), present with craniosynostosis and acanthosis nigricans. There is phenotypic overlap between the signs and symptoms of Crouzon syndrome with acanthosis nigricans and those of the classic Crouzon syndrome; however, skin abnormalities such as pale, flat scars in thick, dark areas of the skin are unique to Crouzon syndrome with acanthosis nigricans.

*Epidemiology*: unknown.

*Eye Findings*: hypertelorism, optic atrophy, proptosis, shallow orbits, and strabismus.

*Inheritance*: AD.

*Known Genes or Gene Locus*: FGFR3.

## Cutis Gyrata Syndrome of Beare and Stevenson[8,16]

*OMIM*: #123790.

*Description*: Beare-Stevenson cutis gyrata syndrome is characterized by craniosynostosis and cutis gyrata, in addition to other signs and symptoms such as acanthosis nigricans, ear defects, anogenital anomalies, and prominent umbilical stump.

*Epidemiology*: unknown; fewer than 20 cases have been reported worldwide.

*Eye Findings*: downslanting palpebral fissures, exophthalmos, hypertelorism, optic atrophy, poor vision, and proptosis.

*Inheritance*: AD.

*Known Genes or Gene Locus*: FGFR2.

## Goldenhar Syndrome[37,38]

*OMIM*: %164210.

*Description*: Persons with Goldenhar syndrome, also commonly used interchangeably with the terms hemifacial microsomia, oculoauricular dysplasia or facioauriculovertebral sequence, often present with facial asymmetry in which the cheekbones, jaws, and the eye on one side of the face are abnormal. The most common signs and symptoms are a partially formed or absent ear, ocular dermoid cysts, and spinal abnormalities. Intelligence is not affected.

*Epidemiology*: incidence of 1/3500−1/5600.

*Eye Findings*: anophthalmia, blepharophimosis, epibulbar dermoid, lipodermoid, microphthalmia, strabismus, and upper eyelid coloboma.

*Inheritance*: AD; de novo mutation.

*Known Genes or Gene Locus*: unknown.

## Gomez-Lopez-Hernandez Syndrome (Cerebello-Trigeminal-Dermal Dysplasia)[39−41]

*OMIM*: %601853.

*Description*: Gomez-Lopez-Hernandez syndrome is characterized by alopecia, trigeminal anesthesia, and rhombencephalosynapsis. Additional symptoms may include brachyturricephaly, mid-face hypoplasia, short stature, and/or intellectual disability. Though the cause is poorly understood, the condition is thought to have a genetic basis with autosomal recessive inheritance. Fewer than 30 cases have been reported worldwide.

*Epidemiology*: unknown.

*Eye Findings*: absent corneal reflexes, corneal opacities, hypertelorism, strabismus, telecanthus, and visual impairment.

*Inheritance*: AR.

*Known Genes or Gene Locus*: unknown.

## Hunter-McAlpine Craniosynostosis Syndrome[8,42−45]

*OMIM*: 601379.

*Description*: This condition, Hunter-McAlpine craniosynostosis syndrome, typically presents with microcephaly due to craniosynostosis, intellectual disability, and developmental delay. Affected individuals often have almond-shaped eyes, ptosis, and a small downturned mouth.

*Epidemiology*: prevalence of <1/1,000,000.

*Eye Findings*: amblyopia, astigmatism, almond-shaped palpebral fissures, ptosis, strabismus, and visual impairment.

*Inheritance*: AD.

*Known Genes or Gene Locus*: 17q23.1-q24.2.

## Jackson-Weiss Syndrome[8,46,47]

*OMIM*: #123150.

*Description*: Jackson-Weiss syndrome typically presents with craniosynostosis, mid-facial hypoplasia, and foot abnormalities. Intelligence is usually normal.

*Epidemiology*: unknown.

*Eye Findings*: hypertelorism, proptosis, ptosis, and strabismus.

*Inheritance*: AD.

*Known Genes or Gene Locus*: FGFR1, FGFR2.

## Lowry MacLean Syndrome[48,49]

*OMIM*: 600252.

*Description*: Lowry MacLean syndrome is associated with craniosynostosis, microcephaly, glaucoma, growth failure, and dysmorphic features including trigonocephaly, cleft palate, and congenital heart defects. Only three cases have been reported worldwide.

*Epidemiology*: unknown.

*Eye Findings*: glaucoma and exotropia.

*Inheritance*: unknown; possible AD.

*Known Genes or Gene Locus*: unknown.

## Muenke Syndrome[8,18,50,51]

*OMIM*: #602849.

*Description*: Muenke syndrome is characterized by coronal craniosynostosis, macrocephaly, mid-face hypoplasia, and developmental delay. Hearing loss and abnormalities of the hands and feet may be present. The syndrome accounts for an estimated 8% of all cases of craniosynostosis.

*Epidemiology*: incidence of 1/30,000.

*Eye Findings*: downslanting palpebral fissures, hypertelorism, proptosis, and ptosis.

*Inheritance*: AD.

*Known Genes or Gene Locus*: FGFR3.

## Opitz Trigonocephaly Syndrome[8,52]

*OMIM*: #211750.

*Description*: Opitz trigonocephaly syndrome, also known as C syndrome, is characterized by trigonocephaly, severe intellectual disability, hypotonia, cardiac defects, redundant skin, and abnormal facial features.

*Epidemiology*: unknown; approximately 70 cases have been reported worldwide.

*Eye Findings*: epicanthal folds, upward slanting palpebral fissures, and strabismus.

*Inheritance*: AD.

*Known Genes or Gene Locus*: CD96.

## Pierre Robin Sequence[53-55]

*OMIM*: %261800.

*Description*: Individuals with Pierre Robin sequence present with micrognathia, glossoptosis, and cleft palate, causing difficulty in breathing and poor feeding in infancy. The primary gene associated with the isolated Pierre Robin sequence is located near the *SOX9* gene on chromosome 17. The associated anomalies may be isolated or part of a syndrome such as campomelic dysplasia or Stickler syndrome.

*Epidemiology*: incidence of 1/8500–1/14,000.

*Eye Findings*: glaucoma, microphthalmia, myopia, and retinal detachment.

*Inheritance*: AD, AR, X-linked, isolated.

*Known Genes or Gene Locus*: 17q24.3-q25.1.

## Pfeiffer Syndrome[2,8,18,56,57]

*OMIM*: #101600.

*Description*: The primary features of Pfeiffer syndrome are craniosynostosis, broad thumbs and great toes, brachydactyly, and variable syndactyly. Cloverleaf skull, conductive hearing loss, and ocular proptosis may also be present. Three clinical subtypes have been identified.

*Epidemiology*: incidence of 1/100,000 (all types).

*Eye Findings*: downslanting palpebral fissures, hypertelorism, proptosis, shallow orbits, and strabismus.

*Inheritance*: AD.

*Known Genes or Gene Locus*: FGFR1, FGFR2.

## Por (Cytochrome P450 Oxidoreductase) Deficiency With Antley-Bixler Phenotype[8,58-62]

*OMIM*: *124015.

*Description*: Severe cytochrome P450 oxidoreductase deficiency is associated with disordered steroidogenesis, skeletal malformations characteristic of ABS, and genital anomalies that result in ambiguous genitalia and infertility. Skeletal abnormalities include craniosynostosis, mid-face retrusion, hydrocephalus, and radio-humeral synostosis.

*Epidemiology*: unknown.

*Eye Findings*: hypertelorism and proptosis.

*Inheritance*: AR.

*Known Genes or Gene Locus*: POR.

## Saethre-Chotzen Syndrome[8,63-65]

*OMIM*: #101400.

*Description*: Saethre-Chotzen syndrome is a craniosynostosis syndrome characterized by facial dysmorphism and hand and foot abnormalities. Brachycephaly, facial asymmetry, hypertelorism, and maxillary hypoplasia are often present. Limb abnormalities may include radioulnar synostosis, brachydactyly, cutaneous syndactyly, and hallux valgus.

*Epidemiology*: incidence of 1/25,000–1/50,000.

*Eye Findings*: coronal synostosis, hypertelorism, lacrimal duct abnormalities, orbital asymmetry, ptosis, shallow orbits, and strabismus.

*Inheritance*: AD.

*Known Genes or Gene Locus*: TWIST1, FGFR2.

## Shprintzen-Goldberg Craniosynostosis Syndrome[8,66-69]

*OMIM*: #182212.

*Description*: Shprintzen-Goldberg syndrome is phenotypically similar to Marfan syndrome and Loeys-Dietz syndrome, sharing the same craniofacial, skeletal, skin, and cardiovascular findings. Additional findings associated with Shprintzen-Goldberg syndrome include intellectual disability and severe hypotonia.

*Epidemiology*: unknown.

*Eye Findings*: downslanting palpebral fissures, exophthalmos, hypertelorism, myopia, ptosis, shallow orbits, strabismus, and telecanthus.

*Inheritance*: AD, though most cases are due to de novo mutation.

*Known Genes or Gene Locus*: SKI.

## Treacher Collins Syndrome[70-73]

*OMIM*: #154500 (TCS 1), #613717 (TCS 2), #248390 (TCS 3).

*Description*: Treacher Collins syndrome presents with extremely variable signs and symptoms, ranging from mild to severe. Characteristic features include downslanting palpebral fissures, eyelid colobomas, micrognathia, and malformation of the ears such as microtia and stenosis/atresia of the external auditory canal. Conductive hearing loss and cleft palate are often associated. Three subtypes of this disorder have been identified.

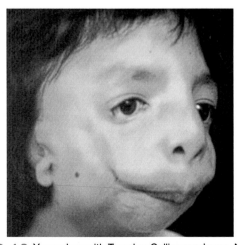

FIG. 4.2 Young boy with Treacher Collins syndrome. Note the coloboma of the lower eyelids, downslanting palpebral fissures, microtia, macrostomia, and hypoplasia of the maxilla and mandible. (Courtesy Molina F. Treacher–Collins syndrome. *Plastic Surgery*. January 1, 2013:828–836.e1. © 2013.)

*Epidemiology*: incidence of 1/50,000.

*Eye Findings*: absent/sparse eyelashes, blepharospasm, cataracts, downslanting palpebral fissures (Fig. 4.2), hypertelorism (Fig. 4.2), iris coloboma, lower/upper eyelid colobomas (Fig. 4.2), lacrimal duct stenosis, microphthalmia, ptosis, strabismus, visual impairment, and visual loss.

*Inheritance*: AD (TCS 1, TCS 2), AR (TCS 2, TCS 3).

*Known Genes or Gene Locus*: TCOF1 (TCS 1), POLR1D (TCS 2), POLR1C (TCS 3).

## REFERENCES

1. Barik M, et al. Novel mutation detection of fibroblast growth factor receptor 1 (FGFR1) gene, FGFR2IIIa, FGFR2IIIb, FGFR2IIIc, FGFR3, FGFR4 gene for craniosynostosis: a prospective study in Asian Indian patient. *J Pediatr Neurosci*. 2015;10(3):207–213.
2. Júnior HM, et al. Pfeiffer syndrome: clinical and genetic findings in five Brazilian families. *Med Oral Patol Oral Cir Bucal*. 2015;20(1):e52–e58.
3. Barroso E, et al. Mild isolated craniosynostosis due to a novel FGFR3 mutation, p.Ala334Thr. *Am J Med Genet A*. 2011;155A(12):3050–3053.
4. Chen CP, et al. Second-trimester molecular prenatal diagnosis of sporadic Apert syndrome following sonographic findings of mild ventriculomegaly and clenched hands mimicking trisomy 18. *Taiwan J Obstet Gynecol*. 2010; 49(1):129–132.
5. Weber B, et al. Prenatal diagnosis of apert syndrome with cloverleaf skull deformity using ultrasound, fetal magnetic resonance imaging and genetic analysis. *Fetal Diagn Ther*. 2010;27(1):51–56.
6. *Antley Bixler Syndrome*. NORD (National Organization for Rare Disorders). 2007. Accessed 6.01.2018.
7. Lahiri S, Ghoshal B, Nandi D. A case of Antley-Bixler syndrome. *J Clin Neonatol*. 2012;1:46–48.
8. Panigrahi I. Craniosynostosis genetics: the mystery unfolds. *Indian J Hum Genet*. 2011;17:48–53. https://doi.org/10.4103/0971-6866.86171.
9. Tomková M, Marohnic CC, Baxová A, Martásek P. Antley-Bixler syndrome or POR deficiency? *Cas Lek Cesk*. 2008; 147:261–265.
10. Barik M, et al. Novel mutation detection of fibroblast growth factor receptor 1 (FGFR1) gene, FGFR2IIIa, FGFR2IIIb, FGFR2IIIc, FGFR3, FGFR4 gene for craniosynostosis: a prospective study in Asian Indian patient. *J Pediatr Neurosci*. 2015;10(3):207–213.
11. Chen CP, et al. Second-trimester molecular prenatal diagnosis of sporadic Apert syndrome following sonographic findings of mild ventriculomegaly and clenched hands mimicking trisomy 18. *Taiwan J Obstet Gynecol*. 2010; 49(1):129–132.
12. Weber B, et al. Prenatal diagnosis of Apert syndrome with cloverleaf skull deformity using ultrasound, fetal magnetic resonance imaging and genetic analysis. *Fetal Diagn Ther*. 2010;27(1):51–56.

13. Anyane-Yeboa K, Gunning L, Bloom AD. Baller-Gerold syndrome craniosynostosis-radial aplasia syndrome. *Clin Genet*. 1980;17:161–166.

14. *Baller-Gerold Syndrome*. Genetics Home Reference. Available at: https://ghr.nlm.nih.gov/condition/baller-gerold-syndrome.

15. Cao DH, et al. Identification of novel compound heterozygous RECQL4 mutations and prenatal diagnosis of Baller-Gerold syndrome: a case report. *Genet Mol Res*. 2015;14:4757–4766.

16. *Beare-Stevenson Cutis Gyrata Syndrome*. Genetics Home Reference. Available at: https://ghr.nlm.nih.gov/condition/beare-stevenson-cutis-gyrata-syndrome.

17. Hall BD, Cadle RG, Golabi M, Morris CA, Cohen MM. Beare-Stevenson cutis gyrata syndrome. *Am J Med Genet*. 1992;44:82–89.

18. Robin NH, Falk MJ, Haldeman-Englert CR. FGFR-related craniosynostosis syndromes. In: Adam MP, et al., eds. *GeneReviews®*. Seattle: University of Washington; 1993.

19. *Carpenter Syndrome*. UNC School of Medicine Division of Plastic and Reconstructive Surgery. Available at: https://www.med.unc.edu/plastic/ptinfo/pediatric-plastic-and-craniofacial-surgery/carpenter-syndrome.

20. *Carpenter Syndrome*. NORD (National Organization for Rare Disorders). 2016. Accessed 6.01. 2018.

21. Twigg SRF, et al. Mutations in multidomain protein MEGF8 identify a Carpenter syndrome subtype associated with defective lateralization. *Am J Hum Genet*. 2012;91:897–905.

22. *Craniometaphyseal Dysplasia*. Genetics Home Reference. Available at: https://ghr.nlm.nih.gov/condition/craniometaphyseal-dysplasia.

23. *Craniometaphyseal Dysplasia*. NORD (National Organization for Rare Disorders). 2005. Accessed 6.01. 2018.

24. Hollway GE, Phillips HA, Adès LC, Haan EA, Mulley JC. Localization of craniosynostosis Adelaide type to 4p16. *Hum Mol Genet*. 1995;4:681–683.

25. Robin NH, Segel B, Carpenter G, Muenke M. Craniosynostosis, Philadelphia type: a new autosomal dominant syndrome with sagittal craniosynostosis and syndactyly of the fingers and toes. *Am J Med Genet*. 1996;62:184–191.

26. Florisson JMG, et al. Boston type craniosynostosis: report of a second mutation in MSX2. *Am J Med Genet A*. 2013;161A:2626–2633.

27. Bashir RA, et al. Lin-Gettig syndrome: craniosynostosis expands the spectrum of the KAT6B related disorders. *Am J Med Genet A*. 2017;173:2596–2604.

28. Hedera P, Innis JW. Possible third case of Lin-Gettig syndrome. *Am J Med Genet*. 2002;110:380–383.

29. Daum S, Le Beau J, Minuit P. Dysplasie telencephalique avec excroissance de l'os frontal. *Sem Hop Paris*. 1958;34:1893–1896.

30. Jabbour JT, Taybi H. Craniotelencephalic dysplasia. *Am J Dis Child*. 1964;108:627–632.

31. Hughes HE, Harwood-Nash DC, Becker LE. Craniotelencephalic dysplasia in sisters: further delineation of a possible syndrome. *Am J Med Genet*. 1983;14:557–565.

32. *Crouzon Syndrome*. NORD (National Organization for Rare Disorders). 2016. Accessed 11.01. 2018.

33. Helman SN, Badhey A, Kadakia S, Myers E. Revisiting Crouzon syndrome: reviewing the background and management of a multifaceted disease. *Oral Maxillofac Surg*. 2014;18:373–379.

34. Arnaud E, Collet C, di Rocco F. *Orphanet: Crouzon Syndrome Acanthosis Nigricans Syndrome*. 2013. Available at: http://www.orpha.net/consor/cgi-bin/OC_Exp.php?Lng=EN&Expert=93262.

35. Barroso E, et al. Mild isolated craniosynostosis due to a novel FGFR3 mutation, p.Ala334Thr. *Am J Med Genet A*. 2011;155A(12):3050–3053.

36. Mir A, Wu T, Orlow SJ. Cutaneous features of Crouzon syndrome with acanthosis nigricans. *JAMA Dermatol*. 2013;149:737–741.

37. Gaurkar SP, Gupta KD, Parmar KS, Shah BJ. Goldenhar syndrome: a report of 3 cases. *Indian J Dermatol*. 2013;58:244.

38. *Oculo-auriculo-vertebral Spectrum*. NORD (National Organization for Rare Disorders). 2007. Accessed 13.01. 2018.

39. Fernández-Jaén A, Fernández-Mayoralas DM, Calleja-Pérez B, Muñoz-Jareño N, Moreno N. Gomez–lopez-hernandez syndrome: two new cases and review of the literature. *Pediatr Neurol*. 2009;40:58–62.

40. Poretti A, Bartholdi D, Gobara S, Alber FD, Boltshauser E. Gomez-Lopez-Hernandez syndrome: an easily missed diagnosis. *Eur J Med Genet*. 2008;51:197–208.

41. Tully HM, et al. Beyond Gómez-López-Hernández syndrome: recurring phenotypic themes in rhombencephalosynapsis. *Am J Med Genet A*. 2012;158A:2393–2406.

42. Hunter AG, McAlpine PJ, Rudd NL, Fraser FC. A 'new' syndrome of mental retardation with characteristic facies and brachyphalangy. *J Med Genet*. 1977;14:430–437.

43. Hunter A, et al. The Hunter–McAlpine syndrome results from duplication 5q35–qter. *Clin Genet*. 2005;67:53–60.

44. *Hunter McAlpine Craniosynostosis*. Orphanet. Available at: http://www.orpha.net/consor/cgi-bin/OC_Exp.php?lng=en&Expert=97340.

45. Thomas JA, et al. Hunter-McAlpine craniosynostosis phenotype associated with skeletal anomalies and interstitial deletion of chromosome 17q. *Am J Med Genet*. 1996;62:372–375.

46. *Jackson-Weiss Syndrome*. Genetics Home Reference. Available at: https://ghr.nlm.nih.gov/condition/jackson-weiss-syndrome.

47. *Jackson Weiss Syndrome*. Orphanet. Available at: http://www.orpha.net/consor/cgi-bin/OC_Exp.php?Expert=1540&lng=EN.

48. Al-Torki NA, Sabry MA, Al-Awadi SA, Al-Tarkeit N. Lowry-Maclean syndrome with osteopenic bones and possible autosomal dominant inheritance in a Bedouin family. *Am J Med Genet*. 1997;73:491–492.

49. Kousseff BG, Ranells JD. Lowry-MacLean syndrome does exist. *Am J Med Genet*. 1994;53:300–301.

50. Abdel-Salam GMH, et al. Muenke syndrome with pigmentary disorder and probable hemimegalencephaly: an expansion of the phenotype. *Am J Med Genet.* 2011;155:207−214.

51. Doherty ES, et al. Muenke syndrome (FGFR3-related craniosynostosis): expansion of the phenotype and review of the literature. *Am J Med Genet.* 2007;143A:3204−3215.

52. Kaname T, et al. Mutations in CD96, a member of the immunoglobulin superfamily, cause a form of the C (opitz trigonocephaly) syndrome. *Am J Hum Genet.* 2007;81:835−841.

53. Benko S, et al. Highly conserved non-coding elements on either side of SOX9 associated with Pierre Robin sequence. *Nat Genet.* 2009;41:359−364.

54. Girard B, Saraux H, Lasfargues G. Ophthalmologic manifestations of the Pierre Robin syndrome. Report of a case of microphthalmia. *Ann Pediatr Paris.* 1990;37:39−43.

55. Tan TY, Kilpatrick N, Farlie PG. Developmental and genetic perspectives on Pierre Robin sequence. *Am J Med Genet.* 2013;163:295−305.

56. Harb E, Kran B. Pfeiffer syndrome: systemic and ocular implications. *Optometry.* 2005;76:352−362.

57. *Pfeiffer Syndrome.* Genetics Home Reference. Available at: https://ghr.nlm.nih.gov/condition/pfeiffer-syndrome.

58. Adachi M, et al. Compound heterozygous mutations of cytochrome P450 oxidoreductase gene (POR) in two patients with Antley-Bixler syndrome. *Am J Med Genet A.* 2004;128A:333−339.

59. *Cytochrome P450 Oxidoreductase Deficiency.* Genetics Home Reference. Available at: https://ghr.nlm.nih.gov/condition/cytochrome-p450-oxidoreductase-deficiency.

60. Flück CE, et al. Mutant P450 oxidoreductase causes disordered steroidogenesis with and without Antley-Bixler syndrome. *Nat Genet.* 2004;36:228−230.

61. Idkowiak J, Cragun D, Hopkin RJ, Arlt W. Cytochrome P450 oxidoreductase deficiency. In: Adam MP, et al., eds. *GeneReviews®.* Seattle: University of Washington; 1993.

62. Miller WL. P450 oxidoreductase deficiency: a new disorder of steroidogenesis with multiple clinical manifestations. *Trends Endocrinol Metab.* 2004;15:311−315.

63. Chun K, et al. Genetic analysis of patients with the Saethre-Chotzen phenotype. *Am J Med Genet.* 2002;110:136−143.

64. de Heer IM, et al. Clinical and genetic analysis of patients with Saethre-Chotzen syndrome. *Plast Reconstr Surg.* 2005;115:1894−1902; discussion 1903−1905.

65. Gallagher ER, Ratisoontorn C, Cunningham ML. Saethre-chotzen syndrome. In: Adam MP, et al., eds. *GeneReviews®.* Seattle: University of Washington; 1993.

66. Doyle AJ, et al. Mutations in the TGF-β repressor *SKI* cause Shprintzen-Goldberg syndrome with aortic aneurysm. *Nat Genet.* 2012;44:1249.

67. Greally MT, et al. Shprintzen-Goldberg syndrome: a clinical analysis. *Am J Med Genet.* 1998;76:202−212.

68. Robinson PN, et al. Shprintzen-Goldberg syndrome: fourteen new patients and a clinical analysis. *Am J Med Genet A.* 2005;135:251−262.

69. Schepers D, et al. The SMAD-binding domain of SKI: a hotspot for de novo mutations causing Shprintzen-Goldberg syndrome. *Eur J Hum Genet.* 2015;23:224−228.

70. Dauwerse JG, et al. Mutations in genes encoding subunits of RNA polymerases I and III cause Treacher Collins syndrome. *Nat Genet.* 2011;43:20.

71. Dixon MJ. Treacher Collins syndrome. *Hum Mol Genet.* 1996;5 Spec No:1391−1396.

72. Katsanis SH, Jabs EW. Treacher Collins syndrome. In: Adam MP, et al., eds. *GeneReviews®.* Seattle: University of Washington; 1993.

73. Vincent M, et al. Treacher Collins syndrome: a clinical and molecular study based on a large series of patients. *Genet Med.* 2016;18:49.

## FURTHER READING

1. *Crouzon Syndrome.* Genetics Home Reference. Available at: https://ghr.nlm.nih.gov/condition/crouzon-syndrome.

# CHAPTER 5

# Genetic Abnormalities of the Cornea

MAYA BITAR • YURIKA HARA • DHRUV SETHI • NATARIO L. COUSER

Genetic conditions affecting the cornea include developmental disorders, corneal dystrophies, and disorders associated with systemic conditions. Developmental disorders include central corneal abnormalities such as Peters anomaly and cornea plana; anomalies of the shape and size of the cornea such as megalocornea and microcornea; peripheral abnormalities such as Axenfeld-Rieger syndrome and sclerocornea. Most carry a poor visual prognosis because they are often associated with other ocular abnormalities such as cataract and glaucoma, they occur in the amblyogenic period, and the treatment is challenging and often fails. Corneal dystrophies are a group of inherited conditions that affect the transparent cornea usually bilaterally, often with characteristic clinical or histopathological findings. These conditions may be classified by their anatomical location within the layers of the cornea and by their genotypes.[1] The different categories according to the second edition of the International Committee for Classification of Corneal Dystrophies (IC3D)[2] include epithelial and subepithelial, epithelial-stromal, stromal, and endothelial corneal dystrophies (Table 5.1). Some dystrophies such as Meesmann corneal dystrophy and Fuchs endothelial corneal dystrophy (FECD) have genotypic heterogeneity as they have been associated with different genes. On the other hand, mutations in one gene, transforming growth factor β (*TGFBI* or *BIGH3*), have been associated with phenotypically different dystrophies. The *TGFBI* gene locus is 5q31; it codes for a protein involved in cell adhesion that is present in the extracellular matrix of different human tissues. Most corneal dystrophies are inherited in an autosomal dominant manner, except for Lisch corneal dystrophy which has been described to be inherited in an X-linked dominant manner, and gelatinous drop—like corneal dystrophy (GDLD), macular corneal dystrophy (MCD), congenital hereditary endothelial dystrophy (CHED), and lattice corneal dystrophy (LCD) type 3 which have been described to be inherited in an autosomal recessive manner.

Epithelial and subepithelial corneal dystrophies include corneal epithelial basement dystrophy (EBMD), Lisch corneal dystrophy, Meesmann dystrophy, and gelatinous drop—like corneal dystrophy. EBMD, the most common of the group, is most commonly sporadic, and when familial often has incomplete penetrance. Clinical findings include a map-dot-fingerprint combination of lesions; individuals affected often present with pain or transient vision changes from recurrent epithelial erosions. Lisch corneal dystrophy, caused by a mutation on chromosome Xp22.3, may be identified by a grayish feather—like lesion.[3] Vision may be affected and pain is typically not a feature of Lisch corneal dystrophy.[3] Meesmann dystrophy is often associated with minor irritation or mild vision changes and small epithelial vesicles are seen.

Epithelial-stromal dystrophies include dystrophies that are mainly in Bowman's layer such as Reis-Bucklers dystrophy (RBCD) and Thiel-Behnke dystrophy (TBCD), and dystrophies that are mainly in the stroma such as lattice corneal dystrophy, granular corneal dystrophy (GCD) type 1 and granular corneal dystrophy type 2, formerly known as Avellino's corneal dystrophy. These anterior corneal dystrophies mentioned can cause pain and irritation from recurrent erosions. RBCD and TBCD have a similar honeycomb reticular pattern that may present with pain and vision changes from recurrent epithelial erosions. Electron microscopy can help differentiate between these conditions by showing "rod-shaped bodies" in RBCD and "curly fibers" in TBCD. The disease-causing mutations in RBCD and TBCD is on chromosome 5q31 and chromosome 10q24, respectively.[4,5] The *BIGH3* gene is involved in RBCD, TBCD, lattice dystrophy type 1, and granular dystrophy type 1 and 2. Granular dystrophy type 1 is autosomal dominant, caused by mutations at chromosome 5q31. The pathology consists of granular hyaline material in the stroma. Clinical features include crumblike opacities that do not reach the limbus and have intervening clear areas.

**TABLE 5.1**
Corneal Dystrophies Classified According to IC3D, Second Edition[2]

| Name | Locus | Gene | Inheritance |
|---|---|---|---|
| **EPITHELIAL AND SUBEPITHELIAL DYSTROPHIES** | | | |
| Epithelial basement membrane dystrophy | 5q31 | *TGFBI* | AD<br>Mostly sporadic |
| Epithelial recurrent erosion dystrophies | Unknown | Unknown | AD |
| Subepithelial mucinous corneal dystrophy | Unknown | Unknown | AD |
| Meesmann corneal dystrophy | 12 q13<br>17q12 | *KRT3*<br>*KRT12* | AD |
| Lisch epithelial corneal dystrophy | Xp22.3 | Unknown | XLD |
| Gelatinous drop—like corneal dystrophy | 1p32 | *TACSTD2* | AR |
| **EPITHELIAL—STROMAL TGFBI DYSTROPHIES** | | | |
| Reis-Bückler corneal dystrophy | 5q31 | *TGFBI* | AD |
| Thiel-Behnke corneal dystrophy | 5q31 | *TGFBI* | AD |
| Lattice corneal dystrophy | 5q31 | *TGFBI* | AD |
| Granular corneal dystrophy type 1 | 5q31 | *TGFBI* | AD |
| Granular corneal dystrophy type 2 | 5q31 | *TGFBI* | AD |
| **STROMAL DYSTROPHIES** | | | |
| Macular corneal dystrophy | 16q22 | *CHST6* | AR |
| Schnyder corneal dystrophy | 1p36 | *UBIAD1* | AD |
| Congenital stromal corneal dystrophy | 12q21.33 | *DCN* | AD |
| Fleck corneal dystrophy | 2q34 | *PIKFYVE* | AD |
| Posterior amorphous corneal dystrophy | 12q21.33 | *DCN*<br>*KERA*<br>*LUM*<br>*EPYC* | AD |
| Central cloudy dystrophy of Francois | Unknown | Unknown | AD |
| Pre-Descemet corneal dystrophy | Xp22.31<br>Unknown | *STS*<br>Unknown | XLR (when associated<br>with x-linked ichthyosis)<br>AD (in isolated corneal dystrophy) |
| **ENDOTHELIAL DYSTROPHIES** | | | |
| Fuchs endothelial corneal dystrophy (FECD) | 1p34.3-p32<br>18q21.2<br>10p11.22<br>20p13 | *COL8A2*<br>*TCF4*<br>*ZEB1*<br>*SLC4A11* | AD (early-onset FECD) |
| Posterior polymorphous corneal dystrophy | 20p11.2-q11.2<br>1p34.3-p32.3<br>10p11.22 | Unknown<br>*COL8A2*<br>*ZEB1* | AD |
| Congenital hereditary endothelial dystrophy | 20p13 | *SLC4A11* | AR |
| X-linked endothelial corneal dystrophy | Xq25 | Unknown | XLD |

*IC3D*, International Committee for Classification of Corneal Dystrophies.

Vision loss is slow and progressive. Lattice dystrophy is characterized by stromal deposition of amyloid. The clinical findings are branching refractile linear abnormalities with a diffused corneal stromal haze, decreased vision, and frequent recurrent erosions. Multiple variants have been described classically: Type I, called Biber-Haah-Dimmer, is linked to chromosome 5q31; Type II, which is familial amyloidosis Finish type (Meretoja syndrome), is linked to chromosome 9q34; Type III with an autosomal recessive pattern; and Type IV, which have been described in Japan and Italy, is related to the *TGFB1* gene.[6-8] Patients with Avellino dystrophy or GCD type 2 have clinical features of granular and lattice dystrophy.

Stromal corneal dystrophies include MCD, Schnyder corneal dystrophy, congenital stromal corneal dystrophy (CSCD), fleck corneal dystrophy, central cloudy dystrophy of Francois, and pre-Descemet corneal dystrophy. These are non-TGFBI dystrophies. Macular corneal dystrophy has an autosomal recessive inheritance. The condition is characterized by glycosaminoglycan accumulation in cornea and can affect the cornea endothelium beginning in childhood. Patients develop diffuse haziness of the cornea with stromal opacities that extend to the limbus, contrary to granular dystrophy. Recurrent erosions are possible. Schnyder corneal dystrophy is inherited in an autosomal dominant manner and is related to a disorder of corneal lipid metabolism with accumulation of cholesterol and phospholipids. Central subepithelial crystals are characteristic of the disease are only present in 50% of cases. Clinical findings progress slowly starting with opacification of the central cornea early in life and then formation of a dense corneal arcus with a gradual decrease in corneal sensation. Patients and family members may have hyperlipoproteinemia. CSCD presents at birth with bilateral diffusely cloudy corneas. Central cloudy dystrophy of Francois is phenotypically identical to the corneal degeneration crocodile shagreen, however, the latter is typically benign.

Endothelial corneal dystrophies include FECD, posterior polymorphous cornea dystrophy (PPCD), and CHED 1, now considered similar to PPCD, and CHED 2. Fuchs dystrophy is a common corneal dystrophy. It is more frequent in females and patients over the age of 50 years. There is a rare early-onset form that is autosomal dominant. The late-onset form can be sporadic or familial. Variations in different genes are associated with FECD. The most common is a single nucleotide polymorphism of transcription factor 4 (*TCF4*) gene.[9]

Pathophysiology of Fuchs involves oxidative stress,[10] unfolded protein response,[11] endothelial cell apoptosis, and formation of guttae that can be seen clinically. Corneal edema develops leading to decreased vision and later on to pain from ruptured epithelial bullae. PPCD has been linked to chromosome 20q11. It presents during childhood, and may be inherited in an autosomal dominant or autosomal recessive manner.[12] Clinical findings may include bands with scalloped edges on the posterior cornea surface and glaucoma from abnormal cells migrating into the angle. Patients are commonly asymptomatic. CHED is conventionally divided into type 1 and 2. CHED 1 is inherited in an autosomal dominant manner, is slowly progressive, lacks nystagmus, and typically does not affect the cornea initially at birth.[13] The latest IC3D removed CHED 1 from the corneal dystrophy classification as it was thought to be the same dystrophy as PPCD. CHED 2, now called just CHED by IC3D, is inherited in an autosomal recessive manner, is stationary, is associated with nystagmus, and does cause clouding and thickening of the cornea at birth. Visual prognosis in CHED 2 is poor.[13] CHED 1 has been mapped to chromosome 20q11.2-q11.2, and CHED 2 has been shown to be caused by mutations in the *SLC4A11* gene on chromosome 20p13.[13-15] Treatment of corneal dystrophies depends on the location of the dystrophy and the symptoms. Conservative treatments include lubrication and bandage contact lens for pain from erosions. Superficial keratectomy and phototherapeutic keratectomy with excimer laser can be used to treat recurrent erosions and to improve vision by debulking anterior opacities. Deeper stromal lesions may require cornea transplantation, either lamellar keratoplasty or penetrating keratoplasty. For endothelial dystrophies, endothelial keratoplasty such as Descemet stripping endothelial keratoplasty and Descemet membrane endothelial keratoplasty can be performed. Unfortunately, many dystrophies can recur after treatment; an exception, for example, is FECD.

Corneal disorders associated with systemic genetic conditions include metabolic diseases, multiple endocrine neoplasia 2a and 2b that can cause prominent corneal nerves, and familial dysautonomia (Riley-Day syndrome). Among the lysosomal storage diseases, mucopolysaccharidosis I H or Hurler syndrome, mucopolysaccharidosis I S or Scheie syndrome, mucopolysaccharidosis IV or Morquio syndrome, and mucopolysaccharidosis VI or Maroteaux-Lamy syndrome present with corneal haze starting at an early age. Mucopolysaccharidoses are autosomal recessive, except

Hunter syndrome, which is X-linked. Fabry disease, a sphingolipidosis, can cause cornea verticillata which is usually asymptomatic. In cystinosis, iridescent crystals are deposited in the corneal stroma starting around 1 year of age and are also found in the uvea. Wilson disease, or hepatolenticular degeneration, has a characteristic Kayser-Fleisher ring of copper deposited in Descemet membrane. This ring can develop later in the disease process so its absence does not rule out the diagnosis of this disease. A sunflower cataract can also be found in Wilson's disease. In Riley-Day syndrome, there is a block of norepinephrine production, causing a decrease in lacrimation and corneal sensation with secondary neurotrophic keratitis and corneal ulcers. Tyrosinemia type 2 can also present with recurrent corneal ulcers. They are described as dendritic and can masquerade as herpetic keratitis. Systemic treatment of many metabolic diseases has progressed, but unfortunately it often does not help the corneal manifestations.

## GENETIC DISORDERS
### Bietti Crystalline Corneoretinal Dystrophy[16,17]
*OMIM*: #210370

*Description*: Bietti crystalline corneoretinal dystrophy (BCD) is caused by a defect in lipid metabolism and is characterized by numerous glistening yellow-white crystals in the posterior pole of the retina alongside retinal pigment epithelium atrophy. It is a progressive disorder with most patients developing decreased vision, nyctalopia, and paracentral scotomata between second and fourth decades of life with blindness by the sixth decade of life.

*Epidemiology*: unknown; BCD represents about 3% of cases of nonsyndromic retinitis pigmentosa; estimated gene frequency of 0.005 in China.

*Eye findings*: peripheral crystalline corneal deposits, retinal degeneration, choroidal vessel sclerosis, decreased ERG in advanced cases

*Inheritance*: AR

*Known genes or gene locus*: CYP4V2

### Bilateral Corneal Dermoids[18,19]
*OMIM*: %304730

*Description*: A corneal dermoid is a choristoma consisting of fibrofatty tissue covered by keratinized epithelium and sometimes contains hair and blood vessels. Dermoids occur sporadically, are unilateral, and straddle the corneal limbus. They can be associated with Goldenhar syndrome (oculoauriculovertebral dysplasia) that is also mostly sporadic. There are rare hereditary forms of corneal dermoids that were described: ring dermoids (discussed later in this chapter) and bilateral corneal dermoids of X-linked recessive inheritance. The latter entity presents as bilateral congenital opaque corneas.

*Epidemiology*: unknown

*Eye findings*: raised whitish plaques and fine blood vessels covering the center of the cornea

*Inheritance*: X-linked recessive

*Known genes or gene locus*: Xq24-qter

### Brittle Cornea Syndrome[20,21]
*OMIM*: #229200, #614170 (type 2)

*Description*: Brittle cornea syndrome is a rare connective tissue disorder that results in the weakening of the cornea. The disorder presents with blue sclerae, corneas subject to rupture after minor trauma, as well as hyperelasticity of the skin and joint hypermobility. Type 2 has been found in individuals with consanguineous parents, and symptoms include abnormal gait, mixed forms of deafness, easily bruised skin, and hypercompliance of tympanic membranes.

*Epidemiology*: unknown

*Eye findings*: blue sclerae, myopia, very thin corneas, corneal rupture spontaneously after minor trauma, keratoconus, keratoglobus

*Inheritance*: AR

*Known genes or gene locus*: ZNF469, PRDM5 (type 2)

### Congenital Stromal Cornea Dystrophy[22]
*OMIM*: # 610048

*Description*: Congenital stromal dystrophy presents with abnormally separated stromal lamellae and amorphous deposition. It is nonprogressive or slowly progressive and causes visual loss.

*Epidemiology*: unknown

*Eye findings*: bilateral diffuse corneal clouding with flakelike opacities in the stroma

*Inheritance*: AD

*Known genes or locus*: DCN

### Cornea Plana[23,24]
*OMIM*: #217300

*Description*: Cornea plana is characterized by a flat corneal curvature (less than 43 D), which usually leads to hyperopia, hazy corneal limbus, and arcus lipoides. It can be associated to sclerocornea. Other manifestations can include corneal thinning and malformations of the iris and pupil.

*Epidemiology*: unknown

*Eye findings*: hyperopia, hazy corneal limbus, corneal opacities, thin cornea, glaucoma

*Inheritance*: AR

*Known genes or gene locus*: KERA

## Corneal Dystrophy and Perceptive Deafness (Harboyan Syndrome)[25,26]

OMIM: #217400

*Description*: This is a rare disorder characterized by congenital corneal clouding similar to CHED with late-onset sensorineural deafness. The corneal stroma can be diffusely edematous and thickened.

*Epidemiology*: unknown

*Eye findings*: neonatal corneal haze, nystagmus

*Inheritance*: AR

*Known genes or gene locus*: SLC4A11

## Congenital Hereditary Endothelial Dystrophy (type 2)[27,28,29]

OMIM: #217700

*Description*: This is a disorder characterized by neonatal thickening and opacification of the cornea. Additionally, findings can include altered morphology of the endothelium and secretion of an abnormal collagen layer at the level of Descemet membrane.

*Epidemiology*: unknown

*Eye findings*: congenital corneal clouding, nystagmus

*Inheritance*: AR

*Known genes or gene locus*: SLC4A11

## Corneal Hypesthesia, Familial[30,31]

OMIM: %122450

*Description*: Familial corneal hypesthesia is a rare disorder that presents with corneal hypesthesia. In one family, it was described with normal skin sensation in the distribution of the trigeminal nerves,[31] whereas in another family, there was additional trigeminal anesthesia.[30] MRI imaging shows hypoplastic trigeminal nerves and Gasserian ganglia.

*Epidemiology*: unknown

*Eye findings*: bilateral corneal hypesthesia, epithelial corneal erosions

*Inheritance*: AD

*Known genes or gene locus*: Unknown

## Corneodermatosseous Syndrome[32,33]

OMIM: 122440

*Description*: Corneodermatoosseous syndrome is a rare disorder that is characterized by medullary narrowing of hand bones, brachydactyly, premature birth, soft teeth and early decay, palmoplantar hyperkeratosis, erythematous scaly skin, erythroderma, and corneal dystrophy.

*Epidemiology*: unknown

*Eye findings*: corneal epithelial changes, photophobia

*Inheritance*: AD

*Known genes or gene locus*: Unknown

## Cystinosis[34,35]

OMIM: #219750, #219800

*Description*: Cystinosis is a lysosomal storage disorder that involves abnormal accumulation of cystine and subsequent crystal formation within tissues. There are three forms: infantile, juvenile, and adult. The classic variant is infantile and it includes nephropathic pathology that leads to Fanconi syndrome. The adult nonnephropathic form, less common, causes corneal pathology without renal involvement. Cysteamine eye drops can diminish the presence of cystine crystals in the cornea while oral cysteamine can help with retinopathy.

*Epidemiology*: prevalence of 1/100,000—1/200,000

*Eye findings*: photophobia, recurrent corneal erosions, iridescent corneal crystals that start in periphery then extend creating hazy cornea (Fig. 5.1), conjunctival crystals, peripheral pigmentary retinopathy that progresses centrally causing constriction of visual fields and can be associated with retinal cystine crystals deposition (Fig. 5.1).

*Inheritance*: AR

*Known genes or gene locus*: CTNS

## Deafness and Myopia Syndrome[36]

OMIM: #221200

*Description*: Deafness and myopia syndrome is a rare disorder that was discovered in a consanguineous Amish family. This disease presents with high myopia and congenital bilateral neurosensory hearing loss. It is characterized by symmetric deterioration of hearing loss and speech recognition with age, and severe to profound hearing impairment.

*Epidemiology*: unknown

*Eye findings*: high myopia in infancy or early childhood (>-6 D)

*Inheritance*: AR

*Known genes or gene locus*: SLITRK6

## Dermochondrocorneal Dystrophy of Francois[37,38]

OMIM: %221800

*Description*: Also known as Francois syndrome, this is a rare disorder that is characterized by development of xanthomatous skin nodules, acquired deformities of extremities, and a corneal dystrophy. Nodules are primarily located on the pinnae, hands, elbows, and nose.

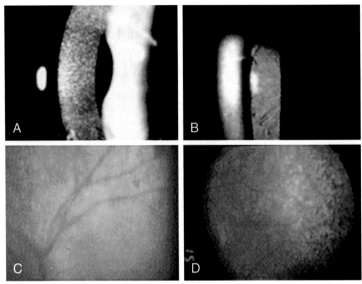

FIG. 5.1 Cystinosis. Crystal deposits in the cornea (A), iris (B), retina (C), and peripheral pigmentary retinopathy (D). (Courtesy Tsilou, Ekaterini, MD; Zhou, Min, MD; Gahl, William, MD, PhD; Sieving, Pamela C., MA, MS; Chan, Chi-Chao, MD. Ophthalmic manifestations and histopathology of infantile nephropathic cystinosis: report of a case and review of the literature. *Surv Ophthalmol.* January 1, 2007;52(1):97—105. © 2007.)

*Epidemiology*: unknown

*Eye findings*: confluent, subepithelial whitish-brown infiltrates of the central cornea with some anterior stromal haze, anterior cortical cataracts; vascular pannus may be present.

*Inheritance*: AR

*Known genes or gene locus*: Unknown

## Epidermolysis Bullosa[39–41]

*OMIM*: #226600

*Description*: This is a severe skin disorder that begins at birth and involves recurrent skin blistering from minor trauma causing scarring and contractures of hands, feet, and joints. There are several genetic subtypes: dystrophic (autosomal recessive and autosomal dominant), junctional, and simplex. Ophthalmic complications are common and are the most severe in the dystrophic recessive and junctional subtypes. Symptoms also involve gastrointestinal strictures, leading to poor nutrition, and patients are at an increased risk of developing squamous cell carcinoma.

*Epidemiology*: prevalence of 6.5/1,000,000

*Eye findings*: corneal abrasions, corneal scarring, eyelid ulcerations, eyelid ectropion, symblepharon, conjunctivitis, cataracts

*Inheritance*: AR, AD

*Known genes or gene locus*: *COL7A1, MMP1*

## Epidermolysis Bullosa Simplex With Muscular Dystrophy[42,43]

*OMIM*: #226670

*Description*: This is a rare disease that presents with early childhood progressive muscular dystrophy and blistering skin changes. This condition can also present with systemic symptoms including growth defects of stature and slow weight gain, anemia, degenerative changes, alopecia, and teeth enamel hypoplasia.

*Epidemiology*: unknown

*Eye findings*: punctate keratitis

*Inheritance*: AR

*Known genes or gene locus*: *PLEC1*

## Epithelial Basement Membrane Corneal Dystrophy (Map-Dot-Fingerprint Corneal Dystrophy)[44,45]

*OMIM*: #121820

*Description*: Epithelial basement membrane corneal dystrophy is associated with bilateral grayish-white dots, flecks, fingerprint lines, or maplike shapes in the epithelium of the cornea. The corneal changes may cause a decrease in vision, lead to painful recurrent erosions, or stay asymptomatic.

*Epidemiology*: 2%—43% in general population

*Eye findings*: map lines-dots-fingerprint lines epithelial corneal changes (Fig. 5.2), recurrent corneal erosions

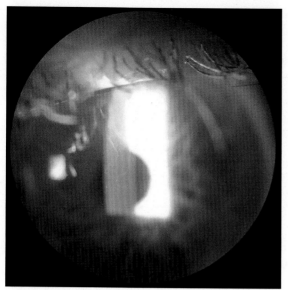

FIG. 5.2 Epithelial basement membrane dystrophy. Slit-beam photograph showing map or fingerprint-like changes in the corneal epithelium. (Courtesy Dr. Maya Bitar, Marshall University School of Medicine.)

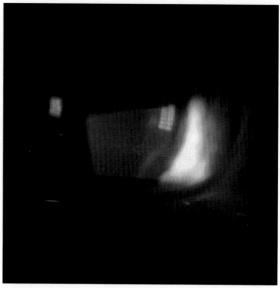

FIG. 5.3 Cornea verticillata. Slit-beam photograph showing whorl-like deposits in the basal layer of the epithelium. (Courtesy Dr. Maya Bitar, Marshall University School of Medicine.)

*Inheritance*: AD
*Known genes or gene locus*: TGFBI

## Fabry Disease (Hereditary Dystopic Lipidosis)[46,47]

*OMIM*: #301500

*Description*: Fabry disease is a disorder of glycophospholipid catabolism where lysosomal enzyme activity of α-galactosidase is deficient or absent. The clinical presentation is systemic with renal failure, cardiac disease, cerebrovascular disease, peripheral neuropathy, and skin lesions. The corneal manifestation is called cornea verticillata. Similar corneal changes can be seen secondary to chronic use of chloroquine and amiodarone medications.

*Epidemiology*: incidence of 1/55,000 males

*Eye findings*: whorl-like lines in the basal corneal epithelium (cornea verticillata) (Fig. 5.3), retinal vessel tortuosity, cataract

*Inheritance*: X-linked
*Known genes or gene locus*: GLA

## Familial Amyloidosis, Finnish Type[48,49]

*OMIM*: #105120

*Description*: This is a rare disorder also known as Meretoja syndrome that is characterized by lattice corneal dystrophy in addition to systemic symptoms including nephrotic syndrome, renal failure, amyloid deposition, cutis laxa, amyloid cardiomyopathy, and cranial neuropathy. The amyloid consists of mutated gelsolin that deposits in the cornea, conjunctiva, sclera, ciliary body, choriocapillaris, ciliary nerves, ciliary vessels, and optic nerve. The onset is often in the third decade, and patients have a characteristic facial mask and nerve palsies.

*Epidemiology*: unknown

*Eye findings*: lattice corneal lines, decreased corneal sensation, lagophthalmos

*Inheritance*: AD
*Known genes or gene locus*: GSN

## Familial Dysautonomia[50,51]

*OMIM*: #223900

*Description*: Familial dysautonomia or Riley-Day syndrome is a disease mainly present in the Ashkenazi Jewish population with symptoms of autonomic dysfunction and defective lacrimation, hypertension, hyperhidrosis, cyclic vomiting, and skin blotching. Additional features include dimished deep tendon reflexes, lack of axon flare after intradermal histamine and lack of fungiform papillae on the tongue.

*Epidemiology*: unknown

*Eye findings*: alacrima, diminished corneal reflex, corneal ulcers with secondary corneal scarring

*Inheritance*: AR
*Known genes or gene locus*: IKBKAP

## Familial Lecithin Cholesterol Acyltransferase Deficiency[52–54]

*OMIM*: 245900

*Description*: Lecithin cholesterol acyltransferase (LCAT) deficiency is a disorder of lipoprotein metabolism which presents typically with diffuse corneal opacities from cholesterol deposits, low HDL, target cell hemolytic anemia, and proteinuria due to renal failure. The corneal changes occur as an early sign before other symptoms of the disorder have developed, and they are usually not visually significant. Papilledema from lipid deposition in the optic nerves occurs rarely but can cause visual loss.

*Epidemiology*: unknown

*Eye findings*: corneal arcus, corneal opacities, papilledema rarely

*Inheritance*: AR

*Known genes or gene locus*: LCAT

## Fish-Eye Disease[55,56]

*OMIM*: #136120

*Description*: Fish-eye disease is a partial LCAT deficiency causing corneal opacities and low HDL. There is no anemia or kidney involvement. It is a rare disorder in which corneal opacities give the appearance of corneas of boiled fish and manifest in adolescence. This disorder is due to a deficiency in high-density lipoprotein lecithin, cholesterol acyltransferase activity causing a failure to esterify HDL cholesterol.

*Epidemiology*: unknown

*Eye findings*: corneal opacities, small dot–like gray-white-yellow, concentrated near the limbus causing progressive decrease in vision.

*Inheritance*: AR

*Known genes or gene locus*: LCAT

## Fleck Corneal Dystrophy[57,58]

*OMIM*: #121850

*Description*: This is a rare cornea dystrophy that can present at birth or within the first 2 years of life. It usually does not affect vision. It can be unilateral or asymmetric. It only affects the stroma. Histologically abnormal keratocytes with intracytoplasmic vesicles containing complex lipids and glycosaminoglycans are seen.

*Epidemiology*: unknown

*Eye findings*: dandruff-like or curvilinear fleck scattered through the corneal stroma. Epithelium, Bowman layer, Descemet membrane, and endothelium are not affected

*Inheritance*: AD

*Known genes or locus*: PIKFYVE (PIK5K3)

## Fuchs Endothelial Corneal Dystrophy[9,59,60]

*OMIM*: #136800

*Description*: FECD involves dysfunction of the corneal endothelium and results in loss of corneal transparency from thickening of Descemet membrane, formation of guttae, and corneal edema. Confocal microscopy shows endothelial cell hypertrophy and polymorphism. Most commonly the disease manifests in the fifth or sixth decade and affect more women than men. It is slowly progressive. There is an infrequent early-onset form with guttae in the first decade of life. Genetics of Fuchs dystrophy is heterogeneous and heritability has been estimated around 40% while it is most commonly sporadic.

*Epidemiology*: this disease affects approximately 4% of adults older than 40 years.

*Eye findings*: corneal endothelial guttata (Fig. 5.4), stromal edema, epithelial microedema and bullae in late stage with secondary erosion and scarring

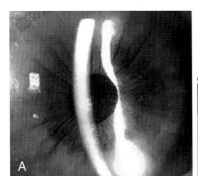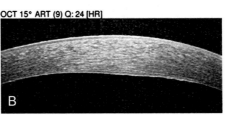

OCT 15° ART (9) Q: 24 [HR]

**FIG. 5.4** Fuchs endothelial corneal dystrophy. (A) Slit-beam photograph showing central endothelial guttae in a beaten metal pattern. (B) Optical coherence tomography showing thickened stroma from corneal edema, irregular Descemet membrane with excrescences corresponding to guttata. (Courtesy Dr. Maya Bitar, Marshall University School of Medicine.)

*Inheritance*: AD in some families

*Known genes or gene locus*: COL8A2 (early onset form), *TCF4* (FECD3), *SLC4A11* (FECD4), *ZEB1* (FECD6)

## Granular Corneal Dystrophy Type 2 (Avellino Corneal Dystrophy/Combined Granular-Lattice Corneal Dystrophy)[61–64,65]

*OMIM*: #607541

*Description*: Avellino corneal dystrophy has clinical and histological characteristics similar to lattice dystrophy in addition to hyaline deposits consistent with granular dystrophy type 1. Patients have decreased vision, and pain may occur from corneal erosions.

*Epidemiology*: prevalence of 11.5/10,000

*Eye findings*: snowflake hyaline changes in anterior stroma, linear amyloid deposits in deeper stroma

*Inheritance*: AD

*Known genes or gene locus*: TGFBI

## Granular Corneal Dystrophy (Groenouw Type I)[66,67]

*OMIM*: #121900

*Description*: Granular dystrophy is a rare corneal disorder consisting of hyaline deposition in the stroma. Findings include crumblike opacities in the center of the cornea with sharp borders or grayish-white granules in a disc-shaped area. Lesions do not extend to the limbus, and are separated by clear spaces but can become confluent with time and erode through Bowman layer causing recurrent erosions. This autosomal dominant disorder can present in the first 10 years of life and is slowly progressive with good vision in childhood. Laser phototherapeutic keratectomy has been found to help visual function and pain from erosions. Corneal graft has a good prognosis with recurrence after many years.

*Epidemiology*: unknown

*Eye findings*: crumblike or granular translucent opacities in stromal layer with clear interval not involving the limbus

*Inheritance*: AD

*Known genes or gene locus*: TGFBI

## Gelatinous Drop–Like Dystrophy[68,69]

*OMIM*: #204870

*Description*: Gelatinous drop–like dystrophy is a form of severe corneal amyloidosis with subepithelial and stromal amyloid deposition. It manifests with blurred vision, foreign body sensation, and photophobia in the first decade of life. By the third decade of life, yellowish gray gelatinous masses form often requiring lamellar keratoplasty, but recurrence is high.

*Epidemiology*: incidence of 1/300,000 in Japan

*Eye findings*: band keratopathy–like or raised yellowish-gray gelatinous masses.

*Inheritance*: AR

*Known genes or gene locus*: TACSTD2

## Ichthyosis Follicularis, Alopecia, and Photophobia Syndrome With or Without Bresheck Syndrome[70,71]

*OMIM*: #308205

*Description*: This syndrome is a rare congenital disorder that can be accompanied by intellectual disability, brain abnormalities, Hirschsprung disease, corneal opacification, kidney dysplasia, cryptorchidism, cleft palate, and skeletal malformations.

*Epidemiology*: unknown

*Eye findings*: photophobia, corneal opacities and erosions, vascularizing keratitis

*Inheritance*: XLR

*Known genes or gene locus*: MBTPS2

## Isolated Congenital Megalocornea[72,73]

*OMIM*: #309300

*Description*: Isolated congenital megalocornea is a rare bilateral nonprogressive disorder in which the corneas are enlarged at birth. It is important to differentiate it from buphthalmos caused by congenital glaucoma which is accompanied by high intraocular pressure and increased axial length. Individuals commonly have normal ocular function other than refractive error. Megalocorneas can also be associated with ocular disorders such as cataract and ectopia lentis and systemic disorders such as Marfan syndrome and Down syndrome.

*Epidemiology*: unknown

*Eye findings*: megalocornea (diameter greater than 13 mm), normal intraocular pressure, astigmatic/myopic refractive errors, mosaic corneal dystrophy, miosis due to decreased function of dilator muscle, arcus juvenilis

*Inheritance*: XLR

*Known genes or gene locus*: CHRDL1

## Keratitis, Hereditary[74,75]

*OMIM*: #148190

*Description*: Hereditary keratitis is a rare disorder with congenital and progressive anterior stromal corneal opacification and peripheral corneal vascularization causing decreased acuity. This may also present with radial defects of iris stroma and foveal hypoplasia.

*Epidemiology*: unknown

*Eye findings*: recurrent stromal keratitis and vascularization, childhood corneal clouding, anterior stromal corneal opacification, foveal hypoplasia, iris stroma radial defects

*Inheritance*: AD

*Known genes or gene locus*: PAX6

## Keratosis Follicularis Spinulosa Decalvans[76,77]

*OMIM*: #308800

*Description*: Keratosis follicularis spinulosa decalvans is a rare genetic skin disorder with widespread keratosis pilaris, cicatricial alopecia of the scalp, eyebrows, and eyelashes. This most commonly affects males, but the inheritance has been noted in X linked and autosomal dominant fashion.

*Epidemiology*: unknown

*Eye findings*: photophobia, blepharitis, conjunctivitis, keratitis, sparse eyelashes/eyebrows

*Inheritance*: X-linked, AD

*Known genes or gene locus*: MBTPS2

## Keratitis-Ichthyosis-Deafness Syndrome[75,78]

*OMIM*: #148210

*Description*: Keratitis-ichthyosis-deafness syndrome (KID syndrome) is a rare disorder that causes ophthalmic corneal epithelial defects including scarring and opacification with sensorineural deafness, lamellar ichthyosis, increased susceptibility to mucocutaneous infections, and squamous cell skin carcinoma.

*Epidemiology*: unknown

*Eye findings*: corneal opacification, corneal epithelial defects, scarring, keratitis, superficial and deep corneal stromal vascularization, photophobia, blindness, trichiasis, keratinized eyelids

*Inheritance*: AD

*Known genes or gene locus*: GJB2

## Lattice Corneal Dystrophy[79,80]

*OMIM*: #122200, #608471

*Description*: An eye disorder in which amyloid deposits form branching fibers creating lattice pattern in the cornea and cause recurrent erosions and vision impairment.

*Epidemiology*: unknown

*Eye findings*: lattice pattern in corneal stroma (Fig. 5.5), recurrent corneal erosions (Fig. 5.5)

*Inheritance*: AD

*Known genes or gene locus*: TGFBI

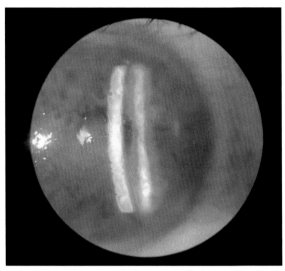

FIG. 5.5 Lattice corneal dystrophy. Slit-lamp photograph showing a branching pattern in the stroma and epithelial scarring secondary to chronic recurrent erosions. (Courtesy Dr. Maya Bitar, Marshall University School of Medicine.)

## Lisch Corneal Dystrophy[81,82]

*OMIM*: %300778

*Description*: This is a rare epithelial corneal dystrophy with onset in childhood. It can be unilateral and can cause decreased vision. It recurs postsuperficial keratectomy. Histology shows vacuolated epithelial cells with PAS positive material.

*Epidemiology*: unknown

*Eye findings*: gray, band-shaped feathery opacities that can appear in whorled patterns, surrounding corneal epithelium is clear.

*Inheritance*: XLD

*Known genes or locus*: Xp22.3

## Macular Corneal Dystrophy (Groenouw Type II)[83,84]

*OMIM*: #217800

*Description*: A rare, severe eye disorder in which corneal opacities form bilaterally in the corneal stroma at 3–9 year of age and eventually lead to visual impairment. It can involve Descemet membrane and the endothelium. Epithelial erosions are not common. The deposits are made of glycosaminoglycans, and there are three types of macular dystrophy based on biochemical differences. The disease can recur on corneal graft.

*Epidemiology*: prevalence of 1–9/100,000

*Eye findings*: gray—white punctate opacities in stromal layer that extent posteriorly and to peripheral cornea with lack of clear spaces between opacities

*Inheritance*: AR

*Known genes or gene locus*: CHST6

## MASS Syndrome (Overlap Connective Tissue Disease)[85,86]

*OMIM*: #604308

*Description*: MASS syndrome is a connective tissue disorder that has many clinical features that overlap with Marfan syndrome and can also result in myopia. MASS is an acronym for its clinical features—mitral valve prolapse, aortic enlargement, and skin and skeletal findings.

*Epidemiology*: unknown

*Eye findings*: myopia

*Inheritance*: unknown

*Known genes or gene locus*: FBN1

## Meesmann Corneal Dystrophy[87,88]

*OMIM*: #122100

*Description*: This corneal dystrophy consists of formation of cysts in corneal epithelium, usually asymptomatic until adolescence or adulthood when the cysts start rupturing on corneal surface, causing irritation and symptoms such as blepharospasm, photophobia, increased lacrimation, foreign body sensation. The cysts are made of degenerated epithelial cell products.

*Epidemiology*: unknown

*Eye findings*: punctate vesicular opacities in corneal epithelium extending to the limbus, corneal sensation may be reduced, recurrent erosions, photophobia

*Inheritance*: AD

*Known genes or gene locus*: KRT3, KRT12

## Megalocornea—Spherophakia—Secondary Glaucoma[89,90]

*OMIM*: #251750

*Description*: A very rare hereditary ocular disease characterized by small spherical lenses, megalocornea, and, in older children, glaucoma. Older children also present morphological features of Marfan syndrome.

*Epidemiology*: unknown

*Eye findings*: megalocornea, spherophakia, deep anterior chamber, myopia, iridodonesis, ectopia lentis

*Inheritance*: AR

*Known genes or gene locus*: LTBP2

## Megalocornea-Intellectual Disability Syndrome[91,92]

*OMIM*: %249310

*Description*: Also known as Neuhauser syndrome, this is a rare intellectual disability syndrome from unknown cause. It is characterized by megalocornea; varying degrees of intellectual disability; and variety of other features including hypotonia, mild facial dysmorphism, seizures, and psychomotor developmental delay.

*Epidemiology*: unknown

*Eye findings*: congenital megalocornea, hypoplasia of the iris, iridodonesis, visual impairment

*Inheritance*: XLR

*Known genes or gene locus*: unknown

## Microcornea Corectopia Macular Hypoplasia[93,94]

*OMIM*: Not listed

*Description*: A very rare disease presenting with microcornea, corectopia, and macular hypoplasia. This disorder has been described in three cases, involving two successive generations in a family.

*Epidemiology*: unknown

*Eye findings*: microcornea, corectopia, macular hypoplasia, nystagmus

*Inheritance*: unknown

*Known genes or gene locus*: unknown

## Microcornea Posterior Megalolenticonus Persistent Fetal Vasculature Coloboma[95,96]

*OMIM*: Not listed

*Description*: Also known as MPPC syndrome, it is a rare disease characterized by bilateral microcornea, posterior megalolenticonus, persistent fetal vasculature, and coloboma.

*Epidemiology*: prevalence of less than one in a million

*Eye findings*: chorioretinal coloboma, microcornea, posterior lenticonus, iris coloboma, retinal dystrophy, microphthalmia

*Inheritance*: unknown

*Known genes or gene locus*: unknown

## Mousa Al Din Al Nassar Syndrome[97,98]

*OMIM*: 271320

*Description*: A rare syndrome that has been described in an inbred Bedouin family and is characterized by spastic ataxia presenting with bilateral congenital cataracts, corneal dystrophy, and nonaxial myopia.

*Epidemiology*: unknown

*Eye findings*: congenital cataract, stromal corneal dystrophy, myopia

*Inheritance*: AR

*Known genes or gene locus*: unknown

## Mucolipidosis Type 4[99,100]

OMIM: #252650

*Description*: An inherited neurodegenerative lysosomal storage disorder characterized by psychomotor delay seen in the first year of life and by progressive vision impairment during the first decade of life with severe vision loss or blindness by adolescence. About 70% of affected individuals have Ashkenazi Jewish ancestry.

*Epidemiology*: incidence of 1/40,000

*Eye findings*: corneal opacity, retinal degeneration, severe vision loss

*Inheritance*: AR

*Known genes or gene locus*: MCOLN1

## Mucopolysaccharidosis Type IH (Hurler Syndrome)[101,102]

OMIM: #607014

*Description*: This is the most severe of the mucopolysaccharidosis type 1 disease and is due to a deficiency of α-iduronidase. Although many clinical findings overlap with the other subtypes of mucopolysaccharidosis type I, clinical features include corneal clouding, gargoyle facies, dwarfism, and progressive mental impairment with onset between 6 and 24 months of age.

*Epidemiology*: incidence of 1/107,000

*Eye findings*: corneal clouding, retinopathy, optic atrophy, glaucoma

*Inheritance*: AR

*Known genes or gene locus*: IDUA

## Mucopolysaccharidosis Type IH/S (Hurler-Scheie Syndrome)[103,104]

OMIM: #607015

*Description*: The intermediate form of mucopolysaccharidosis type I is characterized by corneal clouding, valvular heart disease, joint stiffness, clawlike hands and deafness that can be apparent by mid-teens.

*Epidemiology*: incidence of 1/115,000

*Eye findings*: corneal clouding

*Inheritance*: AR

*Known genes or gene locus*: IDUA

## Mucopolysaccharidosis Type IS (Scheie Syndrome)[105,106]

OMIM: #607016

*Description*: This is the mild form of mucopolysaccharidosis type I, featuring normal intelligence and life expectancy but with corneal clouding and glaucoma.

*Epidemiology*: incidence of 1/500,000

*Eye findings*: corneal clouding, retinopathy, glaucoma

*Inheritance*: AR

*Known genes or gene locus*: IDUA

## Mucopolysaccharidosis Type IVA (Morquio Syndrome A)[107,108]

OMIM: #253000

*Description*: A lysosomal storage disease, with varying severity and age of onset, featuring short stature, corneal clouding, and skeletal and dental abnormalities. Retinopathy also may occur. It is caused by a deficiency of galactosamine-6-sulfatase.

*Epidemiology*: incidence of 1/200,000

*Eye findings*: corneal clouding, Retinopathy (rarely), optic atrophy (rarely)

*Inheritance*: AR

*Known genes or gene locus*: GALNS

## Mucopolysaccharidosis Type IVB (Morquio Syndrome B)[109,110]

OMIM: #253010

*Description*: Skeletal dysplasia and corneal clouding are two characteristic features of this disorder. Retinopathy can also be seen in patients with this disorder. It is caused by a deficiency in β-galactosidase.

*Epidemiology*: incidence of <1/1,000,000

*Eye findings*: corneal clouding, retinopathy

*Inheritance*: AR

*Known genes or gene locus*: GLB1

## Mucopolysaccharidosis Type VI (Maroteaux-Lamy Syndrome)[111,112]

OMIM: #253200

*Description*: A lysosomal storage disorder due to arylsulfatase B deficiency, with manifestations including corneal clouding and glaucoma as well as skeletal abnormalities, hepatosplenomegaly, facial dysmorphism, and cardiac abnormalities. The severity and rate of symptom progression are variable.

*Epidemiology*: incidence of 1/250,000–1/600,000

*Eye findings*: corneal clouding (Fig. 5.6), optic atrophy, glaucoma

*Inheritance*: AR

*Known genes or gene locus*: ARSB

## Mucopolysaccharidosis Type VII (Sly Syndrome)[113,114]

OMIM: #253220

*Description*: A lysosomal storage disorder with varied severity characterized by growth retardation, bone abnormalities, mental impairment, and coarse facies. Corneal opacity can also be a feature in this disorder caused by β-glucuronidase deficiency.

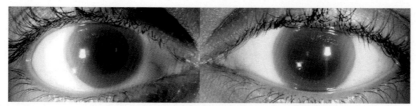

FIG. 5.6 Maroteaux-Lamy syndrome. Bilateral corneal clouding; right eye (left), left eye (right).

*Epidemiology*: incidence of 1/250,000
*Eye findings*: corneal clouding
*Inheritance*: AR
*Known genes or gene locus*: GUSB

## Peters Anomaly[115,116]

*OMIM*: #107250

*Description*: Peters anomaly is an anterior segment dysgenesis in which the anterior segment of the eye develops abnormally due to abnormal migration of neural crest cells causing a posterior corneal defect. Consequently, there is a central corneal opacity at birth often accompanied with iris and lenticular adhesions. Peters anomaly can be associated with other ocular anomalies such as microcornea and with systemic anomalies such as cardiac arrhythmia.

*Epidemiology*: unknown

*Eye findings*: central corneal leukoma, absent Descemet membrane, iris and lens adhesions to posterior cornea, glaucoma

*Inheritance*: AD, AR

*Known genes or gene locus*: PITX3 (anterior segment dysgenesis I), FOXE3 (anterior segment dysgenesis II), FOXC1 (anterior segment dysgenesis III), PITX2 (anterior segment dysgenesis IV), PAX6 (anterior segment dysgenesis V), CYP1B1 (anterior segment dysgenesis VI), PXDN (anterior segment dysgenesis VII), CPAMD8 (anterior segment dysgenesis VIII), B3CLGT (Peters plus syndrome)

## Peters Plus Syndrome (Krause-Kivlin Syndrome)[46,117]

*OMIM*: #261540

*Description*: A genetic condition in which severity differs from person to person and is characterized by Peters anomaly, short stature and shortened limbs, intellectual and developmental delay, and characteristic facial features including cleft palate and malformed ears.

*Epidemiology*: unknown

*Eye findings*: peters anomaly (congenital corneal opacity with posterior leukoma), nystagmus, glaucoma, cataract, coloboma, upslanting palpebral fissures, ptosis, hypertelorism

*Inheritance*: AR
*Known genes or gene locus*: B3GALTL

## Pillay Syndrome (Ophthalmo-Mandibulo-Melic Dysplasia)[118,119]

*OMIM*: %164900

*Description*: A rare disease, characterized by corneal opacities, that leads to complete blindness, limb anomalies, and mastication difficulty due to changes in the mandible including temporomandibular fusion.

*Epidemiology*: unknown

*Eye findings*: corneal opacities, blindness

*Inheritance*: AD

*Known genes or gene locus*: unknown

## Posterior Amorphous Corneal Dystrophy[120,121]

*OMIM*: #612868

*Description*: A Posterior stromal corneal dystrophy that can be congenital and accompanied with iris abnormalities. Electron microscopy shows amorphous extracellular material between the stromal lamellae in the anterior cornea. Vision can be affected.

*Epidemiology*: unknown

*Eye findings*: diffused gray-white sheetlike posterior stromal opacity with interspread areas of lucency, corneal thinning and flattening, hyperopia, iris abnormalities in some cases.

*Inheritance*: AD

*Known genes or locus*: 12q21.33 (LUM, KERA, DCN, EPYC)

## Posterior Embryotoxon[122,123]

*OMIM*: +601920, #118450 (Alagille syndrome)

*Description*: Posterior embryotoxon consists of a thickened and anteriorly displaced Shwalbe's line. While it can be found in around 7% of the general population, it is also often accompanied with other features of anterior segment dysgenesis and systemic syndromes such as Alagille syndrome (where it is present in 95% of cases), deafness, congenital heart defects, and posterior embryotoxon syndrome. Finding of a posterior embryotoxon on clinical exam should alert the clinician to look for glaucoma and involvement of other organs. Alagille syndrome, in addition to the eye, may affect the liver, kidneys, heart, and skeletal system.

*Epidemiology*: prevalence of 1/70,000 (Alagille syndrome)

*Eye findings*: unilateral or bilateral white line anterior to the limbus extending few clock hours on slit-lamp examination (posterior embryotoxon). Alagille syndrome, in addition to posterior embryotoxon, may include anomalous optic disc, band keratopathy, cataracts, chorioretinal atrophy, choroidal folds, deep-set eyes, diffuse fundus hypopigmentation, ectopic pupils, hypertelorism, microcornea, myopia, posterior embryotoxon, retinal pigment clumping, strabismus, upslanting palpebral fissures.

*Inheritance*: AD, de novo

*Known genes or locus*: JAG1 (Type 1), NOTCH2 (Type 2)

### Posterior Polymorphous Corneal Dystrophy[124−126]

OMIM #122000 (PPCD1), #609140 (PPCD2), #609,141 (PPCD3)

*Description*: It is a genetically heterogenous endothelial dystrophy with onset in childhood and rarely at birth. On microscopy, endothelial cells show features of epithelial cells with thickening of Descemet membrane. It is often asymptomatic. It has mostly been described in British and Czech families.

*Epidemiology*: prevalence of 1/100 000 in Czech Republic

*Eye findings*: different distinctive changes in Descemet membrane: vesicular or geographic or bandlike opacities, possible steep corneas, corneal edema in 20% of cases, possible iridocorneal adhesions, high intraocular pressure.

*Inheritance*: AD

*Known genes or locus*: OVOL2 (PPCD1), COL8A2 (PPCD2), ZEB1 (PPCD3)

### Reis-Bucklers Corneal Dystrophy (Corneal Dystrophy of Bowman Layer Type 1)[127−132]

OMIM: #608470

*Description*: This form of corneal dystrophy involves recurring corneal lesions between ages 8 and 20, with degenerative changes in epithelial cells and a disrupted Bowman membrane. Electron microscopy shows "rod-shaped bodies".

*Epidemiology*: unknown

*Eye findings*: subepithelial reticular corneal opacity, peripheral condensation ring separated from limbus with a narrow strip of normal cornea, epithelial erosions causing pain

*Inheritance*: AD

*Known genes or gene locus*: TGFBI

### Ring Dermoid of Cornea[133,134]

OMIM: #180550

*Description*: This is a rare form of corneal dermoid that is bilateral and annular. It was described in a Peruvian and in a Chinese family. It can be associated with glaucoma and cataract. It is characterized by skinlike, yellow-white bumps of tissue that are often elevated and can grow at the edge of the cornea and also on the conjunctiva.

*Epidemiology*: unknown

*Eye findings*: bilateral annular yellow-white tumor at the limbal dermoid with corneal and conjunctival extensions

*Inheritance*: AD

*Known genes or gene locus*: PITX2

### Rutherfurd Syndrome[135,136]

OMIM: %180900

*Description*: A rare oculodental syndrome featuring gingival fibromatosis, noneruption or delayed eruption of teeth, and corneal dystrophy.

*Epidemiology*: unknown

*Eye findings*: dense corneal opacities

*Inheritance*: AD

*Known genes or gene locus*: unknown

### Schnyder Corneal Dystrophy[137−139]

OMIM: #121800

*Description*: This form of corneal dystrophy involves abnormal deposits of cholesterol and phospholipids in the cornea, leading to progressive corneal opacification, glare, and loss of vision usually in the fifth decade. Other manifestations include small iridescent needle-shaped crystals upon slit-lamp examination. Patient and family members should be tested for hyperlipoproteinemia.

*Epidemiology*: unknown

*Eye findings*: cloudy central cornea, dense arcus, central corneal crystals in 50% cases

*Inheritance*: AD

*Known genes or gene locus*: UBIAD1

### Spinocerebellar Degeneration and Corneal Dystrophy[97,140]

OMIM: #271310

*Description*: A Disorder characterized by an atypical combination of spinocerebellar degeneration and corneal dystrophy with manifestations including slow progressive cerebellar abnormalities, corneal opacification, and mental impairment.

*Epidemiology*: unknown
*Eye findings*: epithelial corneal opacity, severe visual impairment
*Inheritance*: AR
*Known genes or gene locus*: unknown

## Thiel Behnke Corneal Dystrophy[129,130,141]

OMIM: 602082

*Description*: This form of rare corneal dystrophy is characterized by progressive honeycomb-like subepithelial corneal opacities with recurrent erosions. Electron microscopy shows "curly fibers." This varies from Reis-Bucklers corneal dystrophy by presenting round edges with dark shadows in the epithelial basal cell layer deposits.

*Epidemiology*: unknown
*Eye findings*: sub Epithelial honeycomb corneal opacities, corneal scarring, corneal erosions causing pain, photophobia
*Inheritance*: AD
*Known genes or gene locus*: TGFBI

## Tyrosinemia, Type II[142,143]

OMIM: #276600

*Description*: A disorder characterized by Accumulation of tyrosine due to deficiency in tyrosine aminotransferase, an enzyme required for the breakdown of tyrosine in tissues and organs. It can cause eye, skin, and intellectual development problems. Skin manifestation consists of hyperkeratotic lesions of the palms soles, and elbows.

*Epidemiology*: prevalence of <1/1,000,000
*Eye findings*: pseudodendritic corneal ulcers that can lead to neovascularization and scarring, conjunctival injection, photophobia
*Inheritance*: AR
*Known genes or gene locus*: TAT

## Wilson Disease[144,145]

OMIM: #277900

*Description*: Also known as hepatolenticular degeneration, this disease is characterized by copper accumulation in the body, especially the liver, kidneys, eyes, and brain. A combination of liver disease and neurological Parkinson-like and psychiatric problems are features of this disease. A characteristic finding is a peripheral golden brown corneal ring at the level of Descemet membrane, but it is not always present. Low serum ceruloplasmin, and high serum and urine copper help establish the diagnosis. The disease can be treated with penicillamine.

*Epidemiology*: prevalence of 1/30,000
*Eye findings*: kayser-Fleischer ring, sunflower cataract
*Inheritance*: AR
*Known genes or gene locus*: ATP7B

## X-Linked Ichthyosis[146–148]

OMIM: #308100

*Description*: Deficiency in steroid sulfatase slows the shedding of skin cells and causes buildup of scales that are typically dark and manifests in only a portion of the body, usually at the trunk or back of the neck. An association with pre-Descemet corneal dystrophy was described.

*Epidemiology*: prevalence of 1/6000 males
*Eye findings*: punctate deep stromal corneal opacities, eyelid scaling, cicatricial ectropion with secondary exposure keratopathy
*Inheritance*: XLR
*Known genes or gene locus*: STS

## Xeroderma Pigmentosum[149,150]

OMIM: 278700

*Description*: Xeroderma pigmentosum is caused by a mutation in a DNA repair gene. It is characterized by increased sensitivity to sunlight and early-age development of carcinoma. Additional clinical findings can include neurologic symptoms such as mental deterioration, low intelligence, microcephaly, and sensorineural deafness.

*Epidemiology*: unknown
*Eye findings*: conjunctivitis, corneal neovascularization, keratitis, microcephaly, eyelid or ocular neoplasms, photophobia
*Inheritance*: AR
*Known genes or gene locus*: XPA, XPC, ERCC2, ERCC3, POLH

## Zellweger Syndrome—Peroxisome Biogenesis Disorder 1A[151,152]

OMIM: #214100

*Description*: The most severe form of the Zellweger spectrum disorder, a peroxisome biogenesis disorder, is characterized by hypotonia, feeding problems, seizures, and hearing and vision loss during infancy. Children with this disorder typically do not survive past their first year of life.

*Epidemiology*: incidence of 1/50,000
*Eye findings*: corneal opacities, cataract, glaucoma, nystagmus, epicanthal folds, upslanting palpebral fissures
*Inheritance*: AR

*Known genes or gene locus*: *PEX1* (PBD1A), *PEX2* (PBD5A), *PEX3* (PBD10 A), *PEX5* (PBD2A), *PEX6* (PBD4A), *PEX10* (PBD6A), *PEX12* (PBD3A), *PEX13* (PBD11 A), *PEX14* (PBD13 A), *PEX16* (PBD8A), *PEX19* (PBD12 A), *PEX26* (PBD7A)

## REFERENCES

1. Auw-Hädrich C, Witschel H. Corneal dystrophies in the light of modern molecular genetic research. *Ophthalmologe*. 2002;99(6):418−426.
2. Weiss J, et al. IC3D classification of corneal dystrophies− edition 2. *Cornea*. 2015;34(10):e32.
3. Lisch W, et al. Lisch corneal dystrophy is genetically distinct from Meesmann corneal dystrophy and maps to xp22.3. *Am J Ophthalmol*. 2000;130(4):461−468.
4. Yee RW, et al. Linkage mapping of Thiel-Behnke corneal dystrophy (CDB2) to chromosome 10q23-q24. *Genomics*. 1997;46(1):152−154.
5. Munier FL, et al. Kerato-epithelin mutations in four 5q31-linked corneal dystrophies. *Nat Genet*. 1997; 15(3):247−251.
6. Edelstein SL, et al. Genotype of lattice corneal dystrophy (R124C mutation in TGFBI) in a patient presenting with features of avellino corneal dystrophy. *Cornea*. 2010; 29(6):698−700.
7. El-Ashry MF, et al. A clinical and molecular genetic study of autosomal-dominant stromal corneal dystrophy in British population. *Ophthalmic Res*. 2005;37(6):310−317.
8. Auw-Hädrich C, Witschel H. Corneal dystrophies in the light of modern molecular genetic research. *Ophthalmologe*. 2002;99(6):418−426.
9. Baratz KH, et al. E2-2 protein and Fuchs's corneal dystrophy. *N Engl J Med*. 2010;363(11):1016−1024.
10. Jurkunas U, Bitar M, et al. Evidence of oxidative stress in the pathogenesis of Fuchs endothelial corneal dystrophy. *Am J Pathol*. 2010;177(5):2278−2289.
11. Engler C, et al. Unfolded protein response in Fuchs endothelial corneal dystrophy: a unifying pathogenic pathway? *Am J Ophthalmol*. 2010;149(2).
12. Héon E, et al. Linkage of posterior polymorphous corneal dystrophy to 20q11. *Hum Mol Genet*. 1995; 4(3):485−488.
13. Kim JH, Ko JM, Tchah H. Fuchs endothelial corneal dystrophy in a heterozygous carrier of congenital hereditary endothelial dystrophy type 2 with a novel mutation in SLC4A11. *Ophthal Genet*. 2015;36(3):284−286.
14. Toma NM, et al. Linkage of congenital hereditary endothelial dystrophy to chromosome 20. *Hum Mol Genet*. 1995;4(12):2395−2398.
15. Vithana EN, et al. Mutations in sodium-borate cotransporter SLC4A11 cause recessive congenital hereditary endothelial dystrophy (CHED2). *Nat Genet*. 2006; 38(7):755−757.
16. Mataftsi A, et al. Bietti's crystalline corneoretinal dystrophy: a cross-sectional study. *Retina*. 2004;24(3): 416−426.
17. Welch RB. Bietti's tapetoretinal degeneration with marginal corneal dystrophy crystalline retinopathy. *Trans Am Ophthalmol Soc*. 1977;75:164.
18. Henkind P, et al. Bilateral corneal dermoids. *Am J Ophthalmol*. 1973;76(6):972−977.
19. Dar P, et al. Potential mapping of corneal dermoids to Xq24-qter. *J Med Genet*. 2001;38(10):719−723.
20. Stein R, Lazar M, Adam A. Brittle cornea: a familial trait associated with blue sclera. *Am J Ophthalmol*. 1968; 66(1):67−69.
21. Ticho U, Ivry M, Merin S. Brittle cornea, blue sclera, and red hair syndrome (the brittle cornea syndrome). *Br J Ophthalmol*. 1980;64(3):175−177.
22. Bredrupey, et al. Congenital stromal dystrophy of the cornea caused by a mutation in the decorin gene. *Invest Ophthal Vis Sci*. 2005;46:420−426.
23. Lehmann OJ, et al. A novel keratocan mutation causing autosomal recessive cornea plana. *Invest Ophthalmol Vis Sci*. 2001;42(13):3118−3122.
24. Pellegata NS, et al. Mutations in KERA, encoding keratocan, cause cornea plana. *Nat Genet*. 2000;25(1): 91−95.
25. Abramowicz MJ, Albuquerque-Silva J, Zanen A. Corneal dystrophy and perceptive deafness (Harboyan syndrome): CDPD1 maps to 20p13. *J Med Genet*. 2002; 39(2):110−112.
26. Harboyan G, et al. Congenital corneal dystrophy: progressive sensorineural deafness in a family. *Arch Ophthalmol*. 1971;85(1):27−32.
27. Callaghan M, et al. Homozygosity mapping and linkage analysis demonstrate that autosomal recessive congenital hereditary endothelial dystrophy (CHED) and autosomal dominant CHED are genetically distinct. *Br J Ophthalmol*. 1999;83(1):115−119.
28. Vithana EN, et al. Mutations in sodium-borate cotransporter SLC4A11 cause recessive congenital hereditary endothelial dystrophy (CHED2). *Nat Genet*. 2006; 38(7):755−757.
29. Pearce WG, Tripathi RC, Morgan GWYN. Congenital endothelial corneal dystrophy. Clinical, pathological, and genetic study. *Br J Ophthalmol*. 1969;53(9):577.
30. Keys CL, Sugar J, Mafee MF. Familial trigeminal anesthesia. *Arch Ophthalmol*. 1990;108(12):1720−1723.
31. Purcell JJ, Krachmer JH. Familial corneal hypesthesia. *Arch Ophthalmol*. 1979;97(5):872−874.
32. Stern JK, et al. Corneal changes, hyperkeratosis, short stature, brachydactyly, and premature birth: a new autosomal dominant syndrome. *Am J Med Genet A*. 1984; 18(1):67−77.
33. Žmegač ZJ, Sarajlić MV. A rare form of an inheritable palmar and plantar keratosis. *Dermatology*. 1965;130(1): 40−52.

34. Lietman PS, et al. Adult cystinosis—a benign disorder. *Am J Med.* 1966;40(4):511–517.
35. Schneider JA, Bradley K, Seegmiller JE. Increased cystine in leukocytes from individuals homozygous and heterozygous for cystinosis. *Science.* 1967;157(3794):1321–1322.
36. Eldridge R, et al. Cochlear deafness, myopia, and intellectual impairment in an Amish family. *Arch Otolaryngol.* 1968;88(1):49–54.
37. Bierly JR, George SP, Volpicelli M. Dermochondral corneal dystrophy (of François). *Br J Ophthalmol.* 1992;76(12):760–761.
38. Caputo R, et al. Dermochondrocorneal dystrophy (François' syndrome): report of a case. *Arch Dermatol.* 1988;124(3):424–428.
39. Sato-Matsumura KC, et al. Toenail dystrophy with COL7A1 glycine substitution mutations segregates as an autosomal dominant trait in 2 families with dystrophic epidermolysis bullosa. *Arch Dermatol.* 2002;138(2):269–271.
40. Varki R, et al. Epidermolysis bullosa. II. Type VII collagen mutations and phenotype–genotype correlations in the dystrophic subtypes. *J Med Genet.* 2007;44(3):181–192.
41. Tong L, et al. The eye in epidermolysis bullosa. *Br J Ophthalmol.* 1999;83(3):323–326.
42. Msalih MA, et al. Lethal epidermolytic epidermolysis bullosa: a new autosomal recessive type of epidermolysis bullosa. *Br J Dermatol.* 1985;113(2):135–143.
43. Varki R, et al. Epidermolysis bullosa. I. Molecular genetics of the junctional and hemidesmosomal variants. *J Med Genet.* 2006;43(8):641–652.
44. Werblin TP, Hirst LW, Stark WJ, et al. Prevalence of map-dot-fingerprint changes in the cornea. *Br J Ophthalmol.* 1981;65(6):401–409.
45. Boutboul S, et al. A subset of patients with epithelial basement membrane corneal dystrophy have mutations in TGFBI/BIGH3. *Hum Mutat.* 2006;27(6):553–557.
46. Kim M, Lee SC, Lee SJ. Spontaneous corneal perforation in an eye with Peters' anomaly. *Clin Ophthalmol.* 2013;7:1535–1537. Kint JA. Fabry's disease: alpha-galactosidase deficiency. *Science.* 1970;167(3922):1268–1269.
47. Romeo G, Childs B, Migeon BR. Genetic heterogeneity of α-galactosidase in Fabry's disease. *FEBS Letters.* 1972;27(1):161–166.
48. Darras BT, et al. Familial amyloidosis with cranial neuropathy and corneal lattice dystrophy. *Neurology.* 1986;36(3):432–435.
49. Purcell JJ, et al. Lattice corneal dystrophy associated with familial systemic amyloidosis (Meretoja's syndrome). *Ophthalmology.* 1983;90(12):1512–1517.
50. Brunt PW, McKusick VA. Familial dysautonomia: a report of genetic and clinical studies, with a review of the literature. *Medicine.* 1970;49(5):343–374.
51. Ziegler MG, Raymond Lake C, Kopin IJ. Deficient sympathetic nervous response in familial dysautonomia. *N Engl J Med.* 1976;294(12):630–633.
52. Nordöy A, Gjone E. Familial plasma lecithin: cholesterol acyltransferase deficiency a study of the platelets. *Scand J Clin Lab Invest.* 1971;27(3):263–268.
53. Teisberg P, Gjone E. Genetic heterogeneity in familial lecithin: cholesterol acyltransferase (LCAT) deficiency. *J Intern Med.* 1981;210(1–6):1–2.
54. Hörven I, et al. Ocular manifestations in familial lecithin: cholesterol acyltransferase deficiency. *Scand J Clin Lab Invest.* 1974;33(suppl 137):89–91.
55. Carlson LA, Philipson B. Fish-eye disease A new familial condition with massive corneal opacities and dyslipoproteinaemia. *Lancet.* 1979;314(8149):921–924.
56. Holmquist L, Carlson LA. Inhibitory effect of normal high density lipoproteins on lecithin: cholesterol acyltransferase activity in fish eye disease plasma. *J Intern Med.* 1987;222(1):15–21.
57. Nicholson D, et al. A clinical and histopathological study of François-Neetens speckled corneal dystrophy. *Am J Ophthalmol.* 1977;83(4):554–560.
58. Li S, et al. Mutations in PIP5K3 are associated with François-Neetens mouchetée fleck corneal dystrophy. *Am J Hum Genet.* 2005;77(1):54–63 [Epub 2005 May 18].
59. Hecker LA, et al. Anterior keratocyte depletion in Fuchs endothelial dystrophy. *Arch Ophthalmol.* 2011;129(5):555–561.
60. Wang Z, et al. Advanced glycation end products and receptors in Fuchs' dystrophy corneas undergoing Descemet's stripping with endothelial keratoplasty. *Ophthalmology.* 2007;114(8):1453–1460.
61. Akiya S, et al. Granular-lattice (Avellino) corneal dystrophy. *Ophthalmologica.* 1999;213(1):58–62.
62. Edelstein SL, et al. Genotype of lattice corneal dystrophy (R124C mutation in TGFBI) in a patient presenting with features of avellino corneal dystrophy. *Cornea.* 2010;29(6):698–700.
63. Holland EJ, et al. Avellino corneal dystrophy: clinical manifestations and natural history. *Ophthalmology.* 1992;99(10):1564–1568.
64. Munier FL, et al. Kerato-epithelin mutations in four 5q31-linked corneal dystrophies. *Nat Genet.* 1997;15(3):247–251.
65. Lee JH, et al. Prevalence of granular corneal dystrophy type 2 (Avellino corneal dystrophy) in the Korean population. *Ophthalm Epidemiol.* 2010;17(3):160–165.
66. Dinh R, et al. Recurrence of corneal dystrophy after excimer laser phototherapeutic keratectomy. *Ophthalmology.* 1999;106(8):1490–1497.
67. Møller HU. Granular corneal dystrophy Groenouw type I: clinical aspects and treatment. *Acta Ophthalmol.* 1990;68(4):384–389.
68. Stock EL, Kielar RA. Primary familial amyloidosis of the cornea. *Am J Ophthalmol.* 1976;82(2):266–271.
69. Tsujikawa M, et al. Identification of the gene responsible for gelatinous drop-like corneal dystrophy. *Nat Genet.* 1999;21(4):420–423.

70. Keyvani K, et al. Ichthyosis follicularis, alopecia, and photophobia (IFAP) syndrome: clinical and neuropathological observations in a 33-year-old man. *Am J Med Genet Part A*. 1998;78(4):371−377.

71. Oeffner F, et al. IFAP syndrome is caused by deficiency in MBTPS2, an intramembrane zinc metalloprotease essential for cholesterol homeostasis and ER stress response. *Am J Hum Genet*. 2009;84(4):459−467.

72. Mackey DA, et al. Description of X-linked megalocornea with identification of the gene locus. *Arch Ophthalmol*. 1991;109(6):829−833.

73. Webb Tom R, et al. X-linked megalocornea caused by mutations in CHRDL1 identifies an essential role for ventroptin in anterior segment development. *Am J Hum Genet*. 2012;90(2):247−259.

74. Pearce WG, et al. Autosomal dominant keratitis: a possible aniridia variant. *Can J Ophthalmol J Canadien D'ophthalmologie*. 1995;30(3):131−137.

75. Wilson GN, Squires RH, Weinberg AG. Keratitis, hepatitis, ichthyosis, and deafness: report and review of KID syndrome. *Am J Med Genet Part A*. 1991;40(3):255−259.

76. Oosterwijk JC, et al. Molecular genetic analysis of two families with keratosis follicularis spinulosa decalvans: refinement of gene localization and evidence for genetic heterogeneity. *Hum Genet*. 1997;100(5):520−524.

77. Oosterwijk JC, et al. Refinement of the localisation of the X linked keratosis follicularis spinulosa decalvans (KFSD) gene in Xp22. 13-p22. 2. *J Med Genet*. 1995;32(9):736−739.

78. Langer K, Konrad K, Wolff K. Keratitis ichthyosis and deafness (KID)-syndrome: report of three cases and a review of the literature. *Br J Dermatol*. 1990;122(5):689−697.

79. Stix B, et al. Hereditary lattice corneal dystrophy is associated with corneal amyloid deposits enclosing C-terminal fragments of keratoepithelin. *Invest Ophthal Vis Sci*. 2005;46(4):1133−1139.

80. Waring III GO, Rodrigues MM, Laibson PR. Corneal dystrophies. I. Dystrophies of the epithelium, Bowman's layer and stroma. *Surv Ophthalmol*. 1978;23(2):71−122.

81. Lisch W, et al. Lisch corneal dystrophy is genetically distinct from Meesmann corneal dystrophy and maps to Xp22.3. *Am J Ophthal*. 2000;130:461−468.

82. Lisch W, et al. A new, band-shaped and whorled microcystic dystrophy of the corneal epithelium. *Am J Ophthal*. 1992;114:35−44.

83. Jonasson F, et al. Macular corneal dystrophy in Iceland: a clinical, genealogic, and immunohistochemical study of 28 patients. *Ophthalmology*. 1996;103(7):1111−1117.

84. Thonar EJ, et al. Absence of normal keratan sulfate in the blood of patients with macular corneal dystrophy. *Am J Ophthal*. 1986;102(5):561−569.

85. Dietz HC, et al. Four novel FBN1 mutations: significance for mutant transcript level and EGF-like domain calcium binding in the pathogenesis of Marfan syndrome. *Genomics*. 1994;17(2):468−475.

86. Glesby MJ, Pyeritz RE. Association of mitral valve prolapse and systemic abnormalities of connective tissue: a phenotypic continuum. *JAMA*. 1989;262(4):523−528.

87. Chen JL, et al. Identification of presumed pathogenic KRT3 and KRT12 gene mutations associated with Meesmann corneal dystrophy. *Mol Vis*. 2015;21:1378−1386.

88. Fine BS, et al. Meesmann's epithelial dystrophy of the cornea. *Am J Ophthal*. 1977;83(5):633−642.

89. Desir J, et al. LTBP2 null mutations in an autosomal recessive ocular syndrome with megalocornea, spherophakia, and secondary glaucoma. *Eur J Hum Genet*. 2010;18:761−767.

90. Desir J, et al. LTBP2 null mutations in an autosomal recessive ocular syndrome with megalocornea, spherophakia, and secondary glaucoma. *Eur J Hum Genet*. 2010;18(7):761−767.

91. Antinolo G, et al. Megalocornea- mental retardation syndrome: an additional case. *Am J Med Genet*. 1994;52(2):196−197.

92. Frank Y, et al. Megalocornea associated with multiple skeletal anomalies: a new genetic syndrome? *J Genet Hum*. 1973;21(2):67−72.

93. Cohn HC, Mondino BJ. Corectopia with nystagmus, absent foveal reflexes and corneal changes. *Acta Ophthalmol (Copenh)*. 1981;59(1):85−93.

94. Ghose S, Mehta U. Microcornea with corectopia and macular hypoplasia in a family. *Jpn J Ophthalmol*. 1984;28(2):126−130.

95. Bowe T, Rahmani S, Yonekawa Y. Endoscopic vitrectomy for microcornea, posterior megalolenticonus, persistent fetal vasculature, coloboma syndrome. *Ophthalmology*. 2017;124(12):1742.

96. Ranchod TM, et al. Microcornea, posterior megalolenticonus, persistent fetal vasculature, and coloboma: a new syndrome. *Ophthalmology*. 2010;117(9):1843−1847.

97. Der Kaloustian VM, et al. Familial spinocerebellar degeneration with corneal dystrophy. *Am J Med Genet*. 1985;20(2):325−339.

98. Mousa AR, et al. Autosomally inherited recessive spastic ataxia, macular corneal dystrophy, congenital cataracts, myopia and vertically oval temporally tilted discs: report of a Bedouin family—a new syndrome. *J Neurol Sci*. 1986;76(1):105−121.

99. Bargal R, et al. Identification of the gene causing mucolipidosis type IV. *Nat Genet*. 2000;26(1):118−121.

100. Amir N, Zlotogora J, Bach G. Mucolipidosis type IV: clinical spectrum and natural history. *Pediatrics*. 1987;79(9):953−959.

101. Caruso RC, et al. Electroretinographic findings in the mucopolysaccharidoses. *Ophthalmology*. 1986;93(12): 1612–1616.

102. Collins ML, Traboulsi EI, Maumenee IH. Optic nerve head swelling and optic atrophy in the systemic mucopolysaccharidoses. *Ophthalmology*. 1990;97(11): 1445–1449.

103. Jensen OA, et al. Hurler-Scheie phenotype: report of an inbred sibship with tapeto-retinal degeneration and electron-microscopic examination of the conjunctiva. *Ophthalmologica*. 1978;176(4):194–204.

104. Schmidt H, et al. Radiological findings in patients with mucopolysaccharidosis I H/S (Hurler-Scheie syndrome). *Pediat Radiol*. 1987;17(5):409–414.

105. Quigley HA, Maumenee AE, Stark WJ. Acute glaucoma in systemic mucopolysaccharidosis I-S. *Am J Ophthal*. 1975; 80(1):70–72.

106. Scheie HG, Hambrick Jr GW, Barness LA. A newly recognized forme fruste of Hurler's disease (gargoylism). *Am J Ophthal*. 1962;53:753–769.

107. Beck M, et al. Fetal presentation of Morquio disease type A. *Prenat Diag*. 1992;12(12):1019–1029.

108. Charrow J, et al. Diagnostic evaluation, monitoring, and perioperative management of spinal cord compression in patients with Morquio syndrome. *Mol Genet Metab*. 2015; 114(1):11–18.

109. Giugliani R, et al. Progressive mental regression in siblings with Morquio disease type B (mucopolysaccharidosis IV B). *Clin Genet*. 1987;32(5):313–325.

110. Trojak JE, et al. Morquio-like syndrome (MPS IVB) associated with deficiency of beta-galactosidase. *Johns Hopkins Med J*. 1980;146(2):75–79.

111. Cantor LB, Disseler JA, Wilson 2nd FM. Glaucoma in the Maroteaux-Lamy syndrome. *Am J Ophthal*. 1989;108(4): 426–430.

112. Jin W-D, et al. Mucopolysaccharidosis type VI: identification of three mutations in the arylsulfatase B gene of patients with the severe and mild phenotypes provides molecular evidence for genetic heterogeneity. *Am J Hum Genet*. 1992;50(4):795–800.

113. Montano AM, et al. Clinical course of Sly syndrome (mucopolysaccharidosis type VII). *J Med Genet*. 2016; 53(6):403–418.

114. Tomatsu S, et al. Mucopolysaccharidosis type VII: characterization of mutations and molecular heterogeneity. *Am J Hum Genet*. 1991;48(1):89–96.

115. Hanson IM, et al. Mutations at the PAX6 locus are found in heterogeneous anterior segment malformations including Peters' anomaly. *Nat Genet*. 1994;6(2): 168–173.

116. Withers SJ, Gole GA, Summers KM. Autosomal dominant cataracts and Peters anomaly in a large Australian family. *Clin Genet*. 1999;55(4):240–247.

117. Kivlin JD, et al. Peters' anomaly as a consequence of genetic and nongenetic syndromes. *Arch Ophthal*. 1986; 104(1):61–64.

118. Norton ME, Scoutt LM, Feldstein VA. *Callen's Ultrasonography in Obstetrics and Gynecology*. 6th ed. Philadelphia, PA: Elsevier; 2008:322.

119. Pillay VK. Ophthalmo-mandibulo-melic dysplasia, an hereditary syndrome. *J Bone Joint Surg Am*. 1964;46: 858–862.

120. Aldave AJ, et al. Linkage of posterior amorphous corneal dystrophy to chromosome 12q21.33 and exclusion of coding region mutations in KERA, LUM, DCN, and EPYC. *Invest Ophthal Vis Sci*. 2010;51:4006–4012.

121. Johnson AT, et al. The pathology of posterior amorphous corneal dystrophy. *Ophthalmology*. 1990;97:104–109.

122. Orssaud C, et al. Relevance of identifying JAG1 mutations in patients with isolated posterior embryotoxon. *J Glaucoma*. 2016;25(12):923–925.

123. Caignec Le, et al. Familial deafness, congenital heart defects, and posterior embryotoxon caused by cysteine substitution in the first epidermal-growth-factor-like domain of Jagged 1. *Am J Hum Genet*. 2002;71:180–186.

124. Davidson AE, et al. Autosomal-dominant corneal endothelial dystrophies CHED1 and PPCD1 are allelic disorders caused by non-coding mutations in the promoter of OVOL2. *Am J Hum Genet*. 2016;98:75–89.

125. Biswas S, Munier FL, Yardley J, et al. Missense mutations in COL8A2, the gene encoding the alpha-2 chain of type VIII collagen, cause two forms of corneal endothelial dystrophy. *Hum Mol Genet*. 2001;10:2415–2423.

126. Liskova P, Tuft SJ, Gwilliam R, et al. Novel mutations in the ZEB1 gene identified in Czech and British patients with posterior polymorphous corneal dystrophy. *Abstr Hum Mutat*. 2007;28:638.

127. Akiya S, Brown SI. The ultrastructure of Reis-Bucklers' dystrophy. *Am J Ophthal*. 1971;72(3):549–554.

128. Hall P. Reis-Bucklers dystrophy. *Arch Ophthal*. 1974; 91(3):170–173.

129. Kobayashi A, Sugiyama K. In vivo laser confocal microscopy findings for Bowman's layer dystrophies (Thiel-Behnke and Reis-Bucklers corneal dystrophies). *Ophthalmology*. 2007;114(1):49–75.

130. Küchle M, et al. Reevaluation of corneal dystrophies of Bowman's layer and the anterior stroma (Reis-Bucklers and Thiel-Behnke types): a light and electron microscopic study of eight corneas and a review of the literature. *Cornea*. 1995;14(4):333–354.

131. Small KW, et al. Mapping of Reis-Bucklers' corneal dystrophy to chromosome 5q. *Am J Ophthal*. 1996;121(4): 384–390.

132. Tanhehco TY, et al. Two cases of Reis-Bücklers corneal dystrophy (granular corneal dystrophy type III) caused by spontaneous mutations in the TGFBI gene. *Arch Ophthalmol*. 2006;124(4):589–593.

133. Mattos J, Contreras F, O'Donnell Jr FE. Ring dermoid syndrome: a new syndrome of autosomal-dominantly inherited, bilateral, annular limbal dermoids with corneal and conjunctival extension. *Arch Ophthal*. 1980; 98(6):1059–1061.

134. Xia K, et al. Mutation in PITX2 is associated with ring dermoid of the cornea. *J Med Genet.* 2004;41(12):e129.
135. Higgs JE, Clayton-Smith J. Rutherfurd syndrome revisited: intellectual disability is not a feature. *Clin Dysmorph.* 2015;24(3):125−127.
136. Houston IB, Shotts N. Rutherfurd's syndrome: a familial oculo-dental disorder. *Acta Paediat Scand.* 1966;55:233−238.
137. Battisti C, et al. Schnyder corneal crystalline dystrophy: description of a new family with evidence of abnormal lipid storage in skin fibroblasts. *Am J Med Genet.* 1998;75(1):35−39.
138. Bron AJ, Williams HP, Carruthers ME. Hereditary crystalline stromal dystrophy of Schnyder. I. Clinical features of a family with hyperlipoproteinaemia. *Br J Ophthalmol.* 1972;56(5):383.
139. Lisch W, et al. Schnyder's dystrophy: progression and metabolism. *Ophthalmic Paediat Genet.* 1986;7(1):45−56.
140. Pryse-Phillips W. *Companion to Clinical Neurology.* 3rd ed. New York, NY: Oxford University Press; 2009:366.
141. Yee RW, et al. Linkage mapping of Thiel-Behnke corneal dystrophy (CDB2) to chromosome 10q23-q24. *Genomics.* 1997;46(1):152−154.
142. Chitayat D, et al. Hereditary tyrosinaemia type II in a consanguineous Ashkenazi Jewish family: intrafamilial variation in phenotype; absence of parental phenotype effects on the fetus. *J Inherit Metab Dis.* 1992;15(2):198−203.
143. Garibaldi LR, et al. Oculocutaneous tyrosinosis: report of two cases in the same family. *Helv Paediat Acta.* 1977;32(2):173−180.
144. Gadoth N, Liel Y. Transient external ophthalmoplegia in Wilson's disease. *Metab Pediat Ophthal.* 1980;4(2):71−72.
145. Gow PJ, et al. Diagnosis of Wilson's disease: an experience over three decades. *Gut.* 2000;46(3):415−419.
146. Basler E, et al. Identification of point mutations in the steroid sulfatase gene of three patients with X-linked ichthyosis. *Am J Hum Genet.* 1992;50(3):483−491.
147. Gillard EF, et al. Deletion of a DNA sequence in eight of nine families with X-linked ichthyosis (steroid sulphatase deficiency). *Nucleic Acids Res.* 1987;15(10):3977−3985.
148. Haritoglou C, et al. Corneal manifestations of X-linked ichthyosis in two brothers. *Cornea.* 2000;19(6).
149. Kraemer KH, Myung ML, Scotto J. Xeroderma pigmentosum: cutaneous, ocular, and neurologic abnormalities in 830 published cases. *Arch Dermatol.* 1987;123(2):241−250.
150. Robbins Jay H, et al. Xeroderma pigmentosum: an inherited disease with sun sensitivity, multiple cutaneous neoplasms, and abnormal DNA repair. *Ann Intern Med.* 1974;80(2):221−248.
151. Hittner HM, Kretzer FL, Mehta RS. Zellweger syndrome: lenticular opacities indicating Carrier status and lens abnormalities characteristic of homozygotes. *Arch Ophthal.* 1981;99(11):1977−1982.
152. Li X, et al. PEX11-beta deficiency is lethal and impairs neuronal migration but does not abrogate peroxisome function. *Mol Cell Biol.* 2002;22(12):4358−4365.

## FURTHER READING

1. El-Ashry MF, et al. A clinical and molecular genetic study of autosomal-dominant stromal corneal dystrophy in British population. *Ophthalm Res.* 2005;37(6):310−317.
2. Hou YC, et al. Phenotype−genotype correlations in patients with TGFBI-linked corneal dystrophies in Taiwan. *Mol Vision.* 2012;18:362.

# CHAPTER 6

# Genetic Abnormalities of the Crystalline Lens

SCOTT R. LAMBERT • PAYTON M. MILLER • JANINE SMITH-MARSHALL • NATARIO L. COUSER

Genetic conditions that affect the crystalline lens generally either disrupt its transparency or alter the natural position by causing displacement. A congenital cataract (Fig. 6.1) is an opacification of the crystalline lens of the eye that occurs during development. They are the primary cause of treatable blindness in children worldwide,[1] with a prevalence of 4.2 per 10,000.[2] Congenital cataracts may be sporadic, can involve all inheritance patterns, be an inherited isolated anomaly (nonsyndromic) (Table 6.1),[3-7] or be associated with a variety of systemic anomalies (syndromic) (Table 6.2).[3] Over 100 genes are associated with inherited congenital cataracts; 35 genes have been reported with isolated congenital cataracts and 15 genes may cause congenital cataracts associated with other eye anomalies but no systemic associations.[3] In developed countries, more than one-half of all bilateral congenital cataracts are associated with hereditary disease. Congenital cataract formation is a clinical component of a wide spectrum of systemic disorders, including inborn errors of metabolism, leukoencephalopathies, and peroxisomal disorders. While these disorders may seem widespread, they are similar in mechanism, as the cataract formation is created by an accumulation of proteins and metabolites in serum that deposit in and opacify the lens. For example, in individuals with hyperferritinemia, cataract formation is the result of opacification due to ferritin accumulation in the crystalline lens.

Ectopia lentis is a dislocation of the natural crystalline lens from the normal position (Figure 6.2). A lens subluxation refers to a partially dislocated lens, while a lens luxation refers to a completely dislocated lens. A single dislocated lens may result from trauma, but individuals with bilateral dislocated lenses will often have an underlying genetic cause. These genetic causes may include homocystinuria, Marfan syndrome, Weill-Marchesani syndrome, Ehlers-Danlos syndrome (EDS), sulfite oxidase deficiency, and mutations in the *LEPREL1* gene and the a disintegrin and metalloproteinase with thrombospondin motifs (ADAMTS) family of genes.[8-11] A sector lens coloboma may be an isolated crystalline lens abnormality or associated with ectopia lentis; lens zonules may be partially visible within the area of reflection between the congenital lens defect and margin of the iris.[12,13]

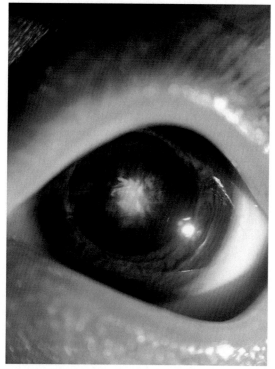

FIG. 6.1 Congenital cataract. Central lens opacity, right eye.

**TABLE 6.1**
**List of Nonsyndromic Cataract Genes by Inheritance Pattern**

| Inheritance Pattern | Genes Associated With Nonsyndromic Congenital Cataracts |
|---|---|
| Autosomal dominant | CHMP4B, CRYBB2, CRYGB, CRYGC, CRYGD, CRYGS, FTL, GJA3, MIP, PRX, RRAGA, TMEM114, UNC45 B, VIM |
| Autosomal recessive | BFSP1, CTPL1, FYOC1, GALK1, GCNT2, LEMD2, LIM2, LONP1, LSS, SIPA1L3, TDRD7, WDR87 |
| Autosomal dominant or recessive | BFSP2, CRYBA1, CRYBB1, CRYBB3, EPHA2, HSF4 |
| De novo | CRYGA, WDR36 |

## GENETIC DISORDERS

### Alport Syndrome[14,15]

*OMIM*: #301050, #203780, #104200.

*Description*: Alport syndrome is a disorder characterized by glomerulonephropathy (that often progresses to end-stage renal disease), bilateral and high-frequency sensorineural hearing loss, ocular dysfunctions, and, in rare cases, aortic aneurism. These findings are a result of the absence of collagen IV network from the epithelial basement membranes, specifically the glomerular basement membrane.

*Epidemiology*: prevalence of 1/50,000.

*Eye Findings*: anterior lenticonus (Fig. 6.3), corneal erosions, myopia, and retinal pigmentary changes (specifically, perimacular flecks).

*Inheritance*: XLD, AR, AD

*Known Genes or Gene Locus*: COL4A5 (X-linked), COL4A4 (AR), COL4A3 (AR and AD).

### Cataract-Microcornea Syndrome[16–18]

*OMIM*: #116200.

*Description*: Cataract-microcornea syndrome is a heterogenetic disorder characterized by congenital cataracts and microcornea (classified by diameters less than 10 mm in both the horizontal and vertical axes) without additional systemic disease or abnormality. The disorder is very rare, with less than 20 pedigrees documented in literature.

*Epidemiology*: unknown.

*Eye Findings*: aphakia (unilaterally), congenital cataracts, congenital posterior polar cataracts, cornea plana, glaucoma, microcornea, myopia, Peters' anomaly, prominent Schwalbe's ring, and sclerocornea

*Inheritance*: AD.

*Known Genes or Gene Locus*: CRYAA, CRYBB1, CRYGD, GJA8.

### Cerebrotendinous Xanthomatosis[19–21]

*OMIM*: #213700.

*Description*: Cerebrotendinous xanthomatosis is a lipid storage disorder characterized by abnormally high plasma cholestanol levels accompanied by the accumulation of cholestanol and cholesterol in tissues, and especially in the brain, Achilles tendons, and lungs. Affected patients present with chronic diarrhea and bilateral cataract formation in early childhood, followed by the onset of progressive neurologic dysfunction and tendon xanthomas in adolescence and early adulthood.

*Epidemiology*: incidence of 1/36,072–1/75,601 amongst South Asians; 1/64,267–1/64,712 amongst East Asians; 1/71,677–1/148,914 amongst North Americans; 1/134,970–1/461,358 amongst Europeans; 1/263,222–1/468,624 amongst Africans.

*Eye Findings*: cataracts (juvenile), palpebral xanthelasmas, optic nerve atrophy, retinal vessel sclerosis, and proptosis.

*Inheritance*: AR.

*Known Genes or Gene Locus*: CYP27A1.

### Chanarin-Dorfman Syndrome[22–25]

*OMIM*: #275630.

*Description*: Chanarin-Dorfman syndrome is a disorder characterized by nonbullous, congenital ichthyosiform erythroderma, fatty-liver-derived hepatosplenomegaly, myopathy, and slight intellectual disorder. Due to a deficiency in the CGI-58 lipase coactivator, affected individuals cannot metabolize neutral lipids. This leads to nonlysosomal and multisystem triglyceride storage.

*Epidemiology*: unknown.

*Eye Findings*: cataracts, ectropion, nystagmus, and strabismus.

*Inheritance*: AR.

*Known Genes or Gene Locus*: ABHD5.

### Congenital Primary Aphakia[25,26]

*OMIM*: #610256.

*Description*: Congenital primary aphakia is the absence of the lens resulting from failure of induction of the lens during embryonic development. Total aplasia, determined histologically, distinguishes congenital

**TABLE 6.2**
**Syndromic Cataract Genes Information**

| Locus | Gene | Inheritance | OMIM | Disease | Gene Product |
|---|---|---|---|---|---|
| 1p36.32 | PEX10 | AR | 614870 | Neonatal adrenoleukodystrophy, Zellweger syndrome | Protein of peroxisomal matrix |
| 1p36.22 | PEX14 | AR | 614887 | Zellweger syndrome | Peroxisomal import machinery |
| 1p36.1p34 | HSPG2 | AR | 224410/25800 | Schwartz–Jampel syndrome type 1/dyssegmental dysplasia | Perlecan protein |
| 1p36p35 | GALE | AR | 230350 | Galactose epimerase deficiency | UDP-galactose-4-epimerase |
| 1p34.1 | POMGNT1 | AR | 253280 | Muscular dystrophy-dystroglycanopathy | Type 2 transmembrane protein that resides in the Golgi apparatus |
| 1p22p21 | ABCD3 | AR | 616278 | Zellweger syndrome 2 | Member of the superfamily of ATP-binding cassette transporters |
| 1p21 | COL11A1 | AD | 604841/154780 | Stickler syndrome type 2, Marshall syndrome | One of the two alpha chains of type XI collagen |
| 1q41 | IARS2 | AR | 616007 | Cataracts, growth hormone deficiency, sensory neuropathy, sensorineural hearing loss, skeletal dysplasia | Aminoacyl-tRNA synthetase |
| 1q41 | RAB3GAP2 | AR | 212720/614225 | Martsolf syndrome, Warburg Micro syndrome | RAB3 protein regulates exocytosis of neurotransmitters and hormones |
| 1q42 | GNPAT | AR | 222765 | Rhizomelic chondrodysplasia punctata type 2 | Enzyme in synthesis of ether phospholipids |
| 2p14p16 | PEX13 | AR | 614883 | Zellweger syndrome | Peroxisomal membrane protein |
| 2q21.3 | RAB3GAP1 | AR | 600118 | Warburg Micro syndrome | Catalytic subunit of a Rab GTPase-activating protein |
| 2q24q31 | LRP2 | AR | 222448 | Donnai-Barrow syndrome | Low-density lipoprotein-related protein 2 |
| 2q33qter | CYP27A1 | AR | 213700 | Cerebrotendinous xanthomatosis | Member of the cytochrome P450 superfamily |
| 2q37 | KCNJ13 | AD | 193230 | Snowflake vitreoretinal degeneration | Member of the inwardly rectifying potassium channel family |
| 3p21.1 | COL7A1 | AR | 226600 | Epidermolysis bullosa dystrophica | Alpha chain of type VII collagen |
| 3p14.3 | FLNB | AD, AR | 150250/272460 | Larsen syndrome/spondylocarpotarsal synostosis syndrome | Member of the filamin family |
| 3q21q22 | CNBP | AD | 602668 | Myotonic dystrophy type 2 | A nucleic acid-binding protein with seven zinc-finger domains |

Continued

**TABLE 6.2**
Syndromic Cataract Genes Information—cont'd

| Locus | Gene | Inheritance | OMIM | Disease | Gene Product |
|---|---|---|---|---|---|
| 3q25 | SLC33A1 | AR | 614482 | Congenital cataracts, hearing loss, neurodegeneration | Required for the formation of O-acetylated (Ac) gangliosides |
| 4p16.1 | HMX1 | AR | 612109 | Oculoauricular syndrome | Transcription factor that belongs to the H6 family of homeobox proteins |
| 4p15.32 | CC2D2A | AR | 612285 | Joubert syndrome 9 | Play a critical role in cilia formation |
| 4p12q12 | SRD5A3 | AR | 612713 | Kahirazi syndrome | Steroid 5-alpha reductase family |
| 4q32q35 | ETFDH | AR | 231680 | Glutaric acidemia | Component of the electron-transfer system in mitochondria |
| 4q35.1 | TRAPPC11 | AR | 615356 | Muscular dystrophy limb girdle 2S | A subunit of the TRAPP tethering complex |
| 5q12.1 | ERCC8 | AR | 216400 | Cockayne syndrome type A | A WD repeat protein |
| 5q14.3 | VCAN | AD | 143200 | Wagner syndrome 1 | A member of the aggrecan/versican proteoglycan family |
| 5q31 | SIL1 | AR | 248800 | Marinesco-Sjögren syndrome | Resident endoplasmic reticulum N-linked glycoprotein |
| 6p24 | TFAP2A | AD | 113620 | Branchiooculofacial syndrome | A transcription factor |
| 6p23 | GCM2 | AD | 146200 | Hypoparathyroidism familial isolated | A homolog of the Drosophila glial cells missing gene |
| 6p21.3 | NEU1 | AR | 256550 | Sialidosis type 2 | A lysosomal enzyme that cleaves terminal sialic acid residues |
| 6q21q23.2 | GJA1 | AD | 164200 | Oculodentodigital dysplasia | A member of the connexin gene family |
| 6q22q24 | PEX7 | AR | 215100 | Rhizomelic chondrodysplasia punctata type 1 | Cytosolic receptor for the set of peroxisomal matrix enzymes |
| 6q24.2 | PEX3 | AR | 614882 | Zellweger syndrome | Involved in peroxisome biosynthesis and integrity |
| 7p15.3 | FAM126 A | AR | 610532 | Hypomyelinating leukodystrophy 5 | Part in the beta-catenin/LEF signaling pathway |
| 7q21.2 | PEX1 | AR | 214100 | Zellweger syndrome | A member of the AAA ATPase family |
| 7q31.1 | CAV1 | AD | 606721 | Partial lipodystrophy, congenital cataracts, neurodegeneration syndrome | Main component of the caveolae plasma membranes |
| 7q34 | AGK | AR | 212350 | Sengers syndrome | A mitochondrial membrane protein involved in lipid and glycerolipid metabolism |

| Location | Gene | Inheritance | OMIM | Disease/Syndrome | Protein |
|---|---|---|---|---|---|
| 8p21.1 | ESCO2 | AR | 268300 | Roberts syndrome | Acetyltransferase activity may be required for the establishment of sister chromatid cohesion |
| 8q13.3 | EYA1 | AD | 601653 | Branchiootorenal syndrome 1 | A member of the EYA family of proteins |
| 8q21.1 | PXMP3 | AR | 614866 | Zellweger syndrome | An integral peroxisomal membrane protein required for peroxisome biogenesis |
| 8q21q22 | CNGB3 | AR | 262300 | Achromatopsia 3 | The beta subunit of a cyclic nucleotide-gated ion channel |
| 8q24.3 | RECQL4 | AR | 268400 | Rothmund-Thompson syndrome | DNA helicase that belongs to the RecQ helicase family |
| 9p13.13 | GALT | AR | 230400 | Galatosemia | Galactose-1-phosphate uridyltransferase |
| 9p24 | VLDLR | AR | 224050 | Cerebellar hypoplasia and mental retardation with or without quadrupedal locomotion 1 | Low-density lipoprotein receptor |
| 9q31q33 | FKTN | AR | 253800 | Muscular dystrophy-dystroglycanopathy | A putative transmembrane protein localized to the cis-Golgi compartment |
| 9q34 | LMX1B | AD | 161200 | Nail-patella syndrome | A member of LIM-homeodomain family of proteins |
| 9q34.1 | POMT1 | AR | 236670 | Muscular dystrophy-dystroglycanopathy A1 | An O-mannosyltransferase |
| 10q11.23 | ERCC6 | AR | 214150/133540 | Cerebrooculofacioskeletal syndrome I/Cockayne syndrome type B | A DNA-binding protein that is important in transcription-coupled excision repair |
| 10q23.31 | PTEN | AD | 158350 | Cowden disease | A tumor suppressor |
| 10q24.3 | ALDH18A1 | AD/AR | 616603/219150 | Cutis laxa AD/cutis laxa AR | A member of the aldehyde dehydrogenase family |
| 10q26 | OAT | AR | 258870 | Gyrate atrophy of choroid and retina | Mitochondrial enzyme ornithine aminotransferase |
| 11p15.3p15.1 | PTH | AD/AR | 146200 | Familial isolated hypoparathyroidism | A member of the parathyroid family of proteins |
| 11q13.4 | LRP5 | AR, AD | 601813/607634 | Exudative vitreoretinopathy 4/osteopetrosis, autosomal dominant 1 | A transmembrane low-density lipoprotein receptor |
| 11q13.2q13.5 | DHCR7 | AR | 270400 | Smith-Lemli-Opitz syndrome | An enzyme that removes the C(7-8) double bond in the B ring of sterols |
| 11q13.4 | CLPB | AR | 616271 | 3-methylglutaconic aciduria with cataracts, neurologic involvement, neutropenia | Member of the ATPases associated with diverse cellular activities (AAA+) superfamily |

*Continued*

**TABLE 6.2**
**Syndromic Cataract Genes Information—cont'd**

| Locus | Gene | Inheritance | OMIM | Disease | Gene Product |
|---|---|---|---|---|---|
| 11q14.2 | FZD4 | AD | 133780 | Retinopathy of prematurity | A member of the frizzled gene family |
| 11q22.3 | MMP1 | AR | 226600 | Epidermolysis bullosa dystrophic | A member of the peptidase M10 family of matrix metalloproteinases |
| 11q22.1q23.2 | CRYAB | AD | 608810 | Myofibrillar myopathy | Members of the small heat shock protein (HSP20) family |
| 11q23.3 | SC5DL | AR | 607330 | Lathosterolosis | Enzyme of cholesterol biosynthesis |
| 11q25 | JAM3 | AR | 613730 | Hemorrhagic destruction of brain, subependymal calcification | Immunoglobulin superfamily gene member |
| 12q13.12 | TUBA1A | AD | 611603 | Lissencephaly | Microtubule constituents of to the tubulin superfamily |
| 12p13.3 | PEX5 | AR | 214110 | Zellweger syndrome | Protein essential for the assembly of functional peroxisomes |
| 12q24 | MVK | AR | 610377 | Mevalonic aciduria | Peroxisomal enzyme mevalonate kinase |
| 13q12 | GJB6 | AD | 129500 | Clouston syndrome | One of the connexin proteins |
| 13q12.3 | B3GALTL | AR | 261540 | Peters plus syndrome | A beta-1,3-glucosyltransferase that transfers glucose to O-linked fucosylglycans on thrombospondin type-1 repeats |
| 13q14.3 | ITM2B | AD | 117300 | Cerebral amyloid angiopathy | A transmembrane protein |
| 13q34 | COL4A1 | AD | 607595 | Cerebral small vessel disease | A type IV collagen alpha protein |
| 14q21.1 | SEC23 A | AR | 607812 | Craniolenticulosutural dysplasia | A member of the SEC23 subfamily of the SEC23/SEC24 family |
| 14q24 | POMT2 | AR | 613150 | Muscular dystrophy-dystroglycanopathy | An O-mannosyltransferase |
| 15q15 | BUB1B | AR | 257300 | Mosaic variegated aneuploidy syndrome 1 | A kinase involved in spindle checkpoint function |
| 15q21.1 | FBN1 | AD | 608328 | Weill-Marchesani syndrome | A member of the fibrillin family of proteins |
| 15q25 | POLG | AD/AR | 157640 | Progressive external ophthalmoplegia with mitochondrial DNA deletions 1 | The catalytic subunit of mitochondrial DNA polymerase |
| 16p13.3p13.2 | GFER | AR? | 613076 | Progressive mitochondrial myopathy, sensorineural hearing loss, developmental delay | Structural and functional homolog of the yeast scERV1 gene |
| 16q21 | NOD2 | AD | 186580 | Blau syndrome | A member of the Nod1/Apaf-1 family |

| Location | Gene | Inheritance | OMIM # | Syndrome | Description |
|---|---|---|---|---|---|
| 16q23 | ADAMTS18 | AR | 267750 | Knobloch syndrome | A member of the ADAMTS (a disintegrin and metalloproteinase with thrombospondin motifs) protein family |
| 16q22q23 | MAF | AD | 601088 | Ayme-Gripp Syndrome | A DNA-binding, leucine zipper-containing transcription factor |
| 17p13.3 | YWHAE | AD | 247200 | Miller-Dieker lissencephaly syndrome | Member of the 14-3-3 family of proteins which mediate signal transduction by binding to phosphoserine-containing proteins |
| 17q12 | PEX12 | AR | 614859 | Zellweger syndrome | Member of the peroxin-12 family |
| 17q21 | WNT3 | AR | 273395 | Tetra-amelia syndrome | Secreted signaling proteins implicated in oncogenesis |
| 17q21.33 | XYLT2 | AR | 605822 | Spondylo-ocular syndrome | An isoform of xylosyltransferase, which belongs to a family of glycosyltransferases |
| 18q12.3 | EPG5 | AR | 242840 | Vici syndrome (immunodeficiency, cleft lip/palate, cataract, hypopigmentation, absent corpus callosum), | A large coiled-coil domain-containing protein that functions in autophagy |
| 18q23 | CTDP1 | AR | 604168 | Congenital cataracts, facial dysmorphism, neuropathy | A protein which interacts with the carboxy-terminus of the RAP74 subunit of transcription initiation factor TFIIF |
| 19q13.1 | MAN2B1 | AR | 248500 | Alpha-mannosidosis | An enzyme that hydrolyzes terminal, nonreducing alpha-D-mannose residues in alpha-D-mannosides |
| 19q13.3 | DMPK | AD | 160900 | Myotonic dystrophy 1 | A serine-threonine kinase |
| 19q13.32 | FKRP | AR | 613153 | Muscular dystrophy-dystroglycanopathy | A protein which is targeted to the medial Golgi apparatus and is necessary for posttranslational modification of dystroglycan |
| 20p11.21q12 | ABHD12 | AR | 612674 | Polyneuropathy, hearing loss, ataxia, retinitis pigmentosa, cataract | An enzyme that catalyzes the hydrolysis of 2-arachidonoyl glycerol |
| 20q13.13q13.2 | SALL4 | AD | 607323 | Duane-radial ray syndrome | A zinc finger transcription factor thought to play a role in the development of abducens motor neurons |
| 20q13.3 | GNAS | AD | 103580/612462/612463 | Pseudohypoparathyroidism type 1A/pseudohypoparathyroidism type 1C/pseudohypoparathyroidism | Multiple transcript variants encoding different isoforms |

Continued

**TABLE 6.2**
**Syndromic Cataract Genes Information—cont'd**

| Locus | Gene | Inheritance | OMIM | Disease | Gene Product |
|---|---|---|---|---|---|
| 21q22.3 | COL18A1 | AR | 267750 | Knobloch syndrome 1 | Alpha chain of type XVIII collagen |
| 22q11.21 | PEX26 | AR | 614872 | Zellweger syndrome | Member of the peroxin-26 gene family |
| 22q12.2 | NF2 | AD | 101000 | Neurofibromatosis type 2 | A protein similar to ezrin, radixin, moesin family of proteins |
| 22q12.3 | LARGE | AR | 613154 | Muscular dystrophy-dystroglycanopathy | A member of the N-acetylglucosaminyltransferase gene family |
| 22q13.1 | MYH9 | AD | 153640 | Fechtner syndrome | A conventional nonmuscle myosin |
| Xp11.4 | BCOR | XL | 300166 | microphthalmia syndromic 2 | An interacting corepressor of BCL6 |
| Xp11.23 | PQBP1 | XL | 309500 | Renpenning syndrome | A nuclear polyglutamine-binding protein that is involved with transcription activation |
| Xp11.23p11.22 | EBP | XL | 302960 | Chondrodysplasia punctata 2 | An integral membrane protein of the endoplasmic reticulum |
| Xp22.3 | ARSE | XL | 302950 | Chondrodysplasia punctata 1 | A member of the sulfatase family |
| Xp22.3 | HCCS | XL | 309801 | Linear skin defects with multiple congenital anomalies | An enzyme that covalently links a heme group to the apoprotein of cytochrome c |
| Xp22 | AIC | XL | 304050 | Aicardi syndrome | Unknown |
| Xp22.13 | NHS | XL | 302350 | Nance-Horan syndrome | A protein containing four conserved nuclear localization signals |
| Xq22 | GLA | XL | 301500 | Fabry disease | A homodimeric glycoprotein that hydrolyzes the terminal alpha-galactosyl moieties from glycolipids and glycoproteins |
| Xq22 | COL4A5 | XL | 301050 | Alport syndrome | One of the six subunits of type IV collagen |
| Xq25q26.1 | OCRL | XL | 309000 | Lowe oculocerebrorenal syndrome | An inositol polyphosphate 5-phosphatase |
| Xq28 | IKBKG | XL | 308300 | Incontinentia pigmenti | Regulatory subunit of the inhibitor of kappaB kinase complex |

AD, autosomal dominant; AR, autosomal recessive; XL, X linked.

Table courtesy and with permission from Messina-Baas O, Cuevas-Covarrubias SA. Inherited congenital cataract: a guide to suspect the genetic etiology in the cataract genesis. *Mol Syndromol.* 2017;8(2):58–78. Copyright © 2017 Karger Publishers, Basel, Switzerland.

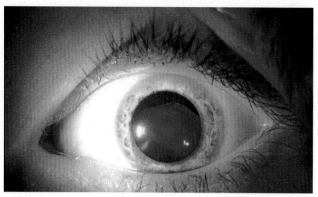

FIG. 6.2 Ectopia lentis with superior lens zonules visible.

primary aphakia from congenital secondary aphakia, in which the lens develops to some degree before being degraded.

*Epidemiology*: unknown.

*Eye Findings*: aniridia, anterior segment aplasia, aphakia, megalocornea, microphthalmia, and sclerocornea.

*Inheritance*: AR.

*Known Genes or Gene Locus*: FOXE3.

## Ectopia Lentis Et Pupillae[27,28]

OMIM: #225200.

*Description*: Ectopia lentis et pupillae is a disorder characterized by bilateral subluxation of the lenses in combination with bilateral displacement of the pupils during development. Disorder presents in the absence of other systemic abnormalities. Typically, lens subluxation and pupil displacement occur in opposite directions.

*Epidemiology*: prevalence of 0.83/10,000 (all congenital ectopia lentis cases); ectopia lentis et pupillae 21.2% of congenital ectopia lentis cases.

*Eye Findings*: abnormal appearing iris, astigmatism, cataract, ectopic lens and pupil, increased axial length, increased corneal diameter, loss of zonular fibers, microspherophakia, myopia, persistent pupillary membrane, retinal detachment, and tilted disk.

*Inheritance*: AR.

*Known Genes or Gene Locus*: ADAMTSL4.

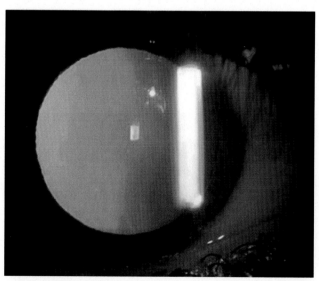

FIG. 6.3 Alport syndrome. Retroilluminated photograph of the lens showing the "oil-drop" appearance of anterior lenticonus. (Courtesy Gregory, Martin C. *Alport syndrome and related disorders. National Kidney Foundation Primer on Kidney Diseases*; January 1, 2018:389–394. © 2018.)

### Ectopia Lentis, Familial[27-29]

*OMIM*: #129600.

*Description*: Familial ectopia lentis is a disorder characterized by stretched zonule fibers leading to dislocation of the lenses of the eyes in the absence of systemic disease. Familial ectopia lentis is a heritable condition of its own and is not used to describe lens dislocation seen in systemic disorders, such as Marfan syndrome.

*Epidemiology*: prevalence of 0.83/10,000 (all congenital ectopia lentis cases).

*Eye Findings*: congenital lens dislocation and narrow angles.

*Inheritance*: AD.

*Known Genes or Gene Locus*: FBN1.

### Ectopia Lentis, Isolated[27-30]

*OMIM*: #225100.

*Description*: Isolated ectopia lentis (Fig. 6.4) is a disorder characterized by dislocation of the lenses of the eyes without associated systemic disorder. The underlying mechanism of disease is production of truncated and dysfunctional ADAMTSL4 protein, which is responsible for anchoring and stabilizing microfibrils that hold the lens in place.

*Epidemiology*: prevalence of 0.83/10,000 (all congenital ectopia lentis cases).

*Eye Findings*: lattice degeneration, lens dislocation, retinal detachment, spherophakia, and staphyloma.

*Inheritance*: AR.

*Known Genes or Gene Locus*: ADAMTSL4.

### Ehlers-Danlos Syndrome[28,31-33]

*OMIM*: #130000, #130010, #130050, #130060, #130070, #130080, #225320, #225400, #225410, #229200, #300049, #601776, #606408, #614170, #614557, #615349, #615539, #616471, #617174, #617821.

*Description*: EDS is a connective tissue disorder that causes patients to have hypermobile joints, hyperextensible skin, and fragility of tissues of multiple different organ systems. EDS is currently categorized into 13 distinct subtypes, with the most common subtypes stemming from defects in collagen components.

*Epidemiology*: prevalence of 1/2500−1/5000.

*Eye Findings*: astigmatism, blue sclera, ectopia lentis, epicanthal folds, fragile globe, hyperopia, keratoconus, keratoglobus, myopia, strabismus, subconjunctival hemorrhage.

*Inheritance*: AD, AR, XLD (#300049).

*Known Genes or Gene Locus*: COL5A1, COL5A2, COL3A1, COL1A1, B4GALT7, COL1A2, PLOD1, ADAMTS2, ZNF469, CHST14, TNXB, PRDMS, FKBP14, B3GALT6, DSE, COL12A1, C1S, FLNA.

### Fine-Lubinsky Syndrome[34-36]

*OMIM*: #601088, %601353.

*Description*: Fine-Lubinsky syndrome is very rare, with less than 10 cases documented in literature. Affected individuals are brachycephalic with distinct craniofacial anomalies (including small and flattened features), intellectual disability, seizures, digital abnormalities, and ocular anomalies. There is still much discrepancy concerning the relationship between Fine-Lubinsky syndrome (for which a locus has not been isolated) and Ayme-Gripp syndrome (#601088/*MAF*), which may be a variant or subset of Fine-Lubinsky syndrome.

*Epidemiology*: unknown.

*Eye Findings*: cataracts, downslanted palpebral fissures, glaucoma, hypertelorism, megalocornea, ptosis, shallow orbits, and trichomegaly.

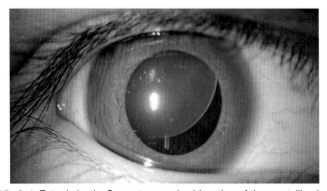

FIG. 6.4 Ectopia lentis. Superotemporal subluxation of the crystalline lens.

*Inheritance*: AR.

*Known Genes or Gene Locus*: MAF.

## Galactokinase Deficiency[37–39]

OMIM: #230200.

*Description*: Galactokinase deficiency is an inborn error of galactose metabolism; patients affected generally have a more mild presentation when compared with patients with classic galactosemia. The disorder manifests through bilateral cataract formation during childhood and involves no additional complications or abnormalities. Cataract formation is driven by accumulation of lactitol in the lens and can be slowed and even reversed with appropriate dietary restriction.

*Epidemiology*: incidence of 1/40,000, according to newborn screening in Berlin from 1991 until 2010.

*Eye Findings*: bilateral cataracts, nystagmus, and pseudotumor cerebri.

*Inheritance*: AR.

*Known Genes or Gene Locus*: GALK1.

## Galactosemia[40]

OMIM: #230400.

*Description*: Galactosemia is an inborn error of galactose metabolism that may present with life-threatening symptoms days after birth, including failure to thrive, hepatic damage, bleeding, and sepsis. These symptoms may be prevented or resolve with a timely application of a lactose/galactose restricted diet. However, untreated galactosemia typically manifests with lasting abnormalities that include developmental delays and apraxia of speech. The majority of females ultimately experience premature ovarian insufficiency even with good dietary management.

*Epidemiology*: incidence of 1/19,000–1/44,000 in Europeans and Americans; 1/480 in the Irish traveler population.

*Eye Findings*: cataracts (typically with an "oil droplet" appearance)

*Inheritance*: AR.

*Known Genes or Gene Locus*: GALT.

## Hallermann-Streiff Syndrome[41,42]

OMIM: %234100.

*Description*: Hallermann-Streiff syndrome is a disorder characterized by brachycephaly with frontal bossing, bird-like facial structure (beaked nose and micrognathia), dental defects, hypotrichosis, and diminished, but proportional, stature. The underlying cause of Hallermann-Streiff is unknown, but researchers have suspected links to laminal defects and also to decreased serum levels of insulin-like growth factor 1 amongst affected individuals.

*Epidemiology*: unknown.

*Eye Findings*: blue sclera, cataracts, distichiasis, downslanting palpebral fissures, enophthalmos, entropion, microphthalmia, nystagmus, ptosis, retinal detachment, and spontaneous cataract absorption.

*Inheritance*: unknown; suspected that rate of causation by sporadic mutation is high.

*Known Genes or Gene Locus*: unknown.

## Homocystinuria[9,28,43,44]

OMIM: #236200, #236250, #236270, #250940.

*Description*: Heritable homocystinuria is an inborn error of metabolism classically characterized by inability to convert homocysteine to cystathionine and, more marginally, by inability to convert homocysteine to methionine. Affected individuals present with light hair coloration, ocular dysfunctions, intellectual disability, and skeletal anomalies in the first or second decade of life. Patients with homocystinuria are also prone to megaloblastic anemia, eczema, seizures, and thromboembolic events.

*Epidemiology*: prevalence of 1.09/100,000.

*Eye Findings*: displacement of the lens that is typically bilateral and in the nasal and/or inferior direction (Fig. 6.5), glaucoma, iris colobomas, myopia, optic atrophy, optic neuropathy, phacodonesis, and retinal scarring.

*Inheritance*: AR.

*Known Genes or Gene Locus*: CBS, MTHFR, MTRR, MTR.

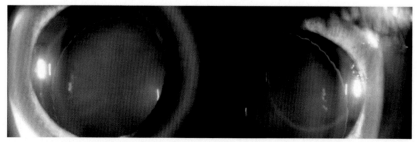

FIG. 6.5 Homocystinuria. Bilateral inferonasal subluxation of crystalline lens; right eye (left), left eye (right).

## Hyperferritinemia Cataract Syndrome[45,46]

*OMIM*: #600886.

*Description*: Hyperferritinemia cataract syndrome is a disorder characterized by increased ferritin concentration in tissues and serum due to the inability of iron regulatory protein to bind and inhibit translation of ferritin mRNA transcripts. Affected individuals present with early onset of cataracts.

*Epidemiology*: prevalence of 1/200,000.
*Eye Findings*: cataracts.
*Inheritance*: AD.
*Known Genes or Gene Locus*: FTL.

## Hypomyelination and Congenital Cataract[47,48]

*OMIM*: #610532.

*Description*: Hypomyelination and congenital cataract syndrome is classified as a congenital leukoencephalopathy. This syndrome is caused by a deficiency in the hyccin membrane protein and is characterized by congenital cataracts and deficiency of myelination in the cerebellum. Affected individuals have delayed development onset at birth and progress toward lower limb wasting, peripheral neuropathy, and psychomotor regression within their first year of life.

*Epidemiology*: unknown.
*Eye Findings*: congenital cataract.
*Inheritance*: AR.
*Known Genes or Gene Locus*: FAM126A.

## Hypoparathyroidism Familial Isolated[49,50]

*OMIM*: #146200.

*Description*: Hypoparathyroidism is an endocrine disorder characterized by presentation of seizures, muscle weakness and tetany, tingling sensations, and dermatological findings (brittle skin, hair, and nails) in early childhood.

*Epidemiology*: incidence of 0.8/100,000 (hypoparathyroidism, acquired and inherited); incidence of isolated inherited hypoparathyroidism is unknown.
*Eye Findings*: cataracts and pseudotumor cerebri.
*Inheritance*: AD.
*Known Genes or Gene Locus*: PTH, GCM2.

## Marfan Syndrome[28,51–53]

*OMIM*: #154700.

*Description*: Marfan syndrome is a connective tissue disorder caused by dysfunction of the fibrillin 1 matrix protein. Affected individuals have characteristically long limbs and digits, hyperflexible joints, increased height, skeletal deformities (particularly of the vertebral column and the anterior chest), and ocular and cardiac abnormalities. Classically, affected individuals are at increased risk of aortic aneurysm and rupture.

*Epidemiology*: incidence of 2/10,000–3/10,000.
*Eye Findings*: ciliary muscle hypoplasia, ectopia lentis, flat corneas, glaucoma, increased axial globe length, iridodonesis, megalocornea, microspherophakia, myopia, and retinal detachment.
*Inheritance*: AD.
*Known Genes or Gene Locus*: FBN1.

## Marinesco-Sjögren Syndrome[54,55]

*OMIM*: #248800.

*Description*: Marinesco-Sjögren syndrome is a hereditary cerebellar ataxia. Characteristic syndrome manifestations include congenital cataracts, progressive myopathy (onset in childhood), skeletal deformities, microcephaly, and hypergonadotrophic hypogonadism.

*Epidemiology*: unknown; about 200 cases documented in literature.
*Eye Findings*: congenital cataracts, epicanthal folds, nystagmus, optic atrophy, and strabismus.
*Inheritance*: AR.
*Known Genes or Gene Locus*: SIL1.

## Marshall Syndrome[56–58]

*OMIM*: #154780.

*Description*: Marshall syndrome is a disorder caused by a splicing mutation in the *COL11A1* transcript. The disorder has been classified as a chondrodysplasia, and manifests through short stature, sensorineural hearing loss, cranial ossification, and distinctive facies (retracted midface, flat nasal bridge, short nose, long philtrum, and anteverted nostrils). There is unresolved discrepancy regarding whether Marshall syndrome is its own entity or a variant of the phenotypically similar Stickler syndrome (OMIM #604841).

*Epidemiology*: unknown.
*Eye Findings*: amblyopia, cataracts, ectopia lentis, glaucoma, hypertelorism, hypotrichosis of the eyelashes, myopia, nystagmus, proptosis, retinal detachment, strabismus, vitreoretinal degeneration, and vitreous humor abnormalities.
*Inheritance*: AD.
*Known Genes or Gene Locus*: COL11A1.

## Martsolf Syndrome[59,60]

*OMIM*: #212720.

*Description*: Martsolf syndrome is a disorder characterized by mild to moderate intellectual disability, hypogonadism, congenital cataracts, microcephaly, and short stature.

*Epidemiology*: unknown; less than 20 cases currently described in literature.

*Eye Findings*: cataracts, hypotelorism, microcornea, microphthalmia, optic nerve atrophy, persistent myotic pupil.

*Inheritance*: AR.

*Known Genes or Gene Locus*: RAB3GAP2.

## MELAS Syndrome[61-63]

OMIM: #540000.

*Description*: MELAS syndrome is a mitochondrial disorder characterized by myopathy, encephalopathy, lactic acidosis, and stroke-like episodes. Presentation usually occurs between ages 2 and 15 years and manifests as seizures, stroke-like episodes followed by hemiparesis, episodes of vomiting, and recurrent headaches.

*Epidemiology*: prevalence of 0.18/100,000.

*Eye Findings*: cataracts, choroidal microangiopathy, cortical blindness, hemianopsia, macular retinal pigment epithelial atrophy, myopathy, ophthalmoplegia, ptosis, and retinal detachment.

*Inheritance*: mitochondrial.

*Known Genes or Gene Locus*: MTTL1, MTTQ, MTTH, MTTK, MTTC, MTTS1, MTND1, MTND5, MTND6, MTTS2.

## Microspherophakia with Hernia[64]

OMIM: 157150.

*Description*: Microspherophakia with hernia is a disorder characterized by the presence of inguinal hernias alongside microspherophakia and, often, additional ocular abnormalities. It has been suggested that microspherophakia with hernia is a disorder of the connective tissue.

*Epidemiology*: unknown; only one affected pedigree documented in literature.

*Eye Findings*: ectopia lentis with dislocation superiorly, exophoria, glaucoma, iridodonesis, myopia, nystagmus, retinal detachment, and vitreous opacities.

*Inheritance*: AD.

*Known Genes or Gene Locus*: unknown.

## Molybdenum Cofactor Deficiency[65-67]

OMIM: #252150, #252160, #615501.

*Description*: Molybdenum cofactor deficiency is an inborn error of metabolism involving deficiency of functional xanthine dehydrogenase and sulfite oxidase (and subsequent depletion of serum uric acid and accumulation of sulfite) due to lack of cofactor. Disorder presents in the week after birth and manifests as intractable seizures, psychomotor retardation, poor feeding, and progressive encephalopathy leading to premature death.

*Epidemiology*: prevalence of 1/100,000−1/200,000.

*Eye Findings*: ectopia lentis, enophthalmos, hypertelorism, myopia, nystagmus, and spherophakia

*Inheritance*: AR.

*Known Genes or Gene Locus*: MOCS1, MOCS2, GPHN.

## Myotonic Dystrophy[68-70]

OMIM: #160900, #602668.

*Description*: Myotonic dystrophy is an adult-onset disorder characterized by myotonia, progressive muscle weakness accompanied by pain and stiffness, early cataract formation, arrhythmias, and endocrine abnormalities. The syndrome is caused by a trinucleotide repeat mutation such that severity is modulated by degree of repeat amplification.

*Epidemiology*: prevalence of 9.65/100,000 for myotonic dystrophy type 1; 0.99/100,000 for myotonic dystrophy type 2.

*Eye Findings*: iridescent cataract and ptosis.

*Inheritance*: AD.

*Known Genes or Gene Locus*: DMPK, ZNF9, CNBP.

## Pseudohypoparathyroidism Type 1A[71-74]

OMIM: #103580.

*Description*: Pseudohypoparathyroidism type 1A is a disorder of endocrine function resulting from loss-of-function mutations in the maternal gene coding for the alpha subunit of a G stimulatory protein associated with parathyroid hormone receptor. Patients present with Albright hereditary osteodystrophy (a collection of developmental and skeletal defects, including truncated fourth and fifth metacarpals) with multihormone resistance, intellectual disability, and early onset obesity.

*Epidemiology*: prevalence of 1.1/100,000 for all pseudohypoparathyroidism subtypes (1A, 1B, 1C, 2) combined.

*Eye Findings*: anisocoria, band keratopathy, cataracts, corneal opacities, macular degeneration, microphthalmia, nystagmus, papilledema, strabismus, and tortuosity of retinal vessels.

*Inheritance*: AD.

*Known Genes or Gene Locus*: GNAS.

## Pseudohypoparathyroidism Type 1C[71,72,74]

OMIM: #612462.

*Description*: Pseudohypoparathyroidism type 1C is clinically indistinguishable from type 1A and manifests as Albright hereditary osteodystrophy, multihormone resistance, intellectual disability, and early onset obesity. Type 1C is distinct from type 1A in that there are decreased cAMP levels without explicit dysfunction of the G stimulatory protein.

*Epidemiology*: prevalence of 1.1/100,000 for all pseudohypoparathyroidism subtypes (1A, 1B, 1C, 2) combined.

*Eye Findings*: anisocoria, cataracts, corneal opacities, macular degeneration, microphthalmia, nystagmus, papilledema, and tortuosity of retinal vessels.

*Inheritance*: AD.

*Known Genes or Gene Locus*: GNAS.

## Pseudopseudohypoparathyroidism[75]

*OMIM*: #612463.

*Description*: Pseudopseudohypoparathyroidism is a disorder that presents much like the pseudohypoparathyroid syndromes but has no associated parathyroid hormone resistance. Patients present with intellectual disability, obesity, and Albright hereditary osteodystrophy. The mutation responsible for pseudopseudohypoparathyroidism is carried on the paternal chromosome, in contrast to that responsible for the pseudohypoparathyroid syndromes.

*Epidemiology*: unknown.

*Eye Findings*: cataracts, nystagmus, and orbital ossification.

*Inheritance*: AD.

*Known Genes or Gene Locus*: GNAS.

## Rhizomelic Chondrodysplasia Punctata Type 1[76,77]

*OMIM*: #215100.

*Description*: Rhizomelic chondrodysplasia punctata type 1 (RCDP1) is a peroxisomal disorder involving increased serum phytanic acid concentrations and decreased serum plasmalogens. RCDP1 is characterized by a distinctive dwarfism (marked by disproportionate shortening of the proximal extremities), punctate calcification of the epiphysis, characteristic facies, delayed development, and severe intellectual disability. Affected individuals are at increased risk for respiratory infections and usually do not live past their first decade of life.

*Epidemiology*: prevalence of <1/100,000.

*Eye Findings*: cataracts, epicanthal folds, hypertelorism, and upslanted palpebral fissures.

*Inheritance*: AR.

*Known Genes or Gene Locus*: PEX7.

## Sengers Syndrome[78–80]

*OMIM*: #212350.

*Description*: Sengers syndrome is a disorder characterized by hypertrophic cardiomyopathy, lactic acidosis, skeletal myopathy, and cataract formation. Sengers presents as two distinct subtypes: a severe congenital form

characterized by death in infancy and a mild, slowly progressing form where death may be delayed up until the patient's 5th decade.

*Epidemiology*: unknown; less than 10 affected pedigrees documented in literature.

*Eye Findings*: congenital cataracts, glaucoma, myopia, nystagmus, and strabismus.

*Inheritance*: AR.

*Known Genes or Gene Locus*: AGK.

## Sulfocysteinuria (Sulfite Oxidase Deficiency)[28,81–83]

*OMIM*: #272300.

*Description*: Sulfocysteinuria is an inborn error of metabolism involving insufficient oxidation of sulfite to sulfate in the body. The infantile subtype presents soon after birth and is characterized by encephalopathy and seizure, followed by severe intellectual disability. The late onset subtype presents between 6 and 18 months and is characterized by developmental delay, dystonia, choreoathetosis, and ataxia.

*Epidemiology*: unknown.

*Eye Findings*: ectopia lentis and spherophakia

*Inheritance*: AR.

*Known Genes or Gene Locus*: SUOX.

## Weill-Marchesani Syndrome[8,28]

*OMIM*: #277600, #608328, #614819.

*Description*: Weill-Marchesani syndrome is a disorder of connective tissues associated with brachydactyly, stiffness of the joints, below average height, abnormalities of the lens, and occasional heart defects.

*Epidemiology*: prevalence of 1/100,000.

*Eye Findings*: cataracts, ectopia lentis, glaucoma, microspherophakia, myopia, and shallow anterior chamber.

*Inheritance*: AD, AR.

*Known Genes or Gene Locus*: ADAMTS10, FBN1, LTBP2.

## Werner Syndrome[84,85]

*OMIM*: #277700.

*Description*: Werner syndrome (WRN) is a progeroid syndrome characterized by rapid premature aging onset after puberty with premature death in the 4th or 5th decade of life. Characteristic features of disorder include bird-like facies and abnormal fat distribution (such that individuals have thin limbs and thick trunks), and individuals are prematurely prone to development of cancerous malignancies. Manifestations of Werner's are a result of diminished DNA repair, replication, and telomerase maintenance because of impaired WRN helicase.

*Epidemiology*: prevalence of 1/200,000 in the United States; 1/20,000–1/40,000 in Japan.

*Eye Findings*: bullous keratopathy (postoperatively) and cataracts.

*Inheritance*: AR.

*Known Genes or Gene Locus*: RECQL2.

## Verloes Van Maldergem Marneffe Syndrome (Microspherophakia-Metaphyseal Dysplasia)[86,87]

*OMIM*: 157151.

*Description*: Verloes Van Maldergem Marneffe syndrome manifests as skeletal dysplasia, ocular abnormalities, and sever dwarfism with characteristic features, including thickened diaphysis, enlarged femoral necks, and relatively normal small distal bones.

*Epidemiology*: unknown; one pedigree documented in literature.

*Eye Findings*: ectopia lentis, high myopia, lens coloboma, microspherophakia, and retinal detachment.

*Inheritance*: AD.

*Known Genes or Gene Locus*: unknown.

## REFERENCES

1. Pi LH, et al. Prevalence of eye diseases and causes of visual impairment in school-aged children in Western China. *J Epidemiol*. 2012;22:37–44.
2. Wu X, Long E, Lin H, Liu Y. Prevalence and epidemiological characteristics of congenital cataract: a systematic review and meta-analysis. *Sci Rep*. 2016;6:28564.
3. Messina-Baas O, Cuevas-Covarrubias SA. Inherited congenital cataract: a guide to suspect the genetic etiology in the cataract genesis. *Mol Syndromol*. 2017;8(2):58–78. https://doi.org/10.1159/000455752.
4. Shiels A, Hejtmancik J. Genetics of human cataract. *Clin Genetics*. 2013;84(2):120–127. https://doi.org/10.1111/cge.12182.
5. Hejtmancik JF. Congenital cataracts and their molecular genetics. *Semin Cell Dev Biol*. 2008;19(2):134–149. https://doi.org/10.1016/j.semcdb.2007.10.003.
6. Huang B, He W. Molecular characteristics of inherited congenital cataracts. *Eur J Med Genet*. 2010;53(6):347–357. https://doi.org/10.1016/j.ejmg.2010.07.001. Epub 2010 Sep. 17.
7. Shiels A, Fielding Hejtmancik J. Mutations and mechanisms in congenital and age-related cataracts. *Exp Eye Res*. 2017;156:95–102. Published online 2016 Jun 19. https://doi.org/10.1016/j.exer.2016.06.011.
8. Faivre L, et al. In frame fibrillin-1 gene deletion in autosomal dominant Weill-Marchesani syndrome. *J Med Genet*. 2003;40(1):34–36.
9. Hafidi Z, et al. Atypical presentation of ectopia lentis in homocystinuria. *J Pediatr*. 2015;166(4):1091.
10. Khan AO, et al. Recessive mutations in LEPREL1 underlie a recognizable lens subluxation phenotype. *Ophthalmic Genet*. 2015;36(1):58–63.
11. Couser NL, McClure J, Evans MW, Haines NR, Burden SK, Muenzer J. Homocysteinemia due to MTHFR deficiency in a young adult presenting with bilateral lens subluxations. *Ophthalmic Genet*. 2017;38(1):91–94.
12. Sabin Sahu, Reena Yadav, Sharad Gupta, and Lila Raj Puri Bilateral ectopia lentis with isolated lens coloboma in Marfan syndrome. *GMS Ophthalmol Cases*. 2016;6: Doc14. Published online 2016 Dec 5. https://doi.org/10.3205/oc000051. PMCID: PMC5144584 PMID: 28028488.
13. Aggarwal A, El-Bash AR, Inker S, Musarella MA. Symmetrical bilateral lens colobomas in two brothers. *J Pediatr Ophthalmol Strabismus*. 2004;41(5):302–304.
14. Haas M. Alport syndrome and thin glomerular basement membrane nephropathy: a practical approach to diagnosis. *Arch Pathol Lab Med*. 2009;133(2):224–232.
15. Levy M, et al. Estimating prevalence in single-gene kidney diseases progressing to renal failure. *Kidney Int*. 2000;58(3):925–943.
16. Salmon JF, et al. Variable expressivity of autosomal dominant microcornea with cataract. *Arch Ophthalmol*. 1988;106:505–510.
17. Stefaniak E, et al. An unusual pedigree with microcornea-cataract syndrome. *J Med Genet*. 1995;32:813–815.
18. Wang KJ, et al. A novel mutation in CRYBB1 associated with congenital cataract-microcornea syndrome: the p.Ser129Arg mutation destabilizes the βB1/βA3-crystallin heteromer but not the βB1-crystallin homomer. *Hum Mutat*. 2011;32(3):2050–2060.
19. Appadurai V, et al. Apparent underdiagnosis of cerebrotendinous xanthomatosis revealed by analysis of ~60,000 human exomes. *Mol Genet Metab*. 2015;116(4):298–304.
20. Salen G, et al. Epidemiology, diagnosis, and treatment of cerebrotendinous xanthomatosis (CTX). *J Inherit Metabolic Dis*. 2017;40(6):771–781.
21. Tibrewal S, et al. Cerebrotendinous xanthomatosis: early diagnosis on the basis of juvenile cataracts. *J Am Assoc Pediatr Ophthalmol Strabismus*. 2017;21(6):505–507.
22. Bruno C, et al. Clinical and genetic characterization of chanarin-dorfman syndrome. *Biochem Biophys Res Commun*. 2008;369(4):1125–1128.
23. Demir B, et al. Chanarin-Dorfman syndrome. *Clin Exp Dermatol*. 2017;42(6):699–701.
24. Redaelli C, et al. Clinical and genetic characterization of Chanarin-Dorfman syndrome patients: first report of large deletions in the ABHD5 gene. *Orphanet J Rare Dis*. 2010;5(33).
25. Anjum I, et al. A mutation in the FOXE3 gene causes congenital primary aphakia in an autosomal recessive consanguineous Pakistani family. *Mol Vis*. 2010;16:549–555.
26. Valleix S, et al. Homozygous nonsense mutation in the FOXE3 gene as a cause of congenital primary aphakia in humans. *Am J Hum Genet*. 2006;79(2):358–364.

27. Fuchs J, et al. Congenital ectopia lentis: a Danish national survey. *Acta Ophthalmol Scand.* 1998;76:20−26.
28. Sadiq M, et al. Genetics of ectopia lentis. *Semin Ophthalomol.* 2013;28(5−6):313−320.
29. Chandra A, et al. A genotype-phenotype comparison of ADAMTSL4 and FBN1 in isolated ectopia lentis. *Investig Ophthalmol Vis Sci.* 2012;53:4889−4896.
30. Neuhann T, et al. ADAMTSL4-associated isolated ectopia lentis: further patients, novel mutations and a detailed phenotype description. *Am J Med Genet.* 2015;167(10): 2376−2381.
31. Brady A, et al. The Ehlers-Danlos syndromes, rare types. *Am J Med Genet.* 2017;175(1):70−115.
32. Joseph A, et al. Characteristics, diagnosis, and management of Ehlers-Danlos syndromes: a review. *JAMA Facial Plast Surg.* 2018;20(1):70−75.
33. Loeys BL. *Aneurysms − Osteoarthritis Syndrome: SMAD3 Gene Mutations.* San Diego, CA: Elsevier Inc.; 2017:63−72.
34. Cole P, et al. Fine-Lubinsky syndrome: managing the rare syndromic synostosis. *J Plastic Reconstr Aesthetic Surg.* 2010;63(1):e70−e72.
35. Letter to the editor: reply to Ayme and Philip. *Am J Med Genet.* 1997;70:334−335.
36. Niceta M, et al. Mutations impairing GSK3-mediated MAF phosphorylation cause cataract, deafness, intellectual disability, seizures, and a down syndrome-like facies. *Am J Hum Genet.* 2015;96(5):816−825.
37. Bzduch V, et al. Cataract and early nystagmus due to galactokinase deficiency. *J Inherit Metabolic Dis.* 2017;40(5): 749−750.
38. Hennermann J, et al. Features and outcome of galactokinase deficiency in children diagnosed by newborn screening. *J Inherit Metabolic Dis.* 2011;34(2):399−407.
39. Rosenberg RN. *Rosenberg's Molecular and Genetic Basis of Neurological and Psychiatric Disease.* 5th ed. San Diego, CA: Elsevier Inc.; 2015:615−626.
40. Murphy M, et al. Genetic basis of transferase-deficient galactosaemia in Ireland and the population history of the Irish travellers. *Eur J Hum Genet.* 1999;7:549−554.
41. Kortum F. Hallermann-Streiff syndrome: no evidence for a link to laminopathies. *Mol Syndromol.* 2011;2(1):27−34.
42. Maka E. Two cases of Hallermann − Streiff syndrome with retinal abnormalities. *J Clin Exp Ophthalmol.* 2015;6(2).
43. Moorthie S, et al. Systematic review and meta-analysis to estimate the birth prevalence of five inherited metabolic diseases. *J Inherit Metabolic Dis.* 2014;37(6):889−898.
44. Mulvihill A, et al. Ocular findings among patients with late-diagnosed or poorly controlled homocystinuria compared with a screened, well-controlled population. *J Am Assoc Pediatr Ophthalmol Strabismus.* 2001;5(5): 311−315.
45. Craig J, et al. Hereditary hyperferritinemia-cataract syndrome: prevalence, lens morphology, spectrum of mutations, and clinical presentations. *Arch Ophthalmol.* 2003; 121(12):1753−1761.
46. Girelli D, et al. Molecular basis for the recently described hereditary hyperferritinemia- cataract syndrome: a mutation in the iron-responsive element of ferritin L-subunit gene. *Blood.* 1995;86:4050−4053.
47. Biancheri R, et al. Hypomyelination and congenital cataract: broadening the clinical phenotype. *Arch Neurol.* 2011;68(9):1191−1194.
48. Numata Y, et al. Epidemiological, clinical, and genetic landscapes of hypomyelinating leukodystrophies. *J Neurol.* 2014;261(4):752−758.
49. Clarke B, et al. Epidemiology and diagnosis of hypoparathyroidism. *Endocrinol Metab.* 2016;101(6): 2284−2299.
50. Mohammadpour M, et al. Advanced cataracts and pseudotumor cerebri as the first presentations of hypoparathyroidism. *Iran J Ophthalmol.* 2013;25(3): 244−248.
51. Judge D, et al. Marfan's syndrome. *Lancet.* 2005;366: 1965−1976.
52. Latasiewicz M, et al. Marfan syndrome: ocular findings and novel mutations − in pursuit of genotype-phenotype associations. *Can Ophthalmol Soc.* 2016;51(2):113−118.
53. Maumenee I. The eye in the Marfan syndrome. *Trans Am Ophthalmol Soc.* 1981;79:684−733.
54. Fogel B, et al. Clinical features and molecular genetics of autosomal recessive cerebellar ataxias. *Lancet Neurol.* 2007;6(3):245−257.
55. Nair P, et al. Marinesco-sjögren syndrome in an Emirati child with a novel mutation in SIL1 affecting the 5′ untranslated region. *Med Princ Pract.* 2016;25(6):580−582.
56. Annunen S, et al. Splicing mutations of 54-bp exons in the COL11A1 gene cause Marshall syndrome, but other mutations cause overlapping Marshall/Stickler phenotypes. *Am J Hum Genet.* 1999;65(4):974−983.
57. Baraitser M. Marshall/Stickler syndrome. *J Med Genet.* 1982;19:139−140.
58. Griffith A, et al. Marshall syndrome associated with a splicing defect at the COL11A1 locus. *Am J Hum Genet.* 1998;62(4):816−823.
59. Aligianis I, et al. Mutation in Rab3 GTPase-activating protein (RAB3GAP) noncatalytic subunit in a kindred with Martsolf syndrome. *Am J Hum Genet.* 2006;78(4): 702−707.
60. Handley M, et al. Mutation spectrum in RAB3GAP1, RAB3-GAP2, and RAB18 and genotype−phenotype correlations in Warburg micro syndrome and Martsolf syndrome. *Hum Mutat.* 2013;34(5):686−696.
61. Sultan H, et al. Retinal detachment and microangiopathy in mitochondrial encephalomyopathy, lactic acidosis, and stroke-like episodes syndrome. *Can J Ophthalmol.* 2017;52(6):e208−e211.
62. Yatsuga S, et al. MELAS: a nationwide prospective cohort study of 96 patients in Japan. *Biochim Biophys Acta (BBA).* 2012;1820(5):619−624.

63. Zhu C, et al. Ophthalmological findings in 74 patients with mitochondrial disease. *Ophthalmic Genet.* 2017; 38(1):67−69.
64. Johnson V, et al. Dominant microspherophakia. *Arch Ophthalmol.* 1971;85:534−542.
65. Nagappa M, et al. Child neurology: molybdenum cofactor deficiency. *Neurology.* 2015;85(23):e175−e178.
66. Reiss J, et al. Molybdenum cofactor deficiency: mutations in GPHN, MOCS1, and MOCS2. *Hum Mutat.* 2011; 32(1):10−18.
67. Zaki M, et al. Molybdenum cofactor and isolated sulphite oxidase deficiencies: clinical and molecular spectrum among Egyptian patients. *Eur J Paediatr Neurol.* 2016; 20(5):714−722.
68. Kamsteeg E, et al. Best practice guidelines and recommendations on the molecular diagnosis of myotonic dystrophy types 1 and 2. *Eur J Hum Genet.* 2012;20:1203−1208.
69. Ranum L, et al. Myotonic dystrophy: RNA pathogenesis comes into focus. *Am J Hum Genet.* 2004;74(5):793−804.
70. Theadom A, et al. Knowledge of sub-types important to understanding the prevalence of myotonic dystrophy. *Neuroepidemiology.* 2016;46:228.
71. Grajewski R, et al. Cataract in pseudohypoparathyroidism. *J Cataract Refract Surg.* 2016;42(7):1094−1096.
72. Levine M. An update on the clinical and molecular characteristics of pseudohypoparathyroidism. *Curr Opin Endocrinol Diabetes Obes.* 2012;19(6):443−451.
73. Liu J, et al. The stimulatory G protein α-subunit $G_s\alpha$ is imprinted in human thyroid glands: implications for thyroid function in pseudohypoparathyroidism types 1A and 1B. *J Clin Endocrinol Metab.* 2003;88(9):4336−4341.
74. Underbjerg L, et al. Pseudohypoparathyroidism − epidemiology, mortality and risk of complications. *Clin Endocrinol.* 2016;84(6):904−911.
75. Klauber S. Primary palpebral and orbital ossification in pseudopseudohypoparathyroidism. *Acta Ophthalmol.* 2002;80(5):543−545.
76. Maines E, et al. Newborn with rhizomelia and difficulty breathing. *Skelet Radiol.* 2017;46:291−292.
77. Sahin N, et al. Type 1 rhizomelic chondrodysplasia punctata with a homozygous PEX7 mutation. *J Pediatr Endocrinol Metab.* 2017;30(8).
78. Haghighi A, et al. Sengers syndrome: six novel AGK mutations in seven new families and review of the phenotypic and mutational spectrum of 29 patients. *Orphanet J Rare Dis.* 2014;9(1):1.
79. Mayr J, et al. Lack of the mitochondrial protein acylglycerol kinase causes Sengers syndrome. *Am J Hum Genet.* 2012; 90(2):314−320.
80. Siriwardena K, et al. Mitochondrial citrate synthase crystals: novel finding in Sengers syndrome caused by acylglycerol kinase (AGK) mutations. *Mol Genet Metab.* 2013; 108(1):40−50.
81. Claerhout H, et al. Isolated sulfite oxidase deficiency. *J Inherit Metabolic Dis.* 2018;41(1):101−108.
82. Johnson J, et al. Isolated sulfite oxidase deficiency: identification of 12 novel SUOX mutations in 10 patients. *Hum Mutat.* 2002;20(1):74.
83. Rocha S, et al. Sulfite oxidase deficiency − an unusual late and mild presentation. *Brain Dev.* 2014;36(2):176−179.
84. Dollfus H, et al. Ocular manifestations in the inherited DNA repair disorders. *Surv Ophthalmol.* 2003;48(1):107−122.
85. Muftuoglu M, et al. The clinical characteristics of Werner syndrome: molecular and biochemical diagnosis. *Hum Genet.* 2008;124(4):369−377.
86. Czarny-Ratajczak M, et al. Severe neonatal spondylometaphyseal dysplasia in two siblings. *Am J Med Genet.* 2009; 149A(10):2166−2172.
87. Verloes A, et al. Microspherophakia-metaphyseal dysplasia: a 'new' dominantly inherited bone dysplasia with severe eye involvement. *J Med Genet.* 1990;27:467−471.

# CHAPTER 7

# Genetic Abnormalities With Glaucoma

O'RESE J. KNIGHT • MONA KALEEM • RAKHI MELVANI • JANA BREGMAN •
THOMAS HUNTER • NATARIO L. COUSER

Glaucoma is an optic neuropathy characterized by progressive visual field loss secondary to elevated intraocular pressure, which results in the death of ganglion cell axons. Glaucoma is defined as primary when it occurs in the absence of an identifiable etiology and as secondary when it results from underlying disease processes or systemic factors. Glaucoma can be further classified based on whether the anterior chamber angle is open or closed.[1] The pathogenesis of glaucoma is multifactorial with genetics playing a central role in several subtypes.

Glaucoma is the leading cause of irreversible blindness and the second leading cause of all types of blindness worldwide after cataracts.[2] Associated clinical exam findings include elevated intraocular pressure (IOP), increased cup-to-disc ratio, retinal nerve fiber layer (RNFL) loss, and visual field deficits in the form of arcuate defects, nasal steps, paracentral scotomas, or generalized depression.[1] Additional pathologic changes may vary based on the specific category of glaucoma. Several genes have been linked to the development of congenital, infantile-, juvenile-, and adult-onset primary open-angle glaucoma (POAG) (Table 7.1). Additionally, there are genetic syndromes, which include glaucoma as a key ophthalmic manifestation.

The most common form of glaucoma is POAG, which affects over 60 million individuals worldwide.[1] Our knowledge of POAG chromosomal loci and candidate genes continues to evolve [3–33] (Table 7.2). POAG is an adult-onset disease that is diagnosed based on the presence of optic nerve damage due to elevated IOP. Other characteristics include the presence of an open and normal appearing anterior chamber angle and the absence of a known underlying cause.[1] Visual field deficits may be detected at the time of diagnosis or with disease progression. Normal-tension glaucoma (NTG) closely resembles POAG clinically, but develops in the presence of normal IOP. Juvenile-onset open-angle glaucoma (JOAG) is the younger corollary to POAG and is diagnosed between the ages of 3 and 35 years.[34] While the pathophysiology of POAG, NTG, and JOAG are not fully understood, unique contributory genetic associations have been identified for each of the three glaucoma subtypes.

Primary congenital glaucoma (PCG), also known as infantile glaucoma, develops within the first year of life. Some sources distinguish PCG from infantile glaucoma, which is diagnosed between 1 and 3 years. While PCG shares a similar mechanism of optic nerve damage, the underlying pathogenesis differs from POAG, NTG, and JOAG in that it is more directly related to structural abnormalities within the anterior chamber angle. Physical findings characteristic of PCG may include buphthalmos, increased corneal diameter, corneal edema, Haab striae, and myopia.[35]

Pigment dispersion syndrome (PDS) and pseudoexfoliation syndrome (PXF) are examples of primary entities that have the potential to cause secondary glaucoma. PDS causes deposition of pigment granules from the iris epithelium onto various ocular surfaces including the anterior chamber angle. Over time, this can obstruct aqueous humor outflow, resulting in secondary glaucoma known as pigment dispersion glaucoma (PDG).[36] In PXF, fibrillary material is deposited systemically with primary ocular disease characterized by accumulation on anterior segment structures. In a mechanism similar to what is observed in PDG, deposition within the anterior chamber angle results in increased resistance to aqueous outflow, elevated IOP, and secondary glaucoma.[37] Key unique genes have been implicated in the underlying pathogenesis of both PDS and PXF.[36–39]

Genetic syndromes that are known to cause glaucoma as a main ophthalmic manifestation include

**TABLE 7.1**

Comparison of Infantile Glaucoma (PCG), Juvenile Open-Angle Glaucoma (JOAG), and Primary Open-Angle Glaucoma (POAG)

| Condition | Age of Onset (years) | Phenotype | Known or Candidate Genes |
|---|---|---|---|
| PCG | 0–3 | Epiphora, blepharospasm, buphthalmos, photophobia, corneal edema, Haab striae, elevated IOP, myopia and/or astigmatism, ONH cupping, enlarged corneal diameter | CYP1B1, MYOC |
| JOAG | 3–35 | Elevated IOP with large fluctuations, myopia, ONH cupping | MYOC, CYP1B1, TIGR |
| POAG | >35 | Elevated IOP, ONH cupping | OPTN, ASB10, WDR36, IL20RB, EFEMP1 |

IOP, intraocular pressure; ONH, optic nerve head.

Armfield X-linked mental retardation syndrome, Lowe oculocerebrorenal syndrome, muscle-eye-brain disease, nail-patella syndrome, Nance-Horan syndrome, and Rubinstein-Taybi syndrome. Genetic mutations involved in the pathogenesis of these disorders tend to affect proteins that are present in several organ systems, thus resulting in multisystem congenital anomalies. Several genetic disorders are associated with the development of both glaucoma and congenital cataracts (Table 7.3). In addition to glaucoma, several of the genetic disorders listed result in additional ocular abnormalities, thus reflecting a degree of anterior segment dysgenesis.

## GENETIC DISORDERS

### Armfield X-Linked Mental Retardation Syndrome[40]

*OMIM*: %300261.

*Description*: Armfield X-linked mental retardation syndrome is characterized by short stature, cleft palate, small hands and feet, seizures, glaucoma, and intellectual disability.

*Epidemiology*: unknown.

*Eye Findings*: cataracts, glaucoma, and strabismus.

*Inheritance*: XLR.

*Known Genes or Gene Locus*: Xq28.

### Hereditary Microcornea, Glaucoma, and Absent Frontal Sinuses[41]

*OMIM*: 156700.

*Description*: Hereditary microcornea, glaucoma, and absent frontal sinuses is a syndrome characterized by thickened skin of the palms and flexor surfaces of the fingers resulting in decreased sensitivity to heat, flat round facies, torus palatinus, and absent frontal sinuses.

*Epidemiology*: unknown.

*Eye Findings*: microcornea, open-angle glaucoma without iridocorneal angle abnormalities, and epicanthal folds.

*Inheritance*: AD.

*Known Genes or Gene Loci*: unknown.

### Juvenile Open-Angle Glaucoma[1,34,42,43]

*OMIM*: #137750, %608695.

*Description*: JOAG presents anytime from childhood to early adulthood, between the ages of 3 and 35 years. JOAG characteristically lacks ocular enlargement, as well as any anterior segment structural abnormality. JOAG differs from POAG in its age of onset and magnitude of elevated IOP, which tends to be more severe and with more dramatic IOP fluctuations.

*Epidemiology*: incidence of 1/50,000.

*Eye Findings*: elevated IOP, myopia, and ONH cupping.

*Inheritance*: AD.

*Known Genes or Gene Locus*: MYOC (accounts for 10%–36% of JOAG), CYP1B1. Locus name: GLC1A, GLC1J-K, GLC1M-N.

### Lowe Oculocerebrorenal Syndrome[44–46]

*OMIM*: #309000.

*Description*: Lowe oculocerebrorenal syndrome is characterized by a proximal renal tubulopathy (low-molecular-weight proteinuria, hypercalciuria, renal tubular acidosis, reduced renal ammonia production), vitamin D–resistant rickets, congenital cataracts, hydrophthalmia, intellectual disability, and growth failure. Physical findings may include facial dysmorphisms

### TABLE 7.2
### Known Glaucoma Chromosomal Loci

| Locus | Identifier | OMIM | Gene |
|---|---|---|---|
| 1p36.2-p36.1 | GLC3B | % 600975 | — |
| 1q24.3 | GLC1A | #137750 | TIGR/MYOC |
| 2p16-p15 | GLC1H | % 611276 | EFEMP1 (candidate) |
| 2cen-q13 | GLC1B | % 606689 | — |
| 2p22.2 | GLC3A | #231300 | CYP1B1 |
| 3p22-p21 | GLC1L | — | — |
| 3q21-q24 | GLC1C | % 601682 | IL20RB (candidate) |
| 4q35.1-q35.2 | GLC1Q | — | — |
| 5q22.1 | GLC1G | #609887 | WDR36 |
| 5q22.1-q32 | GLC1M | % 610535 | — |
| 7q36.1 | GLC1F | #603383 | ASB10 |
| 8q23 | GLC1D | % 602429 | — |
| 9p21.2 | GLC3E | #617272 | TEK |
| 9q22 | GLC1J | % 608695 | — |
| 10p13 | GLC1E | #137760 | OPTN |
| 12q14 | GLC1P | #177700 | TBK1 (candidate) |
| 14q24.3 | GLC3C | % 613085 | — |
| 14q24.3 | GLC3D | #613086 | LTBP2 |
| 15q11-q13 | GLC1I | % 609745 | — |
| 15q22-q24 | GLC1N | % 611274 | — |
| 19q13.33 | GLC1O | #613100 | NTF4 |
| 20p12 | GLC1K | % 608696 | — |

#, molecular basis is currently known for OMIM entry; %, molecular basis is not currently known for OMIM entry.

### TABLE 7.3
### Genetic Syndromes Associated With Glaucoma and Cataracts

| |
|---|
| Armfield X-Linked Mental Retardation syndrome |
| Fine-Lubinsky syndrome |
| Lowe oculocerebrorenal syndrome |
| Marshall syndrome |
| Muscle-eye-brain disease |
| Nail-patella syndrome |
| Nance-Horan syndrome |
| Rubinstein-Taybi syndrome |
| Sengers syndrome |
| Walker-Warburg syndrome |
| Weill-Marchesani syndrome |

system, and kidney involvement are all required for diagnosis.

*Epidemiology*: prevalence of 1/500,000.

*Eye Findings*: glaucoma, congenital cataract, miosis, corneal and conjunctival keloids, microphthalmia, and nystagmus.

*Inheritance*: XLR.

*Known Genes or Gene Locus*: OCRL1.

### Nail-Patella Syndrome (Hereditary Osteo-Onychodysplasia Syndrome)[47]

*OMIM*: #161200.

*Description*: Nail-patella syndrome is characterized by limb and pelvic skeletal abnormalities, distal digital abnormalities, and renal abnormalities. Skeletal and digit abnormalities include absent patellas, dypslastic elbows and iliac horns, hypoplastic and dystrophic nails, hyperextensability of proximal and distal interphalangeal joints, and swan neck deformities. Additionally, sensorineural hearing loss, glaucoma, and gastrointestinal and vasomotor dysfunction may be present. Clinical diagnosis can be made with the following findings: (1) absent or dystrophic nails with triangular lunulae, (2) absent or hypoplastic patellae, (3) elbow abnormalities, and (4) iliac horns.

*Epidemiology*: incidence of 1/50,000.

*Eye Findings*: Lester sign (zone of darker pigmentation of the peripupillary iris), POAG, ocular hypertension, cataract, microcornea, microphakia, keratoconus, ptosis, and strabismus.

*Inheritance*: AD.

*Known Genes or Gene Locus*: LMX1B.

(frontal bossing, deep-set eyes, chubby cheeks, fair complexion), hyporeflexia, hypotonia, and developmental delay. Diagnosis can be established by measurement of decreased activity of phosphatidylinositol 4,5-bisphosphate 5 phosphatase, which is due to a mutation in the *OCRL1* gene. Ocular, central nervous

### Nance-Horan Syndrome (Cataract-Dental Syndrome)[48,49]

*OMIM*: #302350.

*Description*: Nance-Horan syndrome is characterized by congenital cataracts (nuclear sclerotic most common), dysmorphic features, dental anomalies (supernumerary teeth, dental agenesis, diastema), global developmental delay, and intellectual disability. Cataracts are typically dense.

*Epidemiology*: unknown.

*Eye Findings*: congenital cataracts, glaucoma, microphthalmia, microcornea, nystagmus, ptosis, and strabismus.

*Inheritance*: XLD.

*Known Genes or Gene Locus*: NHS.

### Normal-Tension Glaucoma[1]

*OMIM*: #606657.

*Description*: NTG is a subtype of POAG occurring in the presence of normal IOP. NTG accounts for approximately one-third of all POAG cases. Physical findings include structurally normal, open anterior chamber angles, ONH cupping, and thin RNFL due to ganglion cell axon loss. The visual field defects are typically paracentral on presentation, and the optic nerve cupping tends to either be shallow with mild pallor or presents with deep focal notching. Established NTG risk factors include the following: vasospastic systemic conditions such as Raynaud phenomenon and migraine, ischemic vascular disease, and increased diastolic blood pressure.

*Epidemiology*: estimated 30%–40% of POAG cases.

*Eye Findings*: glaucoma with normal IOP.

*Inheritance*: unknown.

*Known Genes or Gene Locus*: OPA1, OPTN, TBK1. Locus name: GLC1E, GLC1P.

### Pigment Dispersion Syndrome[36,38]

*OMIM*: %600510.

*Description*: PDS is an open-angle glaucoma secondary to deposition of pigment granules from the iris epithelium onto various ocular surfaces, including anterior chamber structures. Accumulation of pigment in the trabecular meshwork provides resistance to aqueous outflow leading to elevated IOP. Over time this can result in optic nerve damage characteristic of glaucoma. Affected individuals are classically young myopes. PDS is diagnosed clinically based on the following three criteria: the presence of iris transillumination defects, pigment on the corneal endothelium, and pigment in the trabecular meshwork.

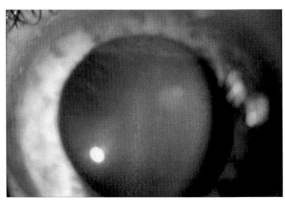

FIG. 7.1 Pigment granule deposition on the corneal endothelium (Krukenberg spindle). (Courtesy Stamper RL, Lieberman MF, Drake MV. Secondary Open Angle Glaucoma, Becker-Shaffer's Diagnosis and Therapy of the Glaucomas. January 1, 2009:266e293. © 2009; From Alward WLM. Color Atlas of Gonioscopy. St Louis: Mosby; 1994.)

*Epidemiology*: incidence of 4.8/100,000 annually of PDS and 1.4/100,000 annually of pigmentary glaucoma in Olmstead County, Minnesota. It is suspected that the true incidences of PDS and PG are higher, as many cases go undiagnosed.

*Eye Findings*: glaucoma, myopia, pigment granules on corneal endothelium (Krukenberg spindle) (Fig. 7.1), iris transillumination defects, midperipheral iris concavity, dense trabecular meshwork pigmentation, pigment deposition anterior/posterior lens surfaces, and zonules (Zentmayer line).

*Inheritance*: AD.

*Known Genes or Gene Locus*: 7q35-q36.

### Primary Congenital Glaucoma[35,50]

*OMIM*: #231300, %600975.

*Description*: Congenital glaucoma is characterized by early onset during the first year of life. Presenting symptoms may include epiphora, blepharospasm, and photophobia. Signs include buphthalmos, increased IOP, increased corneal diameter, corneal edema, Haab striae, myopia and/or astigmatism (most commonly against the rule), and cupping of the ONH.

*Epidemiology*: incidence of 1/10,000.

*Eye Findings*: buphthalmos, elevated IOP, corneal haze, myopia and/or astigmatism, hypoplastic anterior chamber angle structures, Haab striae, corneal enlargement, and ONH cupping.

*Inheritance*: sporadic, AR.

*Known Genes or Gene Locus*: CYP1B1, MYOC, LTBP2, TEK. Locus name: GLC3A-E.

## Primary Open-Angle Glaucoma[2,51]

*OMIM*: #137760, %601682, %602429, #603383, #609887, %611276, #177700.

*Description*: Adult-onset open-angle glaucoma (POAG) is an optic neuropathy characterized by open, structurally normal angles, and progressive visual field loss due to elevated IOP. Symptoms include gradual visual field deficits (typically in the form of arcuate defect, nasal step paracentral scotoma, or generalized depression) beginning peripherally and progressing to central field loss. Physical findings include ONH cupping and RNFL thinning due to ganglion cell axon loss. A diagnosis of POAG can be made if the following criteria are met: (1) evidence of ONH damage from optic disc/RNFL abnormalities and/or reliable and reproducible visual field abnormalities without other causes or explanations for a visual field deficit, (2) adult onset, (3) open and normal appearing anterior chamber angles, and (4) the absence of known secondary causes of open angle glaucoma.

*Epidemiology*: incidence varies based on ethnicity with increased prevalence among African Americans compared to Caucasians. There are estimated to be 60 million suspected cases of POAG worldwide.

*Eye Findings*: elevated IOP, open iridocorneal angles, progressive optic nerve cupping and RNFL thinning (Fig. 7.2), and thin corneas. Loss of visual acuity, optic disc pallor, and afferent pupillary defects are late findings.

*Inheritance*: sporadic, AD.

*Known Genes or Gene Locus: OPTN, ASB10, WDR36 OPTN, ASB10, WDR36, TBK1, NTF4, IL20RB, EFEMP1. Loci associations: ABCA1, AFAP1, ARHGEF12, ATXN2, CAV1/CAV2, CDKN2BAS, FNDC3B, FOXC1, GAS7, GMDS, PMM2, SIX6, TGFBR3, TMCO1, TXNRD2. Locus name: GLC1A-I, GLC1L, and GLC1O-P.*

## Pseudoexfoliation Syndrome[37,39]

*OMIM*: #177650.

*Description*: Pseudoexfoliation syndrome is an age-related condition associated with a fibrillary deposition on the corneal endothelium, iris, trabecular meshwork, zonules, and anterior lens capsule. The pseudoexfoliative material can also be present in other organs, such as the heart, lungs, and kidneys. An association with cardiovascular disease has been suggested. The presence of progressive optic nerve, RNFL, and glaucomatous visual field changes distinguishes pseudoexfoliation glaucoma from pseudoexfoliation syndrome. Pseudoexfoliation glaucoma is the most common form of secondary open-angle glaucoma worldwide.

*Epidemiology*: incidence of 25.9/100,000 annually reported from a defined population (Olmsted County, Minnesota); high prevalence in Scandinavian countries, Ethiopia, South Africa, and among Navajo Indians.

*Eye Findings*: monocular or asymmetric glaucoma, fibrillary deposits on anterior segment structures (conjunctiva, lens, iris, zonules, ciliary processes) (Fig. 7.3), peripapillary iris transillumination defects, increased pigmentation of the trabecular meshwork, pigment anterior to Schwalbe's line (Sampaolesi's line), poor pupillary dilation, and weak zonules.

*Inheritance*: AD.

*Known Genes or Gene Locus: LOXL1.*

## Rubinstein-Taybi Syndrome (Broad Thumb-Hallux Syndrome)[52,53]

*OMIM*: #180849, #613684, #610543.

*Description*: Rubinstein-Taybi syndrome is characterized by growth restriction, facial dysmorphisms, broad thumbs and toes, microcephaly, and intellectual disability. Additional findings may include congenital heart disease, dental anomalies, hirsutism, cataracts,

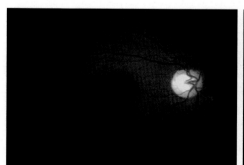
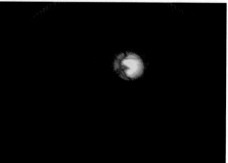

FIG. 7.2 POAG. Bilateral optic nerve cupping; right eye (left), left eye (right).

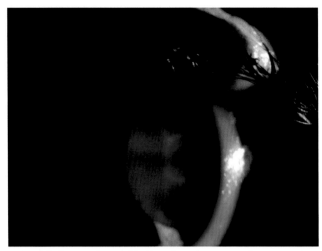

FIG. 7.3 Pseudoexfoliation syndrome. Fibrillary deposits on anterior segment structures (lens).

glaucoma, strabismus, increased risk of tumor formation, recurrent respiratory and ear infection, and premature thelarche in females.

*Epidemiology*: prevalence of 1/100,000–1/125,000.

*Eye Findings*: glaucoma, cataracts, strabismus, iris coloboma, epicanthal folds, ptosis, downward slanting palpebral fissures, heavy and arched eyebrows, long eyelashes, corneal keloids, and nasolacrimal duct obstruction.

*Inheritance*: AD.

*Known Genes or Gene Locus*: CREBBP, EP300.

## REFERENCES

1. Prum BE, Rosenberg LF, Gedde SJ, et al. Primary open-angle glaucoma preferred practice pattern® guidelines. *Ophthalmology*. 2016;123(1):P41–P111.
2. Bonomi L, Marchini G, Marraffa M, et al. Prevalence of glaucoma and intraocular pressure distribution in a defined population: the Egna-Neumarkt study. *Ophthalmology*. 1998;105(2):209–215.
3. Sheffield VC, Stone EM, Alward WL, et al. Genetic linkage of familial open angle glaucoma to chromosome 1q21-q31. *Nat Genet*. 1993;4:47–50.
4. Stone EM, Fingert JH, Alward WL, et al. Identification of a gene that causes primary open angle glaucoma. *Science*. 1997;275:668–670.
5. Akiyama M, Yatsu K, Ota M, et al. Microsatellite analysis of the GLC1B locus on chromosome 2 points to NCK2 as a new candidate gene for normal tension glaucoma. *Br J Ophthalmol*. 2008;92:1293–1296.
6. Charlesworth JC, Stankovich JM, Mackey DA, et al. Confirmation of the adult-onset primary open angle glaucoma locus GLC1B at 2cen-q13 in an Australian family. *Ophthalmologica*. 2006;220:23–30.
7. Stoilova D, Child A, Trifan OC, Crick RP, Coakes RL, Sarfarazi M. Localization of a locus (GLC1B) for adult-onset primary open angle glaucoma to the 2cen-q13 region. *Genomics*. 1996;36:142–150.
8. Keller KE, Yang YF, Sun YY, et al. Interleukin-20 receptor expression in the trabecular meshwork and its implication in glaucoma. *J Ocular Pharmacol Ther*. 2014; 30:267–276.
9. Kitsos G, Eiberg H, Economou-Petersen E, et al. Genetic linkage of autosomal ominant primary open angle glaucoma to chromosome 3q in a Greek pedigree. *Eur J Hum Genet*. 2001;9:452–457.
10. Samples JR, Kitsos G, Economou-Petersen E, et al. Refining the primary open-angle glaucoma GLC1C region on chromosome 3 by haplotype analysis. *Clin Genet*. 2004;65: 40–44.
11. Wirtz MK, Samples JR, Kramer PL, et al. Mapping a gene for adult-onset primary open-angle glaucoma to chromosome 3q. *Am J Hum Genet*. 1997;60:296–304.
12. Wirtz MK, Samples JR, Rust K, et al. GLC1F, a new primary open-angle glaucoma locus, maps to 7q35-q36. *Arch Ophthalmol*. 1999;117:237–241.
13. Trifan OC, Traboulsi EI, Stoilova D, et al. A third locus (GLC1D) for adult-onset primary open-angle glaucoma maps to the 8q23 region. *Am J Ophthalmol*. 1998;126:17–28.
14. Rezaie T, Child A, Hitchings R, et al. Adult-onset primary open-angle glaucoma caused by mutations in optineurin. *Science*. 2002;295:1077–1079.
15. Sarfarazi M, Child A, Stoilova D, et al. Localization of the fourth locus (GLC1E) for adult-onset primary open-angle glaucoma to the 10p15-p14 region. *Am J Hum Genet*. 1998; 62:641–652.
16. Pasutto F, Keller KE, Weisschuh N, et al. Variants in ASB10 are associated with open-angle glaucoma. *Hum Mol Genet*. 2012;21:1336–1349.

17. Bennett SR, Alward WL, Folberg R. An autosomal dominant form of lowtension glaucoma. *Am J Ophthalmol.* 1989;108:238–244.

18. Vithana EN, Nongpiur ME, Venkataraman D, Chan SH, Mavinahalli J, Aung T. Identification of a novel mutation in the NTF4 gene that causes primary open-angle glaucoma in a Chinese population. *Mol Vis.* 2010;16:1640–1645.

19. Fingert JH, Robin AL, Stone JL, et al. Copy number variations on chromosome 12q14 in patients with normal tension glaucoma. *Hum Mol Genet.* 2011;20:2482–2494.

20. Ritch R, Darbro B, Menon G, et al. TBK1 gene duplication and normal-tension glaucoma. *JAMA Ophthalmol.* 2014; 132:544–548.

21. Monemi S, Spaeth G, DaSilva A, et al. Identification of a novel adultonset primary open-angle glaucoma (POAG) gene on 5q22.1. *Hum Mol Genet.* 2005;14:725–733.

22. Mackay DS, Bennett TM, Shiels A. Exome sequencing identifies a missense variant in EFEMP1 Co-Segregating in a family with autosomal dominant primary open-angle glaucoma. *PLoS One.* 2015;10:e0132529.

23. Suriyapperuma SP, Child A, Desai T, et al. A new locus (GLC1H) for adult-onset primary open-angle glaucoma maps to the 2p15-p16 region. *Arch Ophthalmol.* 2007; 125:86–92.

24. Allingham RR, Wiggs JL, Hauser ER, et al. Early adult-onset POAG linked to 15q11-13 using ordered subset analysis. *Investig Ophthalmol Vis Sci.* 2005;46:2002–2005.

25. Crooks KR, Allingham RR, Qin X, et al. Genome-wide linkage scan for primary open angle glaucoma: influences of ancestry and age at diagnosis. *PLoS One.* 2011;6: e21967.

26. Wiggs JL, Lynch S, Ynagi G, et al. A genomewide scan identifies novel early-onset primary open-angle glaucoma loci on 9q22 and 20p12. *Am J Hum Genet.* 2004;74: 1314–1320.

27. Baird PN, Foote SJ, Mackey DA, Craig J, Speed TP, Bureau A. Evidence for a novel glaucoma locus at chromosome 3p21-22. *Hum Genet.* 2005;117:249–257.

28. Fan BJ, Ko WC, Wang DY, et al. Fine mapping of new glaucoma locus GLC1M and exclusion of neuregulin 2 as the causative gene. *Mol Vis.* 2007;13:779–784.

29. Pang CP, Fan BJ, Canlas O, et al. A genome-wide scan maps a novel juvenile-onset primary open angle glaucoma locus to chromosome 5q. *Mol Vis.* 2006;12:85–92.

30. Wang DY, Fan BJ, Chua JK, et al. A genome-wide scan maps a novel juvenile-onset primary open-angle glaucoma locus to 15q. *Investig Ophthalmol Vis Sci.* 2006;47:5315–5321.

31. Pasutto F, Matsumoto T, Mardin CY, et al. Heterozygous NTF4 mutations impairing neurotrophin-4 signaling in patients with primary open-angle glaucoma. *Am J Hum Genet.* 2009;85:447–456.

32. Liu Y, Allingham RR. Major review: molecular genetics of primary open-angle glaucoma. *Exp Eye Res.* 2017;160: 62–84.

33. Porter LF, Urquhart JE, O'Donoghue E, et al. Identification of a novel locus for autosomal dominant primary open angle glaucoma on 4q35.1-q35.2. *Invest Ophthalmol Vis Sci.* 2011;52(11):7859–7865.

34. Johnson AT, Drack AV, Kwitek AE, Cannon RL, Stone EM, Alward WL. Clinical features and linkage analysis of a family with autosomal dominant juvenile glaucoma. *Ophthalmology.* 1993;100(4):524–529.

35. Anderson DR. Primary infantile glaucoma (congenital glaucoma). *Surv Ophthalmol.* 1983;28(1):1–19.

36. Siddiqui Y, Ten Hulzen RD, Cameron JD, Hodge DO, Johnson DH. What is the risk of developing pigmentary glaucoma from pigment dispersion syndrome? *Am J Ophthalmol.* 2003;135(6):794–799.

37. Siordia JA, Franco J, Golden TR, Dar B. Ocular pseudoexfoliation syndrome linkage to cardiovascular disease. *Curr Cardiol Rep.* 2016;18(7):61.

38. Andersen JS, Pralea AM, DelBono EA, et al. A gene responsible for the pigment dispersion syndrome maps to chromosome 7q35-q36. *Arch Ophthalmol.* 1997;115(3): 384–388.

39. Karger RA, Jeng SM, Johnson DH, Hodge DO, Good MS. Estimated incidence of pseudoexfoliation syndrome and pseudoexfoliation glaucoma in Olmsted County, Minnesota. *J Glaucoma.* 2003;12(3):193–197.

40. Armfield K, Nelson R, Lubs HA, et al. X-linked mental retardation syndrome with short stature, small hands and feet, seizures, cleft palate, and glaucoma is linked to Xq28. *Am J Med Genet A.* 1999;85(3):236–242.

41. Holmes LB, Walton DS. Hereditary microcornea, glaucoma, and absent frontal sinuses: a family study. *J Pediat.* 1969;74:968–972.

42. Quigley HA, Broman AT. The number of people with glaucoma worldwide in 2010 and 2020. *Br J Ophthalmol.* 2006; 90(3):262–267.

43. Tielsch JM, Katz J, Singh K, et al. A population-based evaluation of glaucoma screening: the Baltimore eye survey. *Am J Epidemiol.* 1991;134(10):1102–1110.

44. Bailey Jr LC, Olivos IM, Leahey AM, et al. Characterization of a candidate gene for OCRL. *Am J Hum Genet.* 1992; 51(suppl):A4.

45. Levy M, Feingold J. Estimating prevalence in single-gene kidney diseases progressing to renal failure. *Kidney Int.* 2000;58(3):925–943.

46. Nussbaum RL, Suchy SF. The oculocerebrorenal syndrome of Lowe (Lowe syndrome) Ch 252. In: *The Metabolic and Molecular Bases of Inherited Disease.* 8th ed. 2001.

47. Castriota-Scanderbeg A, Dallapiccola B. Nail-patella syndrome. In: *Abnormal Skeletal Phenotypes: From Simple Signs to Complex Diagnoses.* 2005:772–775.

48. Bixler D, Higgins M, Hartsfield J. The Nance-Horan syndrome: a rare X-linked ocular-dental trait with expression in heterozygous females. *Clin Genet.* 1984;26(1): 30–35.

49. Ding X, Patel M, Herzlich AA, Sieving PC, Chan CC. Ophthalmic pathology of Nance-Horan syndrome: case report and review of the literature. *Ophthal Genet.* 2009; 30(3):127–135.

50. Taylor RH, Ainsworth JR, Evans AR, Levin AV. The epidemiology of pediatric glaucoma: the Toronto experience. *J Am Assoc Pediatr Ophthalmol Strabismus.* 1999;3(5): 308–315.

51. Goldwyn R, Waltman SR, Becker B. Primary open-angle glaucoma in adolescents and young adults. *Arch Ophthalmol.* 1970;84(5):579–582.

52. Breuning MH, Dauwerse HG, Fugazza G, et al. Rubinstein-Taybi syndrome caused by submicroscopic deletions within 16p13. 3. *Am J Hum Genet.* 1993;52(2):249.

53. Roelfsema JH, White SJ, Ariyürek Y, et al. Genetic heterogeneity in Rubinstein-Taybi syndrome: mutations in both the CBP and EP300 genes cause disease. *Am J Hum Genet.* 2005;76(4):572–580.

# CHAPTER 8

# Genetic Abnormalities of Ocular Motility

AMY K. HUTCHINSON • HARRISON NGO • EVAN SILVERSTEIN •
NATARIO L. COUSER

Early studies analyzing the connection between human disease with strabismus and nystagmus abnormalities date back to the mid-nineteenth century.[1-3] Ocular motility disorders are a heterogeneous group of conditions that involve an inability to maintain ocular balance and/or execute eye movements efficiently. Maintaining ocular motor control involves a complex interaction between the afferent (signals from the eye to the central nervous system) and efferent (signals from the central nervous system to the eye) visual pathways.[4] The afferent system involves the sensory functions of perceiving objects in our environment, whereas the efferent pathway utilizes supranuclear and infranuclear pathways to control ocular movements. There are six muscles in each eye that control movement (superior, inferior, lateral, and medial rectus muscles, and superior and inferior oblique muscles) with three nerves from the brain that innervate them (cranial nerves III, IV, VI). Since maintaining ocular stability is directly dependent on neural communication, abnormalities such as strabismus, nystagmus, and other eye movement disorders are common in a variety of neurological conditions. As such, isolating the specific ocular movement aberration in the clinical setting can assist in localizing pathology and help formulating a differential diagnosis in complex neurological disease.[1]

## GENETIC DISORDERS
### Aicardi-Goutieres Syndrome[5,6]
OMIM: #225750.

*Description*: Aicardi-Goutieres syndrome presents in infancy and mainly affects the central nervous system, immune system, and the skin. It is characterized by encephalopathy, leukodystrophy, intracranial calcifications, and cerebrospinal fluid (CSF) lymphocytosis.

*Epidemiology*: unknown.

*Eye Findings*: nystagmus and strabismus.

*Inheritance*: AR (Aicardi Goutieres syndrome 1, 2, 3, 4, 5, and 6); AD (Aicardi-Goutieres syndrome 1 and 7).

*Known Genes or Gene Locus*: TREX1 (Aicardi-Goutieres syndrome 1), RNASEH2B (Aicardi-Goutieres syndrome 2), RNASEH2C (Aicardi-Goutieres syndrome 3), RNASEH2A (Aicardi-Goutieres syndrome 4), SAMHD1 (Aicardi-Goutieres syndrome 5), ADAR (Aicardi-Goutieres syndrome 6), IFIH1 (Aicardi-Goutieres syndrome 7).

### Allan-Herndon-Dudley Syndrome[7,8]
OMIM: #300523.

*Description*: Allan-Herndon-Dudley syndrome is an X-linked intellectual disability syndrome associated with hypotonia, muscle hypoplasia, ataxia, spastic paraplegia, and severe cognitive impairment.

*Epidemiology*: unknown.

*Eye Findings*: rotary nystagmus and disconjugate eye movements.

*Inheritance*: X-linked dominant (XLD).

*Known Genes or Gene Locus*: SLC16A2 (MCT8).

### Ataxia-Oculomotor Apraxia Syndrome[9,10]
OMIM: # 208920.

*Description*: Ataxia-occulomotor apraxia syndrome is a childhood onset, AR disorder associated with poorly coordinated and controlled side-to-side eye movement. It is also characterized by chorea, myoclonus, and neuropathy.

*Epidemiology*: unknown.

*Eye Findings*: oculomotor apaxia, nystagmus, hypometric saccades, and external ophthalmoplegia.

*Inheritance*: AR.

*Known Genes or Gene Locus*: APTX, SETX.

## Centronuclear Myopathy[11,12]

*OMIM*: 160150.

*Description*: Centronuclear myopathy is an autosomal dominant disorder that is characterized by progressive muscle weakness ranging from mild to profound. Onset can occur as early as birth to adulthood, although adulthood onset is rare. Nuclei are abnormally positioned centrally in muscle cells.

*Epidemiology*: unknown.

*Eye Findings*: ptosis and limitation of eye movement.

*Inheritance*: AD.

*Known Genes or Gene Locus*: MTMR14.

## Chédiak-Higashi Syndrome[13,14]

*OMIM*: #214500.

*Description*: Chédiak-Higashi syndrome is an AR disorder associated with photosensitivity, reduced ocular and cutaneous pigment, ataxia, peripheral neuropathy, abnormal white blood cells, and decreased clotting.

*Epidemiology*: <500 cases reported.

*Eye Findings*: decreased iris and retina pigmentation, nystagmus, photophobia, strabismus, and macular hypoplasia.

*Inheritance*: AR.

*Known Genes or Gene Locus*: CHS1.

## Childhood-Onset Dystonia with Optic Atrophy and Basal Ganglia Abnormalities[15]

*OMIM*: #617282.

*Description*: Childhood-onset dystonia with optic atrophy and basal ganglia abnormalities is a condition characterized by early onset of involuntary movements and primarily dystonia. Associated optic atrophy with visual impairment may begin at the onset of dystonia or within a few years.

*Epidemiology*: unknown.

*Eye Findings*: optic atrophy and nystagmus.

*Inheritance*: AR.

*Known Genes or Gene Locus*: MECR.

## Christian Syndrome[16,17]

*OMIM*: %309620.

*Description*: Christian syndrome is a rare X-linked disorder characterized by intellectual disability, skeletal dysplasia, and abducens palsy.

*Epidemiology*: unknown.

*Eye Findings*: cranial nerve VI palsy.

*Inheritance*: X-linked.

*Known Genes or Gene Locus*: Locus Xq28.

## Christianson Syndrome[18,19]

*OMIM*: #300243.

*Description*: Christianson syndrome is an X-linked neurodevelopmental and progressive intellectual disability syndrome characterized by microcephaly, impaired ocular movements, severe global developmental delay, developmental regression, hypotonia, abnormal movements, and early-onset seizures of variable types.

*Epidemiology*: unknown.

*Eye Findings*: ophthalmoplegia, deep-set eyes, and bushy eyebrows.

*Inheritance*: XLD.

*Known Genes or Gene Locus*: SLC9A6.

## Chronic Progressive External Ophthalmoplegia[20,21]

*OMIM*: #157640 (AD1), #609286 (AD3).

*Description*: Progressive external ophthalmoplegia is characterized by multiple mitochondrial DNA deletions (PEOA1 and PEOA3 mitochondrial genes) in the skeletal muscle. The most common clinical features include adult onset of weakness of the external eye muscles with exotropia and exercise intolerance.

*Epidemiology*: unknown.

*Eye Findings*: weakness/paralysis of ocular eye muscles (Fig. 8.1), ptosis (Fig. 8.1), and strabismus (Fig. 8.1).

*Inheritance*: AD, AR.

*Known Genes or Gene Locus*: AD: POLG, TWNK, RRM2B, SLC25A4; AR: POLG, RRM2B.

## CK Syndrome[22,23]

*OMIM*: #300831.

*Description*: CK syndrome (CKS) is an X-linked disorder characterized by mild to severe cognitive impairment, seizures, microcephaly, cerebral cortical malformations, dysmorphic facial features, and thin body habitus.

*Epidemiology*: unknown.

*Eye Findings*: strabismus, epicanthal folds, upslanting palpebral fissures, and almond-shaped eyes.

*Inheritance*: X-linked recessive (XLR).

*Known Genes or Gene Locus*: NSDHL.

## Congential Fibrosis of Extraocular Muscles[24,25]

*OMIM*: #135700, #602078, #600638.

*Description*: Congential fibrosis of extraocular muscles (CFEOM) is characterized by bilateral blepharoptosis and ophthalmoplegia with the eyes fixed in an

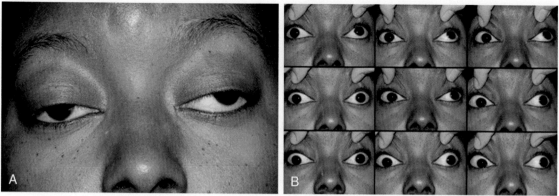

FIG. 8.1 Chronic progressive external ophthalmoplegia. Note the bilateral ptosis and exotropia **(A)**, with significant limitation of ocular motility for both eyes in all gaze positions **(B)**. (Courtesy Fraser, J. Alexander, MD; Biousse, Valérie, MD; Newman, Nancy J., MD. The Neuro-ophthalmology of mitochondrial disease. *Surv Ophthalmol*. July 1, 2010;55(4):299–334. © 2010.)

infraducted position about 20–30° below the horizontal midline. Classic phenotype with bilateral involvement is referred to as CFEOM1. CFEOM2 characterized by bilateral ptosis with eyes fixed in an exotropic position. Affected individuals with CFEOM3 may have unilateral eye involvement, may be able to raise their eyes above midline, or may not have blepharoptosis.

*Epidemiology*: prevalence of 1/230,000.

*Eye Findings*: ptosis and ophthalmoplegia.

*Inheritance*: AD: CFEOM1, CFEOM3A, CFEOM3B; AR: CFEOM2.

*Known Genes or Gene Locus*: KIF21A (CFEOM1, CFEOM3B), PHOX2A (CFEOM2), ARIX, TUBB3 (CFEOM3A).

## Congenital Nystagmus[26–29]

*OMIM*: #310700 (NYS1), %164100 (NYS2), %608345(NYS3), %193003 (NYS4), %300589 (NYS5), #300814 (NYS6), %614826 (NYS7).

*Description*: Congenital nystagmus presents as conjugate, horizontal oscillations of the eyes, in primary or eccentric gaze, often with a preferred head turn or tilt. Other associated features may include mildly decreased visual acuity, strabismus, astigmatism, and occasionally head nodding. It may be present at birth but usually has onset at about 2–3 months of age.

*Epidemiology*: prevalence of 1/5000.

*Eye Findings*: nystagmus (multiple types including horizontal, pendular, jerky, vertical), reduced visual acuity, head turn, and strabismus.

*Inheritance*: AD (NYS2, NYS3, NYS4, NYS6), AR; X-linked (NYS1, NYS5).

*Known Genes or Gene Locus*: FRMD7 (NYS1)

## Dentatorubral-Pallidoluysian Atrophy[30,31]

*OMIM*: #125370.

*Description*: Dentatorubral-pallidoluysian atrophy, commonly known as DRPLA, is a progressive brain disorder that causes involuntary movements, mental and emotional problems, and a decline in thinking ability. The average age of onset of DRPLA is 30 years, but this condition can appear anytime from infancy to mid-adulthood.

*Epidemiology*: prevalence of 2/1,000,000–7/1,000,000 in Japan; rare in other countries.

*Eye Findings*: poor eye movement coordination, corneal endothelial degeneration, optic atrophy, and progressive visual loss.

*Inheritance*: AD.

*Known Genes or Gene Locus*: ATN1.

## Duane Syndrome[32,33]

*OMIM*: %126800 (Type 1), #604356 (Type 2), #617041 (Type 3).

*Description*: Duane syndrome is a disinnervation disorder of eye movement usually associated with limitation of adduction, abduction, or both and retraction of the eye on attempted adduction. Usually only one eye (more commonly the left eye) is affected.

*Epidemiology*: prevalence of 1/1000.

*Eye Findings*: strabismus (Fig. 8.2), eye retraction with palpebral fissure narrowing on adduction (Fig. 8.2), vision loss (uncommon), and amblyopia (uncommon).

*Inheritance*: AD (or sporadic).

*Known Genes or Gene Locus*: chromosome 8q13 (Type 1), CHN1 (Type 2), MAFB (Type 3).

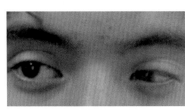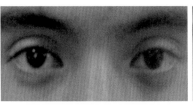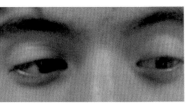

FIG. 8.2 Bilateral Duane syndrome (Type 3). Note the bilateral eye retraction and narrowing of the palpebral fissures with mild limitation on abduction; right gaze (left), forward gaze (middle), left gaze (right). (Courtesy Murillo-Correa, Claudia E., MD; Kon-Jara, Veronica, MD; Engle, Elizabeth C., MD; Zenteno, Juan C., MD, PhD. Clinical features associated with an I126M α2-chimaerin mutation in a family with autosomal-dominant Duane retraction syndrome. *J AAPOS*. June 1, 2009;13(3):245–248. © 2009.)

## Familial Visceral Myopathy with External Ophthalmoplegia[34,35]

*OMIM*: %277320.

*Description*: Familial visceral myopathy with external ophthalmoplegia is an extremely rare AR neuromuscular disease characterized by ocular manifestations of ptosis and diplopia followed by the absence of intestinal peristalsis, leading to abdominal pain, diarrhea, constipation, malabsorption, and progressive intestinal pseudoobstruction.

*Epidemiology*: unknown.

*Eye Findings*: poor eye movement and ptosis.

*Inheritance*: AR.

*Known Genes or Gene Locus*: unknown.

## Fatty Acid Hydroxylase-Associated Neurodegeneration[36,37]

*OMIM*: *611026.

*Description*: Fatty acid hydroxylase-associated neurodegeneration (FAHN) is a progressive disorder of the nervous system (neurodegeneration) due to reduced or eliminated function of the fatty acid 2-hydrolase enzyme. It is characterized by problems with movement and vision that begin during childhood or adolescence.

*Epidemiology*: unknown; few dozen cases reported.

*Eye Findings*: optic atrophy, ophthalmoplegia, reduced visual acuity, strabismus, nystagmus, and supranuclear gaze palsy.

*Inheritance*: AR.

*Known Genes or Gene Locus*: FA2H.

## Gaucher Disease Type 1[38,39]

*OMIM*: #230800.

*Description*: Gaucher disease is an AR lysosomal storage disorder due to deficient activity of an enzyme called beta-glucocerebrosidase. Accumulation of glucocerebroside occurs, and this causes bone disease, hepatosplenomegaly, anemia and thrombocytopenia, and lung disease.

*Epidemiology*: prevalence of 1/50,000–1/100,000 (Gaucher disease type 1 accounts for 90% of individuals affected with Gaucher disease); incidence of 1/450 in Ashkenazi-Jewish population.

*Eye Findings*: macular atrophy, increased vascular permeability, perimacular grayness, brown deposits at limbus, white deposits in anterior segment, strabismus, oculomotor apraxia, supranuclear gaze palsy, hypertelorism, corneal opacities, and nystagmus.

*Inheritance*: AR.

*Known Genes or Gene Locus*: GBA.

## Gaucher Disease Type II[40,41]

*OMIM*: #230900.

*Description*: Gaucher disease type II (GD2) is a rare AR lysosomal disorder presenting with all the symptoms of type I, but it is the acute, neuronopathic form. It is characterized by early onset, typically in the first year after birth with rapid neurodegeneration, marked by severe hypertonia, rigidity, arching (opisthotonus), swallowing impairment, and seizures. Occurs after birth. Infants may present with ichthyosis.

*Epidemiology*: prevalence of <1/100,000.

*Eye Findings*: strabismus and supranuclear gaze palsy.

*Inheritance*: AR.

*Known Genes or Gene Locus*: GBA.

## Gaucher Disease Type IIIA[42,43]

*OMIM*: #231000.

*Description*: Gaucher disease type IIIA is the subacute form Gaucher disease type II that is neuronopathic. It is characterized by having myoclonus and dementia.

*Epidemiology*: prevalence of <1/100,000 (all type III).

*Eye Findings*: strabismus and supranuclear gaze palsy.

*Inheritance*: AR.

*Known Genes or Gene Locus*: GBA.

## Gaucher Disease Type IIIB[44,45]

OMIM: #231005.

*Description*: Gaucher disease type IIIA is the subacute form of Gaucher disease type II that is marked by neurological degeneration. It is characterized by having extensive visceral and bone involvement with massive hepatosplenomegaly and progressive skeletal abnormalities including kyphoscoliosis and barreled chest.

>    *Epidemiology*: prevalence of <1/100,000 (all type III).
>    *Eye Findings*: strabismus and supranuclear gaze palsy.
>    *Inheritance*: AR.
>    *Known Genes or Gene Locus*: GBA.

## Gaucher Disease Type IIIC[39,46]

OMIM: #608013.

*Description*: Gaucher disease type IIIC is the subacute form of Gaucher disease type II that is marked by neurological degeneration. It is characterized by having cardiovascular calcifications.

>    *Epidemiology*: prevalence of <1/100,000 (all type III).
>    *Eye Findings*: strabismus, supranuclear gaze palsy, and corneal opacity.
>    *Inheritance*: AR.
>    *Known Genes or Gene Locus*: GBA.

## Griscelli Syndrome Type 1[47,48]

OMIM: #214450.

*Description*: Griscelli syndrome Type I is a disorder characterized by hypopigmentation of the skin and hair along with severe neurological impairments. It is associated with delayed development, intellectual disability, seizures, weak muscle tone (hypotonia), and eye and vision abnormalities.

>    *Epidemiology*: unknown.
>    *Eye Findings*: iris hypopigmentation and roving eye movements.
>    *Inheritance*: AR.
>    *Known Genes or Gene Locus*: MYO5A.

## Horizontal Gaze Palsy with Progressive Scoliosis 1[49–51]

OMIM: #607313.

*Description*: Horizontal gaze palsy with progressive scoliosis 1 (HGPPS1) is a rare neurologic disorder characterized by eye movement abnormalities apparent from birth and childhood-onset progressive scoliosis. These features are associated with a developmental malformation of the brain stem including hypoplasia of the pons and cerebellar peduncles and defective decussation of certain neuronal systems.

>    *Epidemiology*: unknown.

>    *Eye Findings*: horizontal nystagmus and progressive ophthalmoplegia.
>    *Inheritance*: AR.
>    *Known Genes or Gene Locus*: ROBO3.

## Horizontal Gaze Palsy with Progressive Scoliosis 2[43,52]

OMIM: #617542.

*Description*: Horizontal gaze palsy with progressive scoliosis 2 (HGPPS2) is a rare neurologic disorder characterized by eye movement abnormalities apparent from birth and childhood-onset progressive scoliosis. It is associated with agenesis of the corpus collosum.

>    *Epidemiology*: unknown.
>    *Eye Findings*: horizontal nystagmus.
>    *Inheritance*: AR.
>    *Known Genes or Gene Locus*: DCC.

## Hypomelanosis of Ito[53,54]

OMIM: #300337.

*Description*: Hypomelanosis of Ito is not a distinct disorder but believed to be a chromosomal translocation that can cause eye abnormalities, irregularly spaced teeth, kyphosis, scoliosis, clinodactyly, syndactyly, polydactyly, alopecia, seizures, intellectual disability, and cerebral atrophy. It is characterized by a rare birth defect that causes streaked, whirled, or mottled patches of light-colored skin reflecting pigmentary mosaicism.

>    *Epidemiology*: incidence of 1/8500–1/10,000.
>    *Eye Findings*: iris coloboma, cataract, hypertelorism, epicanthal folds, and strabismus.
>    *Inheritance*: X-linked, AR, AD.
>    *Known Genes or Gene Locus*: Xp11.

## Joubert Syndrome 1[55,56]

OMIM: #213300.

*Description*: Joubert syndrome, also known as Joubert-Boltshauser syndrome, Cerebelloparenchymal disorder IV, and Cerebellooculorenal syndrome, is a rare disorder with multiple modes of inheritance and presents with the absence or underdevelopment of the cerebellar vermis (a part of the brain that controls balance and coordination) and a malformed brain stem. It is commonly characterized by the appearance of a "molar tooth sign" on MRI.

>    *Epidemiology*: prevalence of 1/80,000–1/100,000.

>    *Eye Findings*: pigmentary retinopathy, oculomotor apraxia or difficulty in smooth visual pursuits and jerkiness in gaze tracking, ptosis, chorioretinal coloboma, epicanthal folds, retinal dysplasia (uncommon), and retinal dystrophy (uncommon).

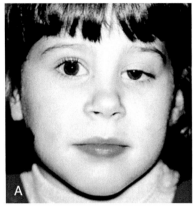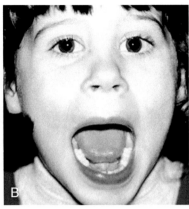

**FIG. 8.3** Marcus Gunn phenomenon. Note the moderate ptosis in the left eye **(A)**, with retraction of the left eyelid upon opening of the mouth **(B)**. (Courtesy Bowling, Brad, FRCSEd(Ophth), FRCOphth, FRANZCO. Eyelids, Kanski's Clinical Ophthalmology; January 1, 2016:1–62. © 2016.)

*Inheritance*: AR (most common), XLR (JBTS 10), AR and AD (JBTS 14,19).

*Known Genes or Gene Locus*: *INPP5E, CEP104, NPHP1, TMEM237, ARMC9, PDE6D, ARL13B, CC2D2A, C5orf42, CEP120, AHI1, CEP41, CSPP1, TMEM67, TCTN3, SUFU, TMEM138, TMEM216, CEP290, TECT1, TCTN2, PIBF1, KIAA0586, KIF7, KATNIP, ZNF423, RPGRIP1L, TMEM231, TMEM107, B9D1, MKS1, B9D2, OFD1.*

## Kearns-Sayre Syndrome[36,45,82]

*OMIM*: #530000.

*Description*: Kearns-Sayre syndrome is a rare disorder that is characterized by progressive external ophthalmoplegia and pigmentary retinopathy with an onset before the age of 20 years. It is also associated with cerebellar ataxia, cardiac conduction block, raised CSF protein content, and proximal myopathy.

*Epidemiology*: unknown.

*Eye Findings*: ptosis, progressive external ophthalmoplegia, and pigmentary retinopathy.

*Inheritance*: mitochondrial.

*Known Genes or Gene Locus*: *MTTL1.*

## Marcus Gunn Phenomenon[57,58]

*OMIM*: 154600.

*Description*: Marcus Gunn phenomenon is a rare disinnervation condition characterized by movement of the upper eyelid in a rapid rising motion (a "wink") each time the jaw moves. The wink phenomenon may be elicited by opening the mouth, thrusting the jaw to the side, jaw protrusion, chewing, smiling, or sucking.

*Epidemiology*: unknown.

*Eye Findings*: unilateral congenital ptosis (Fig. 8.3), elevation of ptotic lid upon movement of lower jaw (Fig. 8.3), amblyopia, and strabismus.

*Inheritance*: possible AD.

*Known Genes or Gene Locus*: unknown.

## Methylmalonic Aciduria and Homocystinuria, CB1D Type[59,60]

*OMIM*: #277410.

*Description*: Methylmalonic aciduria and homocystinuria is a rare genetically heterogeneous disorder of cobalamin (vitamin B12) metabolism. It is characterized by megaloblastic anemia, lethargy, failure to thrive, developmental delay, intellectual deficit, and seizures.

*Epidemiology*: unknown; six reported cases.

*Eye Findings*: nystagmus.

*Inheritance*: AR.

*Known Genes or Gene Locus*: C2orf25 (*MMADHC*).

## Mitochondrial Encephalomyopathy, Lactic Acidosis, and Stroke-like Episodes (MELAS)[61,62]

*OMIM*: #540000.

*Description*: Mitochondrial encephalomyopathy, lactic acidosis, and stroke-like episodes (MELAS) is a genetically heterogeneous mitochondrial disorder that is characterized by a buildup of lactic acid. Most people experience stroke-like episodes that can often involve hemiparesis, seizures, altered consciousness, vision abnormalities, and severe headaches.

*Epidemiology*: unknown.

*Eye Findings*: bilateral cataracts, hemianopsia, cortical blindness, and ophthalmoplegia.

*Inheritance*: mitochondrial.

*Known Genes or Gene Locus*: MTTL1, MTTQ, MTTH, MTTK, MTTC, MTTS1, MTTS2, MTND1, MTND5, MTND6.

## Mitochondrial Neurogastrointestinal Encephalopathy Syndrome (MNGIE)[63,64]

*OMIM*: #603041.

*Description*: Mitochondrial neurogastrointestinal encephalopathy syndrome (MNGIE) is a rare disorder associated with gastrointestinal dysmotility, peripheral neuropathy, ptosis, ophthalmoplegia, and hearing loss. Leukoencephalopathy is considered a hallmark of MNGIE.

*Epidemiology*: unknown.

*Eye Findings*: progressive external ophthalmoplegia and ptosis.

*Inheritance*: AR.

*Known Genes or Gene Locus*: TYMP.

## Moebius Syndrome[22,52,81]

*OMIM*: %157900.

*Description*: Moebius syndrome is a rare neurological disorder of sporadic inheritance that primarily affects muscles that controls facial expression and eye movement (CN VI and VII nuclei).

*Epidemiology*: unknown.

*Eye Findings*: adduction and abduction palsy, conjugated horizontal gaze palsy, Duane retraction syndrome, congenital fibrosis of extraocular muscles, hypertelorism, epicanthal folds, esotropia, exotropia, microphthalmia, and lacrimal duct defects.

*Inheritance*: sporadic.

*Known Genes or Gene Locus*: unknown.

## Oculomotor Apraxia Cogan Type[65,66]

*OMIM*: %257550.

*Description*: Oculomotor apraxia Cogan type is a disorder characterized by defective or absent horizontal voluntary eye movements, and defective or absent horizontal ocular saccadic movements.

*Epidemiology*: unknown.

*Eye Findings*: oculomotor apraxia (defective/absent horizontal eye movements).

*Inheritance*: AR.

*Known Genes or Gene Locus*: unknown.

## Ouvrier-Billson Syndrome[67–69]

*OMIM*: 168885.

*Description*: Ouvrier-Billson syndrome, also called benign paroxysmal tonic upgaze of childhood with ataxia, is a rare syndrome characterized by episodic sustained upward deviation of the eyes and down beating saccades with downgaze; associated with ataxia.

Individuals affected are typically otherwise healthy, and symptoms are typically resolved within 2 years of onset.

*Epidemiology*: unknown.

*Eye Findings*: episodes of an upward tonic ocular deviation.

*Inheritance*: AD.

*Known Genes or Gene Locus*: unknown.

## Schimke X-Linked Mental Retardation Syndrome[70,71]

*OMIM*: 312840.

*Description*: Schimke, X-linked, mental retardation syndrome is a rare disorder characterized by intellectual disability, abnormal involuntary movements, and retarded growth.

*Epidemiology*: unknown.

*Eye Findings*: external ophthalmoplegia.

*Inheritance*: X-linked.

*Known Genes or Gene Locus*: unknown.

## Septo-Optic Dysplasia[72,73]

*OMIM*: #182230.

*Description*: Septo-optic dysplasia is a sporadic disorder characterized by underdevelopment of the optic nerves, abnormal formation of structures along the midline of the brain, and pituitary hypoplasia.

*Epidemiology*: incidence of 1/10,000.

*Eye Findings*: optic nerve hypoplasia, hypoplastic optic discs, nystagmus, and strabismus.

*Inheritance*: AR, AD.

*Known Genes or Gene Locus*: HESX1.

## Spastic Paraplegia[74,75]

*OMIM*: #303350.

*Description*: Spastic paraplegia is a large group of disorders that share the common characteristic of difficulty in walking due to muscle weakness and muscle tightness in the legs.

*Epidemiology*: prevalence of 2/100,000–6/100,000.

*Eye Findings*: nystagmus and optic atrophy.

*Inheritance*: AD, AR, X-linked, mitochondrial.

*Known Genes or Gene Locus*: L1CAM, PLP1, ATL1, SPAST, CYP7B1, NIPA1, SPG7, ALDH18A1, KIF5A, SPG11, RTN2, KIAA0196, HSP60, ZFYVE26, BSCL2, ERLIN2, SPG20, ACP33, SLC16A2, RIPK5, B4GALNT1, DDHD1, KIF1A, REEP1, ZFYVE27, FA2H, PNPLA6, SLC33A1, C19ORF12, GJC2, NT5C2, GBA2, AP4B1, AP5Z1, TECPR2, AP4M1, AP4E1, AP4S1 VPS37A, DDHD2, C12ORF65, CYP2U1, TFG, K1F1C, USP8, WDR48, ARL6IP1, ERLIN1, AMPD2, ENTPD1, ARSI, PGAP1, KLC2, RAB3GAP2, MARS, ZFR, REEP2, CPT1C, IBA57, MAG, CAPN1, FARS2, ATP13A2, UCHL1.

## Spinocerebellar Ataxia, X-Linked 1[76,77]

*OMIM*: #302500.

*Description*: Spinocerebellar ataxia, X-linked 1 is a neurologic disorder characterized by hypotonia at birth, delayed motor development, gait ataxia, difficulty standing, dysarthria, and slow eye movements.

> *Epidemiology*: prevalence of 1/100,000–2/100,000.
> *Eye Findings*: slow eye movements and strabismus.
> *Inheritance*: XLR.
> *Known Genes or Gene Locus*: ATP2B3.

## VACTERL Association with Hydrocephalus[78,79]

*OMIM*: #276950.

*Description*: VACTERL with hydrocephalus is an extremely rare genetic disorder in which the multisystem features of VACTERL (Vertebral abnormalities, Anal Atresia, Cardiac defects, Tracheoesophageal fistula, Esophageal atresia, Renal abnormalities, and Limb abnormalities) association occur in addition to hydrocephalus which is a condition in which accumulation of excessive CSF in the skull causes pressure on the tissues of the brain, resulting in a variety of symptoms.

> *Epidemiology*: unknown.
> *Eye Findings*: downward gaze of eyes and strabismus.
> *Inheritance*: mostly sporadic.
> *Known Genes or Gene Locus*: PTEN.

## Wieacker-Wolff Syndrome[66,80]

*OMIM*: #314580.

*Description*: Wieacker-Wolff syndrome is a severe neurodevelopmental disorder affecting the central and peripheral nervous systems. It is characterized by onset of muscle weakness in utero.

> *Epidemiology*: prevalence of <1/1,000,000.
> *Eye Findings*: ptosis, upslanting palpebral fissures, and oculomotor apraxia.
> *Inheritance*: XLR.
> *Known Genes or Gene Locus*: ZC4H2.

## REFERENCES

1. Shaikh AG, Zee DS. Eye movement research in the twenty-first century-a window to the brain, mind, and more. *Cerebellum US: Springer*; 2017:1473–4230.
2. Estlin JB. Report on the results of one hundred operations for strabismus. *Prov Med J Retrosp Med Sci*. 1842;4(95):303–306.
3. Pomeroy OD. A case of nystagmus, associated with concomitant convergent strabismus, in emmetropic eyes, relieved by correction of the squint. *Trans Am Ophthalmol Soc*. 1875;2:283.
4. Van De Grind WA, Grüsser OJ, Lunkenheimer HU. Temporal transfer properties of the afferent visual system psychophysical, neurophysiological and theoretical investigations. In: Jung R, ed. *Central Processing of Visual Information A: Integrative Functions and Comparative Data. Handbook of Sensory Physiology*. Berlin, Heidelberg: Springer; 1973; 7/3/3 A.
5. Crow YJ, Rehwinkel J. Aicardi-Goutieres syndrome and related phenotypes: linking nucleic acid metabolism with autoimmunity. *Hum Mol Genet*. 2009;18:R130–R136.
6. Rice G, Patrick T, Parmar R, et al. Clinical and molecular phenotype of Aicardi-Goutieres syndrome. *Am J Hum Genet*. 2007;81:713–725.
7. Capri Y, Friesema ECH, Kersseboom S, et al. Relevance of different cellular models in determining the effects of mutations on SLC16A2/MCT8 thyroid hormone transporter function and genotype-phenotype correlation. *Hum Mutat*. 2013;34:1018–1025.
8. Frints Suzanna Gerarda Maria, et al. MCT8 mutation analysis and identification of the first female with Allan–Herndon–Dudley syndrome due to loss of MCT8 expression. *Eur J Hum Genet*. 2008;16(9):1029–1037.
9. Bertini E, des Portes V, Zanni G, et al. X-linked congenital ataxia: a clinical and genetic study. *Am J Med Genet*. 2000;92:53–56.
10. Koeppen AH. Ocular apraxia in recessive ataxia. *Lett Arch Neurol*. 2002;59:874.
11. Banker BQ. The congenital myopathies. In: Engel AG, Banker BQ, eds. *Myology: Basic and Clinical*. New York: McGraw-Hill (Pub.); 1986:1527–1581.
12. Jeannet PY, Bassez G, Eymard B, et al. Clinical and histologic findings in autosomal centronuclear myopathy. *Neurology*. 2004;62:1484.
13. Karim MA, Suzuki K, Fukai K, et al. Apparent genotype-phenotype correlation in childhood, adolescent, and adult Chediak-Higashi syndrome. *Am J Med Genet*. 2002;108:16.
14. Zelickson AS, Windhorst DB, White JG, Good RA. The Chediak-Higashi syndrome: formation of giant melanosomes and the basis of hypopigmentation. *J Invest Dermatol*. 1967;49:575.
15. Heimer G, Keratar JM, Riley LG, et al. MECR mutations cause childhood-onset dystonia and optic atrophy, a mitochondrial fatty acid synthesis disorder. *Am J Hum Genet*. 2016;99:1229–1244.
16. Christian JC, DeMyer WE, Franken EA, Huff JS, Khairi S, Reed TE. X-linked skeletal dysplasia with mental retardation. *Clin Genet*. 1977;11:128–136.
17. Dlouhy SR, Christian JC, Haines JL, Conneally PM, Hodes ME. Localization of the gene for a syndrome of X-linked skeletal dysplasia and mental retardation to Xq27-qter. *Hum Genet*. 1987;75:136–139.
18. Christianson AL, Stevenson RE, van der Meyden CH, et al. X linked severe mental retardation, craniofacial dysmorphology, epilepsy, ophthalmoplegia, and cerebellar atrophy in a large South African kindred is localised to Xq24-q27. *J Med Genet*. 1999;36:759–766.

19. Masurel-Paulet A, Piton A, Chancenotte S, et al. A new family with an SLC9A6 mutation expanding the phenotypic spectrum of Christianson syndrome. *Am J Med Genet.* 2016;170A:2103–2110.

20. Filosto M, Mancuso M, Nishigaki Y, et al. Clinical and genetic heterogeneity in progressive external ophthalmoplegia due to mutations in polymerase-gamma. *Arch Neurol.* 2003;60:1279–1284.

21. Lamantea E, Tiranti V, Bordoni A, et al. Mutations of mitochondrial DNA polymerase gamma-A are a frequent cause of autosomal dominant or recessive progressive external ophthalmoplegia. *Ann Neurol.* 2002;52:211–219.

22. Bianchine JW, Lewis Jr RC. The MASA syndrome: a new heritable mental retardation syndrome. *Clin Genet.* 1974; 5:298–306.

23. McLarren KW, Severson TM, du Souich C, et al. Hypomorphic temperature-sensitive alleles of NSDHL cause CK syndrome. *Am J Hum Genet.* 2010;87:905–914.

24. Hansen E. Congenital general fibrosis of the extraocular muscles. *Acta Ophthal.* 1968;46:469–476.

25. Mackey DA, Chan W-M, Chan C, et al. Congenital fibrosis of the vertically acting extraocular muscles maps to the FEOM3 locus. *Hum Genet.* 2002;110:510–512.

26. Gresty MA, Ell JJ, Findley LJ. Acquired pendular nystagmus. its characteristics, localising value and pathophysiology. *J Neurol Neurosurg Psychiat.* 1982;45:431.

27. Kerrison JB, Koenekoop RK, Arnould VJ, Zee D, Maumenee IH. Clinical features of autosomal dominant congenital nystagmus linked to chromosome 6p12. *Am J Ophthal.* 1998;125:64–70.

28. Mellott ML, Brown Jr J, Fingert JH, et al. Clinical characterization and linkage analysis of a family with congenital X-linked nystagmus and deuteranomaly. *Arch Ophthal.* 1999; 117:1630–1633.

29. Tarpey P, Thomas S, Sarvananthan N, et al. Mutations in FRMD7, a newly identified member of the FERM family, cause X-linked idiopathic congenital nystagmus. *Nat Genet.* 2006;38:1242–1244. Note: Erratum: *Nat Genet.* 2011;43:720.

30. Burke JR, Ikeuchi T, Koide R, et al. Dentatorubral-pallidoluysian atrophy and Haw river syndrome. *Lett Lancet.* 1994;344:1711–1712.

31. Hayashi Y, Kakita A, Yamada M, et al. Hereditary dentatorubral-pallidoluysian atrophy: detection of widespread ubiquitinated neuronal and glial intranuclear inclusions in the brain. *Acta Neuropath.* 1998;96:547–552.

32. Chung M, Stout JT, Borchert MS. Clinical diversity of hereditary Duane's retraction syndrome. *Ophthalmology.* 2000;107:500–503.

33. Gutowski NJ. Duane's syndrome. *Eur J Neurol.* 2000;7: 145–149.

34. Anuras S, Mitros FA, Nowak TV, et al. A familial visceral myopathy with external ophthalmoplegia and autosomal recessive transmission. *Gastroenterology.* 1983;84:346–353.

35. Ionasescu V, Anuras S, Christensen J, Ionasescu R. New familial visceral myopathy with external ophthalmoplegia: clinical pathological and biochemical studies of contractile proteins in fresh and cultured stomach muscle cells. *Abstr Am J Hum Genet.* 1981;33:80A.

36. DiMauro S, Schon EA, Carelli V, Hirano M. The clinical maze of mitochondrial neurology. *Nat Rev Neurol.* 2013; 9:429.

37. Edvardson S, Hama H, Shaag A, et al. Mutations in the fatty acid 2-hydroxylase gene are associated with leukodystrophy with spastic paraparesis and dystonia. *Am J Hum Genet.* 2008;83:643–648.

38. Beutler E. Disease: new molecular approaches to diagnosis and treatment. *Science.* 1992;256:794–799.

39. Bohlega S, Kambouris M, Shahid M, et al. Gaucher disease with oculomotor apraxia and cardiovascular calcification (Gaucher type IIIC). *Neurology.* 2000;54:261.

40. Fried K. Population study of chronic Gaucher's disease. *Isr J Med Sci.* 1973;9:1396–1398.

41. Gupta N, Oppenheim IM, Kauvar EF, et al. Type 2 Gaucher disease: phenotypic variation and genotypic heterogeneity. *Blood Cells Mol Dis.* 2011;46:75.

42. Goker-Alpan O, Schiffmann R, Park JK, Stubblefield BK, Tayebi N, Sidransky E. Phenotypic continuum in neuronopathic Gaucher disease: an intermediate phenotype between type 2 and type 3. *J Pediat.* 2003;143:273–276.

43. Patterson MC, Horowitz M, Abel RB, et al. Isolated horizontal supranuclear gaze palsy as a marker of severe systemic involvement in Gaucher's disease. *Neurology* 1993; 1993:43.

44. Blom S, Erikson A. Gaucher disease—Norrbottnian type. Neurodevelopmental, neurological, and neurophysiological aspects. *Eur J Pediatr.* 1983;140:316.

45. Orrison WW, Robertson Jr WC. Congenital ocular motor apraxia: a possible disconnection syndrome. *Arch Neurol.* 1979;36:29–31.

46. Abrahamov A, Elstein D, Gross-Tsur V, et al. Gaucher's disease variant characterised by progressive calcification of heart valves and unique genotype. *Lancet.* 1995;346:1000.

47. Hurvitz H, Gillis R, Klaus S, et al. A kindred with Griscelli disease: spectrum of neurological involvement. *Eur J Pediatr.* 1993;152:402.

48. Kumar M, Sackey K, Schmalstieg F, et al. Griscelli syndrome: rare neonatal syndrome of recurrent hemophagocytosis. *J Pediatr Hematol Oncol.* 2001;23:464.

49. Chan W-M, Traboulsi EI, Arthur B, Friedman N, Andrews C, Engle EC. Horizontal gaze palsy with progressive scoliosis can result from compound heterozygous mutations in ROBO3. *J Med Genet.* 2006;43:e11.

50. Jen JC, Chan W-M, Bosley TM, et al. Mutations in a human ROBO gene disrupt hindbrain axon pathway crossing and morphogenesis. *Science.* 2004;304:1509–1513.

51. MacDonald DB, Streletz LJ, Al-Zayed Z, Abdool S, Stigsby B. Intraoperative neurophysiologic discovery of uncrossed sensory and motor pathways in a patient with horizontal gaze palsy and scoliosis. *Clin Neurophysiol.* 2004;115:576–582.

52. Verzijl HTFM, van der Zwaag B, Lammens M, ten Donkelaar HJ, Padberg GW. The neuropathology of hereditary congenital facial palsy vs Moebius syndrome. *Neurology.* 2005;64:649–653.

53. Donnai D, Read AP. Hypomelanosis of Ito. *Lett Lancet.* 1992;339:819–820.

54. Montagna P, Procaccianti G, Galli G, Ripamonti L, Patrizi A, Baruzzi A. Familial hypomelanosis of Ito. *Eur Neurol.* 1991;31:345−347.

55. Saraiva JM, Baraitser M. Joubert syndrome: a review. *Am J Med Genet.* 1992;43:726−731.

56. Squires LA, Raymond G, Neumeyer AM, Krishnamoorthy KS, Buyse ML. Dysmorphic features of Joubert syndrome. *Dysmorph Clin Genet.* 1991;5:72−77.

57. Doco-Fenzy M, Mauran P, Lebrun JM, et al. Pure direct duplication (12)(q24.1-q24.2) in a child with Marcus Gunn phenomenon and multiple congenital anomalies. *Am J Med Genet.* 2006;140A:212−221.

58. Falls HF, Kruse WT, Cotterman CW. Three cases of Marcus Gunn phenomenon in 2 generations. *Am J Ophthal.* 1949; 32:53−59.

59. Carmel R, Bedros AA, Mace JW, Goodman SI. Congenital methylmalonic aciduria-homocystinuria with megaloblastic anemia: observations on response to hydroxycobalamin and on the effect of homocysteine and methionine on the deoxyuridine suppression test. *Blood.* 1980;55:570−579.

60. Cooper BA, Rosenblatt DS, Watkins D. Methylmalonic aciduria due to a new defect in adenosylcobalamin accumulation by cells. *Am J Hemat.* 1990;34:115−120.

61. Koenig MK, Emrick L, Karaa A, et al. Recommendations for the management of strokelike episodes in patients with mitochondrial encephalomyopathy, lactic acidosis, and strokelike episodes. *JAMA Neurol.* 2016;73:591.

62. Pavlakis SG, Phillips PC, DiMauro S, De Vivo DC, Rowland LP. Mitochondrial myopathy, encephalopathy, lactic acidosis, and strokelike episodes: a distinctive clinical syndrome. *Ann Neurol.* 1984;16:481−488.

63. Hirano M, Silvestri G, Blake DM, et al. Mitochondrial neurogastrointestinal encephalomyopathy (MNGIE): clinical, biochemical, and genetic features of an autosomal recessive mitochondrial disorder. *Neurology.* 1994;44:721.

64. Taanman J-W, Daras M, Albrecht J, et al. Characterization of a novel TYMP splice site mutation associated with mitochondrial neurogastrointestinal encephalomyopathy (MNGIE). *Neuromusc Disord.* 2009;19:151−154.

65. Cogan DG. Heredity of congenital ocular motor apraxia. *Trans Am Acad Ophthal Otolaryng.* 1972;76:60−63.

66. Wieacker P, Wolff G, Wienker TF, Sauer M. A new X-linked syndrome with muscle atrophy, congenital contractures, and oculomotor apraxia. *Am J Med Genet.* 1985;20:597−606.

67. Ahn JC, Hoyt WF, Hoyt CS. Tonic upgaze in infancy: a report of three cases. *Arch Ophthal.* 1989;107:57−58 [PubMed: 2910287, related citations].

68. Deonna T, Roulet E, Meyer HU. Benign paroxysmal tonic upgaze of childhood: a new syndrome. *Neuropediatrics.* 1990;21:213−214. [PubMed: 2290484, related citations].

69. Ouvrier RA, Billson F. Benign paroxysmal tonic upgaze of childhood. *J Child Neurol.* 1988;3:177−180.

70. Schimke RN, Horton WA, Collins DL, Therou L. A new X-linked syndrome comprising progressive basal ganglion dysfunction, mental and growth retardation, external ophthalmoplegia, postnatal microcephaly and deafness. *Am J Med Genet.* 1984;17:323−332.

71. Tarpey PS, Smith R, Pleasance E, et al. A systematic, large-scale resequencing screen of X-chromosome coding exons in mental retardation. *Nat Genet.* 2009;41:535−543.

72. Dattani MT, Martinez-Barbera J-P, Thomas PQ, et al. Mutations in the homeobox gene HESX1/Hesx1 associated with septo-optic dysplasia in human and mouse. *Nat Genet.* 1998;19:125−133.

73. Webb EA, Dattani MT. Septo-optic dysplasia. *Eur J Hum Genet.* 2010;18:393−397.

74. Dick KJ, Eckhardt M, Paisan-Ruiz C, et al. Mutation of FA2H underlies a complicated form of hereditary spastic paraplegia (SPG35). *Hum Mutat.* 2010;31:E1251−E1260.

75. Fink JK, Heiman-Patterson T, Bird T, et al. Hereditary spastic paraplegia: advances in genetic research. *Neurology.* 1996;46:1507−1514.

76. Aicardi J, Barbosa C, Andermann E, et al. Ataxia-ocular motor apraxia: a syndrome mimicking ataxia-telangiectasia. *Ann Neurol.* 1988;24:497−502.

77. Young ID, Moore JR, Tripp JH. Sex-linked recessive congenital ataxia. *J Neurol Neurosurg Psychiat.* 1987;50:1230−1232.

78. Evans JA, Stranc LC, Kaplan P, Hunter AGW. VACTERL with hydrocephalus: further delineation of the syndrome(s). *Am J Med Genet.* 1989;34:177−182.

79. Reardon W, Zhou X-P, Eng C. A novel germline mutation of the PTEN gene in a patient with macrocephaly, ventricular dilatation, and features of VATER association. *J Med Genet.* 2001;38:820−823.

80. Hirata H, Nanda I, van Riesen A, et al. ZC4H2 mutations are associated with arthrogryposis multiplex congenita and intellectual disability through impairment of central and peripheral synaptic plasticity. *Am J Hum Genet.* 2013; 92:681−695.

81. Webb BD, Shaaban S, Gaspar H, et al. HOXB1 founder mutation in humans recapitulates the phenotype of Hoxb1-/- mice. *Am J Hum Genet.* 2012;91:171−179.

82. Yamashita S, Nishino I, Nonaka I, Goto Y. Genotype and phenotype analyses in 136 patients with single large-scale mitochondrial DNA deletions. *J Hum Genet.* 2008; 53:598.

## FURTHER READING

1. Schulman JA, Shults WT, Jones Jr JM. Monocular vertical nystagmus as an initial sign of chiasmal glioma. *Am J Ophthalmol.* 1979;87:87.

# CHAPTER 9

# Genetic Abnormalities of the Optic Nerve and Color Vision

DANIELA TOFFOLI • MICHAELA MATHEWS • TAWANY ALMEIDA • NATARIO L. COUSER

Genetic abnormalities affecting the optic nerve not only include the primary inherited optic neuropathies but also encompass conditions that primarily affect the brain, retina, or other components of the visual pathway and subsequently lead to the common end stage of optic nerve atrophy.[1] Optic atrophy can also be a manifestation of various inherited disorders of amino acid metabolism and heritable neurodegenerative diseases. Dyschromatopsia, or the inability to perceive some colors, can be a symptom of a heritable or acquired optic neuropathy, or be the manifestation of a primary genetic defect without optic nerve dysfunction. Congenital causes of color vision deficiency may result from mutations in genes that code for the expression of the cone photopigments or the cone cyclic GMP-gated ion channels, associated with the phototransduction cascade.[2]

Many hereditary optic neuropathies lead to irreversible vision loss secondary to optic nerve dysfunction.[3] Dominant optic atrophy (DOA) and Leber hereditary optic neuropathy (LHON) are the most common inherited optic neuropathies. DOA is an autosomal dominant disorder resulting in mitochondrial dysfunction. Up to 70% of cases of DOA are associated with mutations in the *OPA1* gene (3q28-q29) which encodes a nuclear GTPase protein localizing to the inner mitochondrial membrane.[4–6] DOA is characterized by bilateral optic nerve degeneration associated with color vision dysfunction, central or paracentral scotomas, and typically slowly progressive moderate visual loss.[7] LHON, first described by Theodor Leber in 1871,[8] is a maternally inherited mitochondrial disorder characterized by bilateral, sequential, acute, or subacute loss of central vision. It is the most common mitochondrial genetic disease, and primarily affects young adult males. The classic form of LHON exclusively involves the optic nerves,[9] but "Leber plus" disease has been described with associated manifestations including movement disorders, multiple sclerosis-like illness, and deformities of the vertebral column.[10] Three mitochondrial mt(mt)DNA point mutations, m.3460G>A in MT-ND1, m.11778G>A in MT-ND4, and m.14484T>C in MT-ND6 account for approximately 90% of cases in the Caucasian population.[11] Gene therapy studies for LHON are currently underway and thus far have demonstrated favorable safety outcomes.[12,13]

Color vision defects can arise secondary to optic neuropathy or from an inherited defect directly affecting the cone photoreceptor cells of the retina. In a person with trichromatic color vision, all three subtypes of cone photoreceptors function normally. These three types are S, for short wavelength-sensitive (approximately 420 nm) "blue" cones; M, for medium wavelength-sensitive (approximately 530 nm) "green" cones; and L, for long wavelength-sensitive (approximately 560 nm) "red" cones. Dichromatic color vision is classified as the absence of one type of functioning cones. The nomenclature is based on whether the first (Greek: prot-), i.e., red; the second (deuter-), i.e., green; or the third (trit-),i.e., blue photoreceptors are missing. Anomalous trichromacy describes defective color vision due to an anomalous photoreceptor and is usually a less severe defect of color vision. Red-green color vision defects, the most common amongst the different color vision anomalies, have an X-linked recessive inheritance pattern and are therefore more prevalent in males. Blue-yellow defects are much more rare and have an autosomal inheritance pattern. Cone monochromacy is characterized by the absence of two types of photoreceptors. As an isolated mutation, only blue, S cones remain functional. Monochromacy can also result from a combination of two separate dichromatic mutations, leaving only one functional type of cone photoreceptors. Achromatopsia, inherited in an autosomal recessive (AR) pattern and often presenting in the first few months of life, is characterized by loss of function of all cone photoreceptor types. Most affected individuals have poor visual acuity, nystagmus, and total absence of color vision.[14,15]

In summary, the molecular basis of many, but not all, optic neuropathies and color vision defects have been well described. Additional genetic associations are found on an ongoing basis. Therefore, this chapter can only provide a snapshot of the wide genetic variety of optic nerve and color vision disorders. Optic neuropathy and color vision defects may be the only manifestation of a gene mutation or may be a component of a complex heritable disease. As such, they can provide important clues to help diagnose the underlying genetic defect, find and predict associated systemic dysfunction, and guide management.

## GENETIC DISORDERS

### 3-Methylglutaconic Aciduria, Type 1[16–18]
*OMIM*: #250950.

*Description*: Type I methylglutaconic aciduria is a rare disorder of leucine metabolism, which is characterized by two different main presentations. Childhood onset is associated with the nonspecific finding of psychomotor retardation. Adult onset is characterized by a progressive neurodegenerative disorder with ataxia, spasticity, and sometimes dementia. Brain imaging shows white matter lesions in adult onset disease. Some patients who have been identified by newborn screening remain asymptomatic.

*Epidemiology*: unknown; 20 reported cases.
*Eye Findings*: optic atrophy.
*Inheritance*: AR.
*Known Genes or Gene Locus*: AUH.

### Achromatopsia/Rod Monochromacy[14,15,19,20]
*OMIM*: #216900.

*Description*: Achromatopsia/rod monochromacy is non-progressive, complete color blindness, due to loss of function of retinal cone photoreceptors. The underlying genetic defects result in disruption of the retinal phototransduction pathway, causing the cone photoreceptors to hyperpolarize in response to light. Onset of symptoms is within the first weeks of life.

*Epidemiology*: prevalence of 1/30,000.
*Eye Findings*: absence of color vision, poor visual acuity, blindness in bright light (hemeralopia), nystagmus, and photophobia.
*Inheritance*: AR.
*Known Genes or Gene Locus*: CNGA3 (achromatopsia 2), CNGB3 (achromatopsia 3), GNAT2 (achromatopsia 4), PDE6C (achromatopsia 5), PDE6H (achromatopsia 6), ATF6 (achromatopsia 7).

### Arts Syndrome (Mental Retardation, X-Linked, Syndromic 18)[21,22]
*OMIM*: #301835.

*Description*: Arts syndrome (mental retardation, X-linked, syndromic 18) is an X-linked disorder characterized by intellectual disability, early-onset hypotonia, ataxia, delayed motor development, hearing impairment, and optic atrophy. Affected individuals have an increased susceptibility to infections, especially of the upper respiratory tract, leading to death in childhood in most affected individuals. The defect is a loss-of-function PRPS1 mutation, resulting in decreased enzyme activity. The same mutation can also cause X-linked recessive Charcot-Marie-Tooth disease-5 (CMTX5; OMIM #311070) and X-linked deafness-1 (DFNX1; OMOM #304500). There are also considerable phenotypic similarities between Arts syndrome and CMTX5. Arts syndrome is extremely rare with only a few families with this disorder having been described in the medical literature.

*Epidemiology*: unknown; less than 20 cases have been described in the literature since 1999.
*Eye Findings*: optic atrophy and nystagmus.
*Inheritance*: XLR.
*Known Genes or Gene Locus*: PRPS1.

### Autosomal Dominant Cerebellar Ataxia Deafness and Narcolepsy (ADCADN)[23,24]
*OMIM*: #604121.

*Description*: Autosomal Dominant Cerebellar Ataxia Deafness and Narcolepsy (ADCADN) is characterized by adult onset progressive cerebellar ataxia, narcolepsy/cataplexy, sensorineural deafness, and dementia. In some cases it is also associated with optic atrophy, sensory neuropathy, psychosis, and depression.

*Epidemiology*: unknown; 24 cases described since 1995.
*Eye Findings*: optic atrophy.
*Inheritance*: AD.
*Known Genes or Gene Locus*: DNMT1.

### Behr Syndrome[25–27]
*OMIM*: #210000.

*Description/Phenotype*: Behr syndrome is characterized by early-onset primary optic atrophy associated with spinocerebellar degeneration. Symptoms start in early childhood and consist of poor vision, ataxia, spasticity, intellectual disability, and peripheral neuropathy. These may result in lower limb contractures and developmental delay. Hearing loss and gastrointestinal dysmotility has also been observed in patients with *OPA1* mutations. Nerve biopsy may show chronic neuropathy with axonal degeneration and regeneration. Symptoms stabilize after a period of progression.

*Epidemiology*: unknown.

*Eye Findings*: optic atrophy and nystagmus.

*Inheritance*: AR.

*Known Genes or Gene Locus*: OPA1 (homozygous or compound heterozygous mutation).

## Blue Cone Monochromacy[28–30]

OMIM: #303700.

*Description*: Blue cone monochromacy is a rare, stationary syndrome with the absence of functional L (long wavelength sensitive/red) and M (medium wavelength sensitive/green) cones. Vision depends on the remaining S (short wavelength sensitive/blue) cones and rods. Some families with progressive decline in visual function have been described.

*Epidemiology*: prevalence of 1/100,000.

*Eye findings*: reduced visual acuity, pendular nystagmus, photophobia, myopia, and macular pigment epithelial changes.

*Inheritance*: XLR.

*Known Genes or Gene Locus*: OPN1LW, OPN1MW.

## CADASIL (Cerebral Arteriopathy, Autosomal Dominant, with Subcortical Infarcts and Leukoencephalopathy), Type 1 and Type 2[31,32]

OMIM: #125310, #616779.

*Description*: Cerebral arteriopathy, autosomal dominant, with subcortical infarcts and leukoencephalopathy (CADASIL) is a progressive disorder of the small arterial vessels of the brain and manifests with migraine, strokes, and white matter lesions. Recurrent strokes may result in tonic-clonic seizures, Parkinson-like symptoms, and multi-infarct dementia in relatively young adults. Acute loss of vision due to ischemic optic neuropathy has been described. Two separate underlying genetic mutations have been described. CADASIL 2 differs from CADASIL 1 by later age of onset.

*Epidemiology*: prevalence of 2/100,000.

*Eye Findings*: acute ischemic optic neuropathy.

*Inheritance*: AD.

*Known Genes or Gene Locus*: CADASIL Type I: NOTCH3; CADASIL Type 2: HTRA1.

## Charcot-Marie-Tooth Disease (CMT)[33–35]

OMIM: #302800, #118200, #118210.

*Description*: Charcot-Marie-Tooth (CMT) disease constitutes a clinically and genetically heterogeneous group of hereditary motor and sensory peripheral neuropathies. Numerous gene mutations cause CMT. Based on electrophysiology and histopathology, CMT has been divided into primary peripheral demyelinating type 1 and primary peripheral axonal type 2. CMT type 1 neuropathies are characterized by severely reduced motor nerve conduction velocity. Nerve biopsy shows segmental demyelination and remyelination with "onion bulb" formations. CMT type 2 neuropathies are characterized by chronic axonal degeneration and regeneration on nerve biopsy and normal nerve conduction velocity. Spinal CMT (OMIM #158590) is characterized by exclusive motor involvement and sparing of sensory nerves. CMT 4 is characterized by abnormal folding of myelin sheaths resulting in a demyelinating hereditary motor and sensory neuropathy.

*Epidemiology*: prevalence of 1/2500.

*Eye Findings*: slowing of visually evoked potential responses, Argyll Robertson pupils, nystagmus, optic nerve atrophy, and early onset glaucoma have been described in individuals with CMT4B2.

*Inheritance*: AD, AR, XLD.

*Known Genes or Gene Loci*: CMT1: PMP22 (CMT1A, CMT1E), MPZ (CMT1B), LITAF (CMT1C), EGR2 (CMT1D), NEFL (CMT1F). CMT2: MFN2, KIF1B (CMT2A); RAB7A (CMT2B); LMNA (CMT2B1); TRPV4 (CMT2C); BSCL2, GARS (CMT2D); NEFL (CMT2E); HSPB1 (CMT2F); MPZ (CMT2I, CMT2J); GDAP1 (CMT2K); HSPB8 (CMT2L). Certain DNM2 gene mutations also cause a form of CMT2. CMT4: GDAP1 (CMT4A), MTMR2 (CMT4B1), SBF2 (CMT4B2), SH3TC2 (CMT4C), NDRG1 (CMT4D), EGR2 (CMT4E), PRX (CMT4F), FGD4 (CMT4H), and FIG4 (CMT4J).

Intermediate forms of the disorder can be caused by alterations in genes including *DNM2*, *MPZ*, *YARS*, and *GDAP1*. CMTX is caused by mutations in genes including *GJB1* (CMTX1) and *PRPS1* (CMTX5).

## Chondrodysplasia Punctata 2 X-Linked Dominant, Conradi-Hunermann Syndrome[36]

OMIM: #302960.

*Description*: Chondrodysplasia punctata 2 is a clinical abnormality that manifests radiologically as spots, known as stipplings, near the ends of bones and cartilage. More than 95 percent of cases occur in females. The mutation is usually lethal in males. Symptoms consist of midface hypoplasia, cataract, dwarfism, congenital ichthyosis, and alopecia.

*Epidemiology*: incidence of <1/400,000.

*Eye Findings*: downslanting palpebral fissures, cataracts, nystagmus, microphthalmos, and glaucoma. Optic atrophy may occur as a consequence of glaucoma.

*Inheritance*: XLD.
*Known Genes or Gene Locus*: EBP.

## Deuteranopia/Deuteranomaly[37,38]

OMIM: #303800.

*Description*: Deuteranopia is charaterized by the absence of the green photoreceptors. Discrimination of color hues is similarly affected as in protanopia, in that affected individuals perceive the red and green parts of the spectrum as greyish-yellow. In contrast to protanopia, color intensity is relatively preserved. Deuteranomaly is caused by a shift in spectral sensitivity of the green photoreceptors closer to the red spectrum. It is by far the most common type of color vision deficiency. It results in mild decrease of red-green hue discrimination.

*Epidemiology*: the highest frequency in individuals of northern European descent: Deuteranopia in 1%–5% of males, Deuteranomaly in 8%–15% of males, 0.5% of females.

*Eye Findings*: abnormal red-green hue discrimination; usually normal visual acuity and optic nerve appearance.

*Prevalence*: XLR.
*Known Genes or Gene Locus*: OPN1MW.

## Costeff Syndrome/3-Alpha Methylglutaconic Aciduria Type III (MGCA3)[16,39–41]

OMIM: #258501.

*Description*: Costeff syndrome is also known as optic atrophy plus syndrome manifests with early-onset bilateral optic atrophy and later-onset spastic paraparesis, choreoathetosis, and ataxia. Patients present with visual disturbance as early as infancy, with more pronounced vision loss in early childhood. Delayed developmental milestones and ataxia are also observed early on with spastic paraparesis developing in the second decade. Elevated urinary levels of 3-methylglutaconic acid and 3-methylglutaric acid may help in early diagnosis. This syndrome is largely found among Iraqi Jews with few affected individuals having ever been identified outside of this population.

*Epidemiology*: prevalence of 1/10,000 among the Iraqi Jewish population.

*Eye Findings*: optic atrophy and decreased visual acuity.

*Inheritance*: AR.
*Known Genes or Gene Locus*: OPA3.

## Enhanced S-Cone Syndrome[42,43]

OMIM: #268100.

*Description*: Enhanced S-cone syndrome is a rare AR disorder occurring due to an excess number of "S" or short-wavelength cones. Evidence suggests that mutations in the NR2E3 gene, which normally suppresses cone differentiation during embryogenesis, lead to a decrease in the number of rods but an increase in the number of cones, particularly those expressing the S cone opsin. Patients present with nyctalopia with or without reduced vision from the first decade of life.

*Epidemiology*: unknown.

*Eye Findings*: decreased vision, with fundus examination showing foveal schisis, intraretinal macular cysts, retinal pigment epithelial changes along the vascular arcades and nummular pigment deposition outside the vascular arcades, and subretinal white dots.

*Inheritance*: AR.
*Known Genes or Gene Locus*: NR2E3.

## GAPO Syndrome (Growth Retardation, Alopecia, Pseudoanodontia, and Optic Atrophy)[44–46]

OMIM: #230740.

*Description*: GAPO is a rare syndrome characterized by growth retardation, alopecia, pseudoanodontia, and in some patients, progressive optic atrophy. Approximately 38 patients have been reported in the literature. GAPO syndrome is believe to be caused by defects in extracellular matrix homeostasis with abnormal accumulation of extracellular material leading predominantly to connective tissue abnormalities, venous malformations, and heart, lung, and ocular abnormalities. Life expectancy is decreased with many patients suffering from interstitial lung disease and atherosclerosis.

*Epidemiology*: prevalence of <1/1,000,000.

*Eye Findings*: strabismus, optic atrophy, glaucoma, megalocornea, nystagmus, ptosis, and keratoconus.

*Inheritance*: AR.
*Known Genes or Gene Locus*: ANTXR1.

## GM1 Gangliosidosis, Type II[47]

OMIM: #230600.

*Description*: GM1 gangliosidosis is a lysosomal storage disorder resulting from deficient β-galactosidase enzyme activity leading to GM1 ganglioside accumulation, particularly in the central nervous system. There are three main types, with significant overlap of clinical features, including type 1, infantile-onset form; type 2, late infantile or juvenile-onset form; and type 3, adult-onset form. Type 2 GM1 gangliosidosis develops between 7 months and 3 years of age and presents with hypotonia, milestone regression, and seizures. Hepatosplenomegaly and cardiomyopathy may occasionally occur.

*Epidemiology*: prevalence of 1/100,000–1/200,000; increased prevalence in Brazil and the Roma population.

*Eye Findings*: occasionally cherry red spot, few cases of optic atrophy reported.

*Inheritance*: AR.

*Known Genes or Gene Locus*: GLB1.

## Krabbe Disease[48]

OMIM: #245200.

*Description*: Krabbe disease is a neurological disorder, generally presenting in infancy and characterized by irritability, severe developmental regression, hypotonia, spasticity, seizures, and early death. Later onset forms also exist. It is considered to be one of the leukodystrophies as it is a disorder resulting from demyelination and dysmyelination. In this disease, the lysosomal enzyme galactosylceramidase is defective, leading to accumulation of galactosylceramide in macrophages with resultant globoid cell production. Psychosine, a byproduct of galactosylceramide, is toxic to oligodendrocytes ultimately leading to central nervous system demyelination. Optic nerve and chiasmal thickening have been noted on neuroimaging, believed to be secondary to globoid cell accumulation.

*Epidemiology*: prevalence of 1/100,000 (US)

*Eye Findings*: nystagmus, ocular flutter, optic atrophy, and blindness.

*Inheritance*: AR.

*Known Genes or Gene Locus*: GALC.

## Leber Hereditary Optic Neuropathy[9,12,13,49–58]

OMIM: #535000.

*Description*: LHON is a maternally inherited mitochondrial optic neuropathy generally presenting in adolescence or early adulthood with bilateral, sequential, acute, or subacute vision loss. Penetrance is variable and exhibits considerable gender bias with 50% of males and 10% of females developing disease. Occasionally extraocular manifestations such as dystonia, myoclonus, ataxia, and multiple sclerosis-like disease may develop, termed "LHON plus" disease. Three mitochondrial mtDNA point mutations: m.3460G>A in MT-ND1, m.11778G>A in MT-ND4, and m.14484T>C in MT-ND6 account for approximately 90% of cases in the Caucasian population and are responsible for 46.5% and 38.3% of LHON cases in two cohorts of Chinese Han populations.

*Epidemiology*: prevalence of 1/30,000–1/50,000.

*Eye Findings*: Patients present with acute or subacute loss of central vision, first in one eye and then within weeks to months in the second eye, although bilateral simultaneous loss of vision can occur. Poor vision is accompanied by dyschromatopsia and large central scotomas on visual field testing. Visual outcome is typically poor with most patients progressing to legal blindness. Visual improvement can occur, typically in patients harbouring the m.14484T>C mutation. In asymptomatic carriers, the optic nerves frequently show hyperemia, microangiopathy, and telangiectatic vessels (Fig. 9.1). Following disease onset, the temporal aspect of the optic nerves becomes pale, a result of mostly papillomacular bundle retinal ganglion cell involvement. Optical coherence tomography shows a thickened temporal retinal nerve fiber layer (RNFL) in asymptomatic carriers, progressing to temporal RNFL atrophy.

*Inheritance*: mitochondrial.

*Known Genes or Gene Locus*: MTND1, MTND4, MTND5, MTND6.

*Special note*: Stealth BioTherapeutics has gained fast track designation for elamipretide, an eye drop for LHON. This Food and Drug Administration-approved designation serves to hasten the regulatory review of drugs intended to treat serious medical conditions that have few other treatment options, in this case LHON. Clinical trials are in progress.

## Metachromatic Leukodystrophy[59]

OMIM: #250100.

*Description*: Metachromatic leukodystrophy results from deficiency of the lysosomal enzyme arylsulfatase A, leading to sulfatide accumulation and abnormal myelin production. Metachromatic leukodystrophy has an infantile-onset form which is the most common, as well as juvenile- and adult-onset forms. Patients with the infantile form present prior to in the second year of life with milestone regression, muscle weakness progressing to rigidity, seizures, and gait abnormalities.

*Epidemiology*: prevalence of 1/40,000–1/160,000. The condition is more common in certain genetically isolated populations: 1/75 in a small group of Jews who immigrated to Israel from southern Arabia (Habbanites), 1/2500 in the western portion of the Navajo Nation, and 1/8000 among Arab groups in Israel.

*Eye Findings*: optic atrophy, blindness, nystagmus, and macular cherry red spots.

*Inheritance*: AR.

*Known Genes or Gene Locus*: ARSA.

## MICPCH Syndrome[60,61]

OMIM: #300749.

*Description*: MICPCH syndrome, microcephaly with pontine and cerebellar hypoplasia, is an X-linked dominant genetic disorder affecting mostly females, likely because most males do not survive to birth. Patients

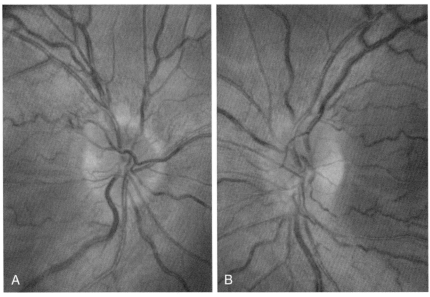

FIG. 9.1 Leber hereditary optic neuropathy. Swelling of the right **(A)** and left **(B)** optic discs involving the retinal nerve fiber layer with atrophy of the temporal fibers of the papillomacular bundle. (Courtesy Sadun, Alfredo; Kim, Alice. Leber's hereditary optic neuropathy, Ocular Disease: Mechanisms and Management; January 2, 2010:330–336. © 2010.)

have severe psychomotor retardation, often without independent ambulation or speech, axial hypotonia, deafness, and various dysmorphic features including a flat nasal bridge, long philtrum, large ears, and severe microcephaly.

*Epidemiology*: unknown.

*Eye Findings*: epicanthal folds, hypertelorism, optic nerve hypoplasia, and strabismus.

*Inheritance*: XLD.

*Known Genes or Gene Locus*: CASK.

## Morning Glory Disc Anomaly[62–64]

*OMIM*: #120430.

*Description*: Morning glory disc anomaly is a congenital malformation of the optic nerve characterized by an enlarged optic disk opening and excavation of the peripapillary fundus with outward radiating papillary vessels, the appearance of which resembles the morning glory flower. Morning glory syndrome is reported to be more prevalent in females and is unilateral in the vast majority of cases. Associations with basal encephalocele, moyamoya disease and PHACE syndrome have been well described in the literature, and it is recommended that all patients with morning glory disc anomaly undergo brain magnetic resonance imaging and angiography.

*Epidemiology*: unknown.

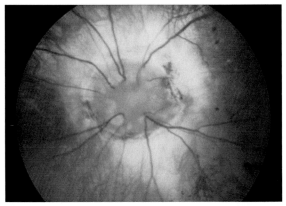

FIG. 9.2 Morning glory disc anomaly. Note the funnel-shaped fundus excavation accompanied by central glial tufts. (Courtesy Brodsky, Michael C. Congenital Optic Disc Anomalies, Ophthalmology; January 2, 2014:871–874.e1. © 2014.)

*Eye Findings*: visual acuity is variable although it is generally poor, ranging from 20/100 to counting fingers. The optic disk appears anomalous, incorporated within a funnel-shaped fundus excavation accompanied by central glial tufts and peripapillary chorioretinal pigmentary changes (Fig. 9.2). Associated findings include amblyopia, strabismus, cataract, nystagmus, and serous retinal detachments.

*Inheritance*: AD.

*Known Genes or Gene Locus*: PAX6 among some pedigrees.

## Moyamoya Disease[65-68]

*OMIM*: #252350 (MYMY1), #607151 (MYMY2), #614042 (MYMY5), #300845 (MYMY4), #615750 (MYMY6), #608796 (MYMY3).

*Description*: Moyamoya disease is a chronic, occlusive cerebrovascular disease most commonly found in East Asia, particularly in Japan where it was first identified, and Korea. It is a disorder involving progressive stenosis and occlusion of terminal portions of the internal carotid artery with development of a compensatory network of vascular collaterals at the base of the brain. Such vascular collaterals resemble a "puff of smoke," explaining the use of the term moyamoya, which means puff of smoke in Japanese. Patients with this disease are at risk of transient ischemic attacks and stroke.

*Epidemiology*: incidence of 0.94/100,000 individuals in Japan; worldwide incidence unknown.

*Eye Findings*: morning glory disc anomaly, ocular ischemic syndrome (reported in one patient with both neurofibromatosis and moyamoya disease), homonymous visual field defects as a result of stroke.

*Inheritance*: AR (MYMY6 with achalasia and MYMY1); XLR (MYMY4); suspected AD pattern for other subtypes.

*Known Genes or Gene Locus*: MYMY1, MYMY1; MYMY2, RNF213; MYMY3, MYMY3; MYMY4, MYMY4; MYMY6 with achalasia, GUCY1A3.

## Myoclonic Epilepsy with Ragged Red Fibers (MERRF)[69]

*OMIM*: #545000.

*Description*: Myoclonic epilepsy with ragged red fibers (MERRF) is a mitochondrial multisystem disorder characterized by myoclonus, epilepsy, ataxia, weakness, and dementia. Onset is in childhood, after normal early development. Associated nonocular findings include hearing loss, short stature, and cardiomyopathy.

*Epidemiology*: unknown.

*Eye Findings*: optic atrophy and occasionally pigmentary retinopathy.

*Inheritance*: mitochondrial.

*Known Genes or Gene Locus*: MTTK is the most common gene associated with MERRF with the most common variant in greater than 80% occurring due to an A-to-G transition at position 8344 (m.8344A>G). Other genes include: MTTL1, MTTH, MTTS1, MTTS2, MTTF, MTND5.

## Optic Atrophy[7,70-76,89]

*OMIM*: #165500 (optic atrophy 1), #616732 (optic atrophy 10), #165300 (optic atrophy 3), #616289 (optic atrophy 9), #311050 (optic atrophy 2), #258500 (optic atrophy 6), #617302 (optic atrophy 11), #605293 (optic atrophy 4), #616648 (optic atrophy 8), #610708 (optic atrophy 5), #612989 (optic atrophy 7).

*Description*: Several genetic causes of optic atrophy are known. Optic atrophy may be an isolated manifestation or be part of syndrome. Dominant optic atrophy (DOA) is the most common hereditary optic neuropathy. It is inherited in an autosomal dominant fashion with up to 70-90% of cases resulting from mutations in the OPA1 nuclear gene (on chromosome 3q29), which encodes a mitochondrial inner membrane protein. DOA presents in the first or second decade of life with slowly progressive bilateral vision loss, dyschromatopsia particularly in the blue-yellow axis, cecocentral scotomas and primarily temporal disc pallor and RNFL loss. The OPA1 (*605290), OPA3 (*606580), and DNM1L (*603850) genes; and the loci for OPA4 at 18q12.2-q12.3 and OPA8 at 16q21-q22 are known to be associated with DOA. Optic atrophy 3 (# 165300) is strongly associated with cataracts.

*Epidemiology*: prevalence of 1/30,000; in Denmark, prevalence is 1/10,000 due to a founder effect.

*Eye Findings*: decreased vision, dyschromatopsia, central or cecocentral scotomas, primarily temporal optic nerve pallor (Fig. 9.3), and cataract (OPA3).

*Inheritance*: AD: optic atrophy 1, 3, 5, and 8; AR: optic atrophy 6, 7, 9, 10, and 11; X-linked: optic atrophy 2.

*Known Genes or Gene Locus*: optic atrophy 1, OPA1; optic atrophy 10 with or without ataxia, mental retardation, and seizures, RTN4IP1; optic atrophy 6, unknown; optic atrophy 11, YME1L1; optic atrophy 7, TMEM126A; optic atrophy 5, DNM1L; optic atrophy 8, unknown; optic atrophy 4, unknown; optic atrophy 3 with cataract, OPA3; optic atrophy 9, ACO2; optic atrophy 2, unknown.

| Disorder/Phenotype | OMIM | Inheritance | Chromosomal Location | Known Gene |
|---|---|---|---|---|
| Optic atrophy 1 | #165500 | AD | 3q29 | OPA1 |
| Optic atrophy 2 | %311050 | XL | Xp11.4-p11.21 | — |
| Optic atrophy 3 with cataract | #165300 | AD | 19q13.32 | OPA3 |
| Optic atrophy 4 | %605293 | ?AD | 18q12.2-q12.3 | — |
| Optic atrophy 5 | #610708 | AD | 12p11.21 | DNM1L |
| Optic atrophy 6 | %258500 | AR | 8q21-q22 | — |
| Optic atrophy 7 | #612989 | AR | 11q14.1 | TMEM126 A |
| Optic atrophy 8 | %616648 | AD | 16q21-q22 | — |
| Optic atrophy 9 | #616289 | AR | 22q13.2 | ACO2 |
| Optic atrophy 10 with or without ataxia, mental retardation, and seizures | #616732 | AR | 6q21 | RTN4IP1 |
| Optic atrophy 11 | #617302 | AR | 10p12.1 | YME1L1 |

## PEHO Syndrome (Progressive Encephalopathy with Edema, Hypsarrhythmia, and Optic Atrophy)[77]

*OMIM*: #260565.

*Description*: PEHO syndrome is a severe AR neurodevelopmental disorder characterized by extreme cerebellar atrophy due to almost total loss of granule neurons. Patients present in early infancy with dysmorphic features, progressive encephalopathy, seizures, hypotonia, and poor fixation. Optic atrophy is noted by 2 years of age.

*Epidemiology*: prevalence in Finland has been estimated at 1/78,000; a few patients have been described from other countries including the Netherlands, Spain, and France.

*Eye Findings*: visual fixation is absent from birth or lost in first months of life, presents with extinguished

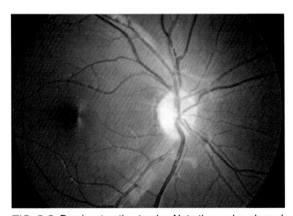

FIG. 9.3 Dominant optic atrophy. Note the wedge-shaped atrophy in the temporal region of the optic disc, right eye. (Courtesy Scanga, Hannah L., MS, CGC; Nischal, Ken K., MD, FRCOphth. Genetics and Ocular Disorders. *Pediatric Clinics of N. Am.* June 1, 2014;61(3), 555–565. © 2014.)

visual evoked potentials, optic atrophy occurs by 2 years of age.

*Inheritance*: AR.

*Known Genes or Gene Locus*: ZNHIT3.

## Pelizaeus-Merzbacher Disease (PMD)[78]

*OMIM*: #312080.

*Description*: PMD is a disease of hypomyelination, arising due to defective or absent production of proteolipid protein, a transmembrane protein found in the myelin sheath. Patients generally present in early infancy with hypotonia, stridor, nystagmus, and head titubations. Patients have delayed milestone development and ultimately limb hypotonia is replaced by spasticity. This genetic disorder is a member of the group of disorders known as leukodystrophies. Leukodystrophy diseases cause degeneration of myelin. This degeneration leads to visual compromises such as optic atrophy and nystagmus.

*Epidemiology*: prevalence of 1/300,000–1/500,000.

*Eye Findings*: optic atrophy and nystagmus.

*Inheritance*: XLR.

*Known Genes or Gene Locus*: PLP1.

## Pontocerebellar Hypoplasia[79]

*OMIM*: #2774709 (Type 2A), #614969 (Type 7), #615809 (Type 9), #612389 (Type 2B), #617026 (Type 2F), #617695 (Type 11), #613811 (Type 2D), #611523 (Type 6), #608027 (Type 3), 614678 (Type 1B), #615803 (Type 10), #607596 (Type 1A), #614961 (Type 8),#615851 (Type 2E), 277470 (Type 2A), #225753 (Type 4), #610204 (Type 5), #612390 (Type 2C).

*Description*: Pontocerebellar hypoplasia (PCH) is a group of conditions affecting the brain characterized by underdevelopment of the cerebellum and pons.

Prenatal atrophy of the cerebellum, pons, and olivary nuclei is followed by atrophy of the cerebral cortex and basal ganglia. Although there is a spectrum of disease severity, the eight different subtypes of PCH include profound global developmental delay and other neurological symptoms based on subtype. Neurological features include hypotonia, feeding and swallowing difficulties, microcephaly, seizures, and extrapyramidal dyskinesias.

*Epidemiology*: unknown.

*Eye Findings*: poor visual fixation, optic atrophy, strabismus, nystagmus, oculomotor apraxia, retinal dystrophy, coloboma, cortical blindness, epicanthal folds, prominent supraorbital ridges, upslanting or downslanting palpebral fissures.

*Inheritance*: AR.

*Known Genes or Gene Locus*: VRK1. PCH1A, *VRK1*; PCH1B, *EXOSC3*; PCH1C, *EXOSC8*; PCH2—(Type 2A) *TSEN54*, (Type 2B) *TSEN2*, (Type 2F) *TSEN15*, (Type 2E) *VPS53*, (Type 2C) *TSEN34*, (Type 2D) *SEPSECS*; PCH3, *PCLO*; PCH4, *TSEN54*; PCH5, *TSEN54*; PCH6, *RARS2*; PCH7, *TOE1*; PCH8, *CHMP1A*; PCH9, *AMPD2*; PCH10, *CLP1*; PCH11, *TBC1D23*.

## Protanopia/Protanomaly[80]

*OMIM*: #303900.

*Description/00*: Protanopia is caused by the absence of L (long wavelength sensitive), "red" cone photoreceptors. Only wavelengths from 400 to 650 nm can be perceived, resulting in pure reds appearing black and the inability to distinguish between blue and purple. Symptoms overlap with Deuteranopia in that all shades in the spectrum from orange to green appear greyish-yellow.

*Epidemiology*: 1% of males.

*Eye Findings*: normal retina and optic nerve appearance.

*Inheritance*: X-linked.

*Known Genes or Gene Locus*: OPN1LW.

## Renal Coloboma Syndrome[81,82]

*OMIM*: #120330.

*Description*: Renal coloboma syndrome presents with renal and optic nerve abnormalities. Patients have hypoplastic and malfunctioning kidneys and optic nerve colobomas (Fig. 9.4). Additionally, they may present with hearing loss, as well as central nervous system and other genitourinary abnormalities. Mutations in the *PAX2* gene, which is critical for the eye, ear, central nervous system, and urogenital development are responsible for the features seen in renal coloboma syndrome. Of note, optic nerve colobomas are believed to

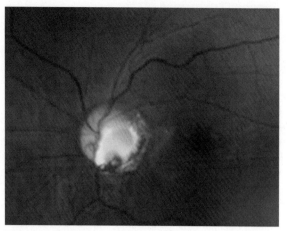

FIG. 9.4 Optic nerve coloboma. (Courtesy Dr. Vikram Brar, Virginia Commonwealth University School of Medicine.)

occur due to abnormal closure of the optic fissure, a critical step in embryogenesis mediated by functions of the *PAX2* gene.

*Epidemiology*: unknown; at least 60 cases have been reported in the scientific literature.

*Eye Findings*: optic nerve and retinal coloboma, scleral staphyloma, morning glory anomaly, excavation of optic disc, orbital cyst, microphthalmia, decreased vision, nystagmus, retinal detachments, and possible macular abnormalities.

*Inheritance*: AD.

*Known Genes or Gene Locus*: PAX2.

## Septo-Optic Dysplasia (de Morsier Syndrome)[83]

*OMIM*: #182230.

*Description*: Septo-optic dysplasia is a syndrome characterized by developmental midline brain defects as well as other central nervous system malformations. Abnormalities including uni- or bilateral optic nerve hypoplasia, corpus callosum dysgenesis, septum pellucidum agenesis, pituitary gland dysfunction and ectopia, and various white and grey matter changes are characteristic. Patients present with decreased uni- or bilateral vision, developmental delay, hormone deficiencies, focal deficits, and seizures.

*Epidemiology*: incidence of 1/10,000.

*Eye Findings*: optic nerve hypoplasia and "double ring sign," and nystagmus.

*Inheritance*: AD, AR, sporadic.

*Known Genes or Gene Locus*: HESX1.

### Tritanopia/Tritanomaly[84–88]

*OMIM*: #190900.

*Description*: Tritanopia is caused by absence of the S or (short-wavelength) blue cones, resulting in defective blue-green color vision. It is the rarest of the dichromatic color deficiencies. To affected individuals, blue appears green and purple appears deep red. Tritanomaly is caused by dysfunction of the S-cone opsin photopigment. Affected individuals have difficulty distinguishing between blue and green and yellow/orange and pink hues.

*Epidemiology*: prevalence of 1/2000–1/20,000.

*Eye Findings*: abnormal blue-green color vision and normal retinal appearance.

*Inheritance*: AD.

*Known Genes or Gene Locus*: OPN1SW.

## REFERENCES

1. Newman NJ, Biousse V. Hereditary optic neuropathies. *Eye*. 2004;18:1144–1160.
2. Behbehani R. Clinical approach to optic neuropathies. *Clin Ophthalmol (Auckl NZ)*. 2007;1(3):233–246.
3. Lee K, Couser NL. Genetic testing for eye diseases: a comprehensive guide and review of ocular genetic manifestations from anterior segment malformation to retinal dystrophy. *Curr Genet Med Rep*. 2016;4:41–48.
4. Alexander C, Votruba M, Pesch UEA, et al. OPA1, encoding a dynamin-related GTPase, is mutated in autosomal dominant optic atrophy linked to chromosome 3q28. *Nat Genet*. 2000;26(2):211–215.
5. Amati-Bonneau P, Guichet A, Olichon A, et al. OPA1 R445H mutation in optic atrophy associated with sensorineural deafness. *Ann Neurol*. 2005;58(6):958–963.
6. Ferré M, Bonneau D, Milea D, et al. Molecular screening of 980 cases of suspected hereditary optic neuropathy with a report on 77 novel OPA1 mutations. *Hum Mutat*. 2009;30(7):E692–E705.
7. Lenaers G, Hamel C, Delettre C, et al. Dominant optic atrophy. *Orphanet J Rare Dis*. 2012;7:46. https://doi.org/10.1186/1750-1172-7-46.
8. Leber T. Ueber hereditaere und congenital angelegte Sehnervenleiden. *Graefes Arch Clin Exp Ophthalmol*. 1871;17:249–291.
9. Yu-Wai-Man P1, Turnbull M, Chinnery PF. Leber hereditary optic neuropathy. *J Med Genet*. 2002;39(3):162–169.
10. Nikoskelainen EK, Marttila RJ, Huoponen K, et al. Leber's "plus": neurological abnormalities in patients with Leber's hereditary optic neuropathy. *J Neurol Neurosurg Psychiat*. 1995;59(2):160–164.
11. Mackey DA, Oostra RJ, Rosenberg T, et al. Primary pathogenic mtDNA mutations in multigeneration pedigrees with Leber hereditary optic neuropathy. *Am J Hum Genet*. 1996;59:481–485.
12. Guy J, Feuer WJ, Davis JL, et al. Gene therapy for Leber hereditary optic neuropathy: low- and medium-dose visual results. *Ophthalmology*. 2017;124(11):1621–1634.
13. Vignal C, Uretsky S, Fitoussi S, et al. Safety of rAAV2/2-ND4 gene therapy for Leber hereditary optic neuropathy. *Ophthalmology*. February 6, 2018. pii:S0161-6420(17)33673-4.
14. Wissinger B, Gamer D, Jagle H, et al. CNGA3 mutations in hereditary cone photoreceptor disorders. *Am J Hum Genet*. 2001;69:722–737.
15. Simunovic MP. Acquired color vision deficiency. *Surv Ophthalmol*. 2015.
16. Anikster Y, Kleta R, Shaag A, Gahl WA, Elpeleg O. Type III 3-methylglutaconic aciduria(optic atrophy plus syndrome, or Costeff optic atrophy syndrome): identification of the OPA3 gene and its founder mutation in Iraqi Jews. *Am J Hum Genet*. 2001;69:1218–1224.
17. Greter J, Hagberg B, Steen G, Sodenhjelm U. 3-Methylglutaconic aciduria: report on a sibship with infantile progressive encephalopathy. *Eur J Pediat*. 1978;129:231–238.
18. Wortmann SB, Kremer BH, Graham A, et al. 3-methylglutaconic aciduria type I redefined: a syndrome with late-onset leukoencephalopathy. *Neurology*. 2010;75:1079–1083.
19. Harrison R, Hoefnagel D, Hayward JN. Congenital total color blindness. *Arch Ophthal*. 1960;64:685–692.
20. Thiadens AAHJ, Den Hollander AI, Roosing S, et al. Homozygosity mapping reveals PDE6C mutations in patients with early-onset cone photoreceptor disorders. *Am J Hum Genet*. 2009;85(2):240–247.
21. de Brouwer APM, Williams KL, Duley et al. Arts syndrome is caused by loss-of-function mutations in PRPS1. *Am J Hum Genet*. 2007;81:507–518.
22. Arts WFM, Loonen MCB, Sengers RCA, Slooff JL. X-linked ataxia, weakness, deafness, and loss of vision in early childhood with a fatal course. *Ann Neurol*. 1993;33:535–539.
23. Winkelmann J, Lin L, Schormair B, et al. Mutations in DNMT1 cause autosomal dominant cerebellar ataxia, deafness and narcolepsy. *Hum Mol Genet*. 2012;21:2205–2210.
24. Melberg A, Hetta J, Dahl N, et al. Autosomal dominant cerebellar ataxia deafness and narcolepsy. *J Neurol Sci*. 1995;134:119–129.
25. Carelli V, Sabatelli M, Carrozzo R, et al. 'Behrsyndrome' with OPA1 compound heterozygote mutations. *Brain*. 2015;138:e321.
26. Behr C. Die komplizierte, hereditaer-familiaere Optikusatrophie des Kindesalters: ein bisher nicht beschriebener Symptomenkomplex. *Klin Monatsbl Augenheilkd*. 1909;47:138–160.
27. Thomas PK, Workman JM, Thage O. Behr's syndrome: a family exhibiting pseudodominant inheritance. *J Neurol Sci*. 1984;64:137–148.
28. Nathans J, Davenport CM, Maumenee IH, et al. Molecular genetics of human blue cone monochromacy. *Science*. 1989;245(4920):831–838.
29. Nathans J, Maumenee IH, Zrenner E, et al. Genetic heterogeneity among blue-cone monochromats. *Am J Hum Genet*. 1993;53(5):987–1000.

30. Gardner JC, Michaelides M, Holder GE, et al. Blue cone monochromacy: causative mutations and associated phenotypes. *Mol Vis.* 2009;15:876–884.

31. Kalimo H, Viitanen M, Amberla K, et al. CADASIL: hereditary disease of arteries causing brain infarcts and dementia. *Neuropath Appl Neurobiol.* 1999;25:257–265.

32. Rufa A, De Stefano N, Dotti MT, et al. Acute unilateral visual loss as the first symptom of cerebral autosomal dominant arteriopathy with subcortical infarcts and leukoencephalopathy. *Arch Neurol.* 2004;61:577–580.

33. Baets J, De Jonghe P, Timmerman V. Recent advances in Charcot-Marie-Tooth disease. *Curr Opin Neurol.* 2014;27(5):532–540. https://doi.org/10.1097/WCO. 0000000000000131 (review).

34. Alajouanine T, Castaigne P, Cambier J, Escourolle R. Maladie de Charcot-Marie: etude anatomo-clinique d'une observation suivie pendant 65 ans. *Presse Med.* 1967;75: 2745–2750.

35. Kiwaki T, Umehara F, Takashima H, et al. Hereditary motor and sensory neuropathy with myelin folding and juvenile onset glaucoma. *Neurology.* 2000;55:392–397.

36. Derry JMJ, Gormally E, Means GD, et al. Mutations in a delta(8)-delta(7) sterol isomerase in the tattered mouse and X-linked dominant chondrodysplasia punctata. *Nat Genet.* 1999;22:286–290.

37. Deeb SS. The molecular basis of variation in human color vision. *Clin Genet.* 2005;67(5):369–377.

38. Drummond-Borg M, Deeb SS, Motulsky AG. Molecular patterns of X chromosome-linked color vision genes among 134 men of European ancestry. *Proc Nat Acad Sci.* 1989;86:983–987.

39. Costeff H, Gadoth N, Apter N, Prialnic M, Savir H. A familial syndrome of infantile optic atrophy, movement disorder, and spastic paraplegia. *Neurology.* 1989;39: 595–597.

40. Yahalom G, Anikster Y, Huna-Baron R, et al. Costeff syndrome: clinical features and natural history. *J Neurol.* 2014;261(12):2275–2282.

41. Chitayat D, Chemke J, Gibson KM, et al. 3-Methylglutaconic aciduria: a marker for as yet unspecified disorders and the relevance of prenatal diagnosis in a 'new' type ('type 4'). *J Inherit Metab Dis.* 1992;15:204–212.

42. Hull S, Arno G, Sergouniotis PI, et al. Clinical and molecular characterization of enhanced S-cone syndrome in children. *JAMA Ophthalmol.* 2014;132(11):1341–1349.

43. Yzer S, Barbazetto I, Allikmets R, et al. Expanded clinical spectrum of enhanced S-cone syndrome. *JAMA Ophthalmol.* 2013;131(10):1324–1330.

44. Hae Hyun Rim P. Ophthalmic aspects of GAPO syndrome: case report and review. *Ophthal Genet.* 2005;26:143–147.

45. Stranecky V, Hoischen A, Hartmannova H, et al. Mutations in ANTRX1 cause GAPO syndrome. *Am J Hum Genet.* 2013; 92(5):792–799. https://doi.org/10.1016/j.ajhg.2013.03. 023. Epub 2013 Apr 18.

46. Troxell TN, Piccinin MA, Smith CM, Parsons ME, Drew GS. GAPO syndrome: a rare genodermatosis presenting with unique features. *Int J Dermatol.* 2018 (epub ahead of print).

47. Brunetti-Pierri N, Scaglia F. GM1 gangliosidosis: review of clinical, molecular, and therapeutic aspects. *Mol Genet Metab.* 2008;94(4):391–396. https://doi.org/10.1016/j. ymgme.2008.04.012.

48. Brodsky MC, Hunter JS. Positional ocular flutter and thickened optic nerves as sentinel signs of Krabbe disease. *J AAPOS.* 2011;15(6):595–597. https://doi.org/10.1016/ j.jaapos.2011.05.024.

49. Carelli V, Carbonelli M, de Coo IF, et al. International consensus statement on the clinical and therapeutic management of Leber Hereditary Optic Neuropathy. *J Neuro-Ophthalmol.* 2017;37:371–381.

50. Chinnery PF, Andrews RM, Turnbull DM, Howell NN. Leber hereditary optic neuropathy: does heteroplasmy influence the inheritance and expression of the G11778A mitochondrial DNA mutation? *Am J Med Genet.* 2001;98: 235–243.

51. Dai Y, Wang C, Nie Z, et al. Mutation analysis of Leber's hereditary optic neuropathy using a multi-gene panel. *Biomed Rep.* 2018;8(1):51–58. https://doi.org/10.3892/ br.2017.1014. Epub 2017 November 8.

52. *FDA Fast-tracks Topical Drops for LHON;* December 19, 2017. Retrieved from: https://www.aao.org/headline/fda-fast-tracks-topical-drops-lhon.

53. Ji Y, Liang M, Zhang J, et al. Mitochondrial ND1 variants in 1281 Chinese subjects with Leber's hereditary optic neuropathy. *Invest Ophthalmol Vis Sci.* 2016;57: 2377–2389.

54. Jia X, Li S, Xiao X, Guo X, Zhang Q. Molecular epidemiology of mtDNA mutations in 903 Chinese families suspected with Leber hereditary optic neuropathy. *J Hum Genet.* 2006;51:851–856.

55. Jiang P, Liang M, Zhang J, et al. Prevalence of mitochondrial ND4 mutations in 1281 Han Chinese subjects with Leber's hereditary optic neuropathy. *Invest Ophthalmol Vis Sci.* 2015;56:4778–4788.

56. Jurkute N, Yu-Wai-Man P. Leber hereditary optic neuropathy: bridging the translational gap. *Curr Opin Ophthalmol.* 2017;28:403–409. https://doi.org/10.1097/ ICU.0000000000000410.

57. Liang M, Jiang P, Li F, et al. Frequency and spectrum of mitochondrial ND6 mutations in 1218 Han Chinese subjects with Leber's hereditary optic neuropathy. *Invest Ophthalmol Vis Sci.* 2014;55:1321–1331.

58. Yu-Wai-Man P, Votruba M, Burté F, La Morgia C, Barboni P, Carelli V. A neurodegenerative perspective on mitochondrial optic neuropatheis. *Acta Neuropathol.* 2016;132: 789–806. https://doi.org/10.1007/s00401-016-1625-2.

59. Libert J, Van Hoof F, Toussaint D, Roozitalab H, Kenyon KR, Green WR. Ocular findings in metachromatic leukodystrophy. *Arch Ophthalmol.* 1979;97:1495–1504.

60. Moog U, Kutsche K, Kortum F, et al. Phenotypic spectrum associated with CASK loss-of-function mutations. *J Med Genet.* 2011;48:741–751.

61. Najm J, Horn D, Wimplinger I, et al. Mutations of CASK cause an X-linked brain malformation phenotype with microcephaly and hypoplasia of the brainstem and cerebellum. *Nat Genet.* 2008;40:1065–1067.

62. Ceynowa DJ, Wickstrom R, Olsson M, et al. Morning glory disc anomaly in childhood - a population-based study. *Acta Ophthalmol.* 2015;93:626−634. https://doi.org/10.1111/aos.12778.

63. Lenhart PD, Lambert SR, Newman NJ, et al. Intracranial vascular anomalies in patients with morning glory disk anomaly. *Am J Ophthalmol.* 2006;142:644−650.

64. Muslubas IS, Hocaoglu M, Arf S, Karacorlu M. A case of morning glory syndrome associated with persistent hyperplastic primary vitreous and Peters' anomaly. *GMS Ophthalmol Cases.* 2017;7. https://doi.org/10.3205/oc000053. Doc02.

65. Barrall J, Summers CG. Ocular ischemic syndrome in a child with moyamoya disease and neurofibromatosis. *Surv Ophthalmol.* 1996;40(6):500−504.

66. Kim JS. Moyamoya disease: epidemiology, clinical features, and diagnosis. *J Stroke.* 2016;18(1):2−11. https://doi.org/10.5853/jos.2015.01627.

67. Noda S, Hayasaka S, Setogawa T, Matsumoto S. Ocular symptoms of moyamoya disease. *Am J Ophthalmol.* 1987; 103:812−816.

68. Baba T, Houkin K, Kuroda S. Novel epidemiological features of moyamoya disease. *Neurol Neurosurg Psychiatry.* 2008;79:900−904.

69. DiMauro S, Hirano M. MERRF: Myoclonic epilepsy associated with ragged red fibers. In: *Gene Reviews.* June 3, 2003.

70. Carelli V, Schimpf S, Fuhrmann N, et al. A clinically complex form of dominant optic atrophy (OPA8) maps on chromosome 16. *Hum Mol Genet.* 2011;20:1893−1905.

71. Chun BY, Rizzo 3rd FJ. Dominant optic atrophy: updates on the pathophysiology and clinical manifestations of the optic atrophy 1 mutation. *Curr Opin Ophthalmol.* 2016;27(6):475−480.

72. Neuhann T, Rautenstrauss B. Genetic and phenotypic variability of optic neuropathies. *Expert Rev Neurother.* 2013; 13(4):357−367. https://doi.org/10.1586/ern.13.19.

73. Lenaers Guy, et al. Dominant optic atrophy. *Orphanet J Rare Dis.* 2012;7:46.

74. Kerrison JB, Arnould VJ, Ferraz Sallum JM, et al. Genetic heterogeneity of dominant optic atrophy, Kjer type: identification of a second locus on chromosome 18q12.2-12.3. *Arch Ophthal.* 1999;117:805−810.

75. Reynier P, Amati-Bonneau P, Verny C, et al. OPA3 gene mutations responsible for autosomal dominant optic atrophy and cataract. *J Med Genet.* 2004;41:e110.

76. Garcin R, Raverdy P, Delthil S, Man HX, Chimenes H. Sur une affection heredo-familiale associant cataracte, atrophie optique, signes extra-pyramidaux et certains stigmates de la maladie de Friedreich. (Sa position nosologique par rapport au syndrome de Behr, au syndrome de Marinesco-Sjogren et a la maladie de Friedreich avec signes oculaires.). *Rev Neurol.* 1961;104:373−379.

77. Riikonen R. The PEHO syndrome. *Brain Dev.* 2001;23(7): 765−769.

78. Hobson GM, Garbern JY. Palizaeus-Merzbacher disease, Palizaeus-Merzbacher-like disease 1, and related hypomuelinating disorders. *Semin Neurol.* 2012;32(1):62−67. https://doi.org/10.1055/s-0032-1306388 [Epub 2012 Mar 15].

79. Rudnick-Schoneborn S, Barth PG, Zerres K. Pontocerebellar hypoplasia. *Am J Med Genet C.* 2014;166C(2): 173−183. https://doi.org/10.1002/ajmg.c.31403 [Epub 2014 June 12].

80. Nathans J, Piantanida TP, Eddy RL, Shows TB, Hogness DS. Molecular genetics of inherited variation in human color vision. *Science.* 1986;232:203−210.

81. Eccles MR, Schimmenti LA. Renal-coloboma syndrome: a multi-system developmental disorder cuased by PAX2 mutations. *Clin Genet.* 1999;56:1−9.

82. Schimmenti LA. Renal coloboma syndrome. *Eur J Hum Genet.* 2011;19(12):1207−1212. https://doi.org/10.1038/ejhg.2011.102 [Epub 2011 Jun 8].

83. Ryabets-Lienhard A, Stewart C, Borchert M, Geffner ME. The optic nerve hypoplasia spectrum. *Adv Pediatr.* 2016;63(1): 127−146. https://doi.org/10.1016/j.yapd.2016.04.009.

84. Gunther KL1, Neitz J, Neitz M. A novel mutation in the short-wavelength-sensitive cone pigment gene associated with a tritancolor vision defect. *Vis Neurosci.* 2006;23:403−409.

85. Weitz CJ, et al. Human tritanopia associated with two amino acid substitutions in the blue-sensitive opsin. *Am J Hum Genet.* 1992;50(3):498−507.

86. Weitz CJ, Went LN, Nathans J. Human tritanopia associated with a third amino acid substitution in the blue-sensitive visual pigment. *Am J Hum Genet.* 1992;51(2): 444−446.

87. Went LN, Pronk N. The genetics of tritan disturbances. *Hum Genet.* 1985;69:255−262.

88. Wright WD. The characteristics of tritanopia. *J Ophthal Soc Am.* 1952;42:509−521.

89. Yu-Wai-Man P, Votruba M, Burté F, et al. A neurodegenerative perspective on mitochondrial optic neuropathies. *Acta Neuropathol.* 2016;132(6):789−806.

## FURTHER READING

1. Gunay-Aygun M, Huizing M, Anikster Y. OPA3-Related 3-methylglutaconic aciduria [Updated 2013 December 19]. In: Adam MP, Ardinger HH, Pagon RA, et al., eds. *GeneReviews® [Internet].* Seattle (WA): University of Washington, Seattle; July 28, 2006:1993−2018. Available from: https://www.ncbi.nlm.nih.gov/books/NBK1473/.

2. Ijlst L, Loupatty FJ, Ruiter JPN, Duran M, Lehnert W, Wanders RJA. 3-Methylglutaconic aciduria type I is caused by mutations in AUH. *Am J Hum Genet.* 2002;71: 1463−1466 [Note: Erratum: *Am J Hum Genet* 2003;73:709].

3. Kelberman D, Dattani MT. Genetics of septo-optic dysplasia. *Pituitary.* 2007;10(4):393−407.

4. Newman NJ. Hereditary optic neuropathies: from the mitochondria to the optic nerve. *Am J Ophthalmol.* 2005;140(3): 517−523.

5. Pelizaeus-merzbacher. In: Post TW, ed. *UpToDate.* Waltham, MA: UpToDate Inc.; 2018. http://cursoenarm.net/UPTODATE/contents/mobipreview.htm?32/19/33072.

6. Verdura E, Herve D, Scharrer E, et al. Heterozygous HTRA1 mutations are associated with autosomal dominant cerebral small vessel disease. *Brain.* 2015;138(Pt 8):2347−2358.

# CHAPTER 10

# Neurocutaneous Syndromes (Phakomatoses)

SUMA P. SHANKAR • JENNIFER HUMBERSON • RAKHI MELVANI • NATARIO L. COUSER

The phakomatoses are a group of systemic disorders with primarily neurocutaneous manifestations. Some phakomatoses have a known inheritance pattern with germline mutations, others have somatic mutations only.[1] Several phakomatoses have been categorized (Table 10.4)[2–4]; the most common include neurofibromatosis type 1 and type 2, tuberous sclerosis, Sturge-Weber syndrome (SWS), and von Hippel-Lindau (VHL) disease.

Neurofibromatosis type 1 (NF1), also called von Recklinghausen disease, affects 1 in 3000 to 4000 people worldwide and is caused by mutations in the *NF1* gene located at chromosome 17q11.[5] It is inherited in an autosomal dominant pattern; half are new mutations. The diagnostic criteria involves two or more of the following: six or more café-au-lait spots 1.5 cm or larger in postpubertal individuals or 0.5 cm or larger in prepubertal individuals, two or more neurofibromas of any type (or one or more plexiform neurofibroma), freckling in the axilla or groin, optic nerve or pathway glioma, two or more Lisch nodules, a distinctive bony lesion (dysplasia of the sphenoid bone or dysplasia or thinning of long bone cortex), a first-degree relative with the disorder (Table 10.1). Additional ocular features include plexiform neurofibroma involving the upper eyelid causing ptosis, refractive errors, amblyopia, glaucoma, and prominent corneal nerves.[6,7]

Neurofibromatosis type 2 (NF2) is caused by mutations in *NF2* gene located at chromosome 22q12.2,[8] inherited in an autosomal dominant pattern, of which 50% are new mutations.[9] NF2 is rarer than NF1, and characteristic features include bilateral acoustic neuromas (vestibular schwannomas) by the age of 30 years and meningiomas. However, ocular findings such as cortical wedge cataracts, retinal hamartoma, thickened optic nerves, and oculomotor nerve palsy may be first presenting features in childhood.[10]

Tuberous sclerosis affects 1 in 6000 to 12,000 individuals, caused by mutations in the *TSC1* gene on chromosome 9q34 or the *TSC2* gene on chromosome 16p13.3, the latter being responsible for the majority of cases.[11] It is inherited in an autosomal dominant pattern and about 50%–70% result from new mutations. Clinical features may include seizures, intellectual disability, and facial angiofibromas (called the Vogt triad). Other features include cortical tubers, subependymal nodules, and astrocytomas in the brain; shagreen patches, hypopigmented macules, periungual fibromas, and astrocytic hamartomas in the retina. Other ocular features include angiofibromas of eyelids, refractive errors, retinal depigmented lesions, retinal colobomas, and optic nerve hamartomas.[12,13]

SWS, also called encephalotrigeminal angiomatosis, is a sporadic, nonfamilial disease that includes hemangiomas of face, eyelid, brain, and choroid; a port-wine

---

**TABLE 10.1**
**Clinical Diagnostic Criteria for Neurofibromatosis Type 1 (NF1)**

**Diagnostic Criteria: ≥2 of the Following Features Must be Present to Diagnose NF1:**

>6 café au lait macules, with greatest dimension >5 mm in prepubertal individuals and >15 mm in postpubertal individuals

>2 neurofibromas of any type or 1 plexiform neurofibroma

Axillary or inguinal freckling

Optic glioma

>2 iris hamartomas

>1 distinctive bony lesion

A first-degree relative with NF1

stain (nevus flammeus) typically in the V1 or V2 region of the face; and seizures.[14] It is caused by somatic mosaic mutations in the *GNAQ* gene on chromosome 9q21.[15] Other features may include developmental delays and glaucoma; managing intraocular pressure in this syndrome may be challenging.[16,17]

Von Hippel-Lindau disease affects 1 in 36,000 individuals. This disorder is caused by mutations in the *VHL* gene, a tumor-suppressor gene located on chromosome 3p25.[18] It is inherited in an autosomal dominant pattern; however, VHL-associated tumors usually show a somatic mutation in addition to the germline VHL mutation fitting with the two-hit hypothesis of tumor suppressor genes. Features include retinal capillary hemangiomas, hemangioblastomas of the central nervous system, pheochromocytoma, and renal cell carcinoma.[19] Genetic counseling for this condition should consider discussing that at-risk family members undergo testing with eye exams, urinary catecholamines, and radiologic imaging.[19]

## GENETIC DISORDERS
### Ataxia-Telangiectasia (Louis-Bar Syndrome)[20-22]

*OMIM*: #208900

*Description*: Ataxia-telangiectasia is associated with progressive cerebellar ataxia and neurologic degeneration, oculocutaneous telangiectasias, pulmonary disease (recurrent sinopulmonary infection, bronchiectasis), hypogonadism, oculomotor abnormalities, immune deficiency, and predisposition to malignancy secondary to chromosomal fragility. Persistent elevation of serum α-fetoprotein is found in more than 95% of A-T patients.

*Epidemiology*: incidence of 1/40,000–1/100,000

*Eye findings*: oculocutaneous telangiectasias (Fig. 10.1), oculomotor abnormalities (such as apraxia)

*Inheritance*: AR (homozygous or compound heterozygous mutation)

*Known genes or gene locus*: ATM

*Diagnostic criteria*: A clinical diagnosis can be established in the presence of early-onset, progressive ataxia and oculocutaneous telangiectasias; identification of mutations on both ATM gene alleles may provide a molecular diagnosis. Progressive cerebellar ataxia along with one or more of the following may assist in establishing a diagnosis: (1) ocular or facial telangiectasia, (2) serum IgA at least 2 SD below normal for age, (3) α fetoprotein at least 2 SD above normal for age, or (4) increased radiation-induced chromosomal breakage in cultured cells.

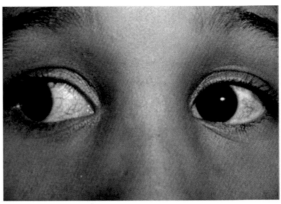

FIG. 10.1 Ataxia-telangiectasia. Tortuous conjunctival vessels on the bulbar conjunctiva. (Courtesy Bielory, Leonard; Bielory, Brett P; Wagner, Rudolph S. Allergic and Immunologic Eye Disease, Pediatric Allergy: Principles and Practice. Published January 1, 2016. Pages 482–497.e3. © 2016.)

### Klippel-Trenaunay-Weber[23-26]

*OMIM*: %149000

*Description*: Klippel-Trenaunay-Weber syndrome is characterized by capillary, venous, and lymphatic malformation with limb hypertrophy. Other findings include nevus flammeus, soft tissue and bone hypertrophy, lymphedema, and risk of thrombosis and coagulopathy.

*Epidemiology*: prevalence of 2/100,000–5/100,000

*Eye findings*: conjunctival telangiectasia, diffuse choroidal hemangioma (rare), glaucoma, persistent fetal vasculature, heterochromia iridum, phacomatosis cesioflammea, ocular melanocytosis, strabismus

*Inheritance*: Isolated cases

*Known genes or gene locus*: mosaic *PIK3CA* pathogenic variants

*Diagnostic criteria*: A clinical diagnosis can be established based on the presence of the following key features: capillary malformation, venous malformation, and limb hypertrophy.

### Neurofibromatosis Type I (von Recklinghausen Disease)[5-7, 27-29]

*OMIM*: #162200

*Description*: Neurofibromatosis type 1 is associated with café au lait macules, axillary and inguinal freckling, neurofibromas, osseous dysplasia, iris hamartomas, hypertension, below average height, scoliosis, seizures, neurologic abnormalities, and learning disabilities. NF1 patients are at higher risk for several types of tumors and malignancies, including astrocytomas and brainstem gliomas. Benign neurofibromas are at risk for malignant transformation.

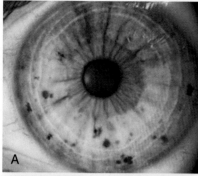
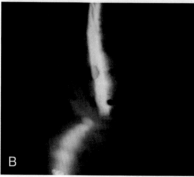

FIG. 10.2 Neurofibromatosis Type 1. **(A)** Pigmented iris hamartomas. **(B)** Slit-lamp examination showing differentiation from iris freckles. Iris freckles are flat and have a lace-work structure. Lisch nodules are raised, round, fluffy, and light brown. (Courtesy Habif, Thomas P., MD, Cutaneous manifestations of internal disease, Clinical Dermatology. Published January 1, 2016. Pages 986–1008. © 2016.)

*Epidemiology*: incidence of 1/3000–1/4000

*Eye findings*: lisch nodules (iris hamartomas) (Fig. 10.2), choroidal nodules, glaucoma, optic nerve glioma, plexiform neurofibromas involving the orbit

*Inheritance*: AD, inherited or de novo mutations

*Known genes or gene locus*: NF1

## Neurofibromatosis Type II[8,30–33]

*OMIM*: #101000

*Description*: Neurofibromatosis type 2 is characterized by predisposition to several neural tumors, the most common of which include vestibular schwannomas (bilateral), other cranial nerve schwannomas, meningiomas, and spinal tumors such as intrinsic ependymomas (Table 10.2). Other findings include peripheral neuropathy, cataracts, epiretinal membranes, retinal hamartomas, and tumors and plaques of the skin.

**TABLE 10.2**
**Clinical Diagnostic Criteria for Neurofibromatosis Type II (NF2)**

| **Diagnostic criteria: A Clinical Diagnosis of NF2 Can be Made if ≥1 of the Following Criteria Exist:** |
|---|
| Bilateral vestibular schwannomas diagnosed before the age of 70 years |
| Unilateral vestibular schwannoma diagnosed before the age of 70 years with family history of first-degree relative with NF2 |
| >2 of the following: meningioma, nonvestibular schwannoma, neurofibroma, glioma, cerebral calcification, cataract; and either family history of first-degree relative with NF2 or unilateral vestibular schwannoma (negative LZTR1 testing) |
| Multiple meningiomas and unilateral vestibular schwannoma or >2 of the following: nonvestibular schwannoma, neurofibroma, glioma, cerebral calcification, cataract |
| *NF2* gene mutation identified from blood sample or from 2 separate tumors |

*Epidemiology*: incidence of 1/30,000

*Eye findings*: cataracts (early onset, typically posterior subcapsular), epiretinal membranes, optic nerve gliomas, meningiomas, retinal hamartomas

*Inheritance*: AD

*Known genes or gene locus*: NF2, inherited or de novo mutations

## Sturge-Weber Syndrome (Cerebrofacial Angiomatosis)[14,16,17,34]

*OMIM*: #185300

*Description*: Sturge-Weber syndrome is a congenital vascular disorder characterized by facial capillary malformation (port-wine stain) (Fig. 10.3) and leptomeningial vascular malformation (angioma). SWS primarily affects the brain and eye, causing neurologic symptoms such as intellectual disability, seizures, neurologic deficits, visual field deficits, glaucoma, and hydrocephalus.

*Epidemiology*: incidence of 1/20,000–1/50,000

*Eye findings*: choroidal hemangioma (diffuse), episcleral and conjunctival vascular malformations, iris heterochromia, glaucoma, visual field defects, increased risk of choroidal effusion with surgical treatment of glaucoma

*Inheritance*: Isolated cases

*Known genes or gene locus*: Somatic mutations in *GNAQ*

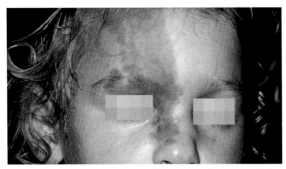

FIG. 10.3 Sturge-Weber syndrome. Involvement of the entire V1 area puts the patient at high risk of having Sturge-Weber syndrome. (Courtesy Habif, Thomas P., MD, Vascular tumors and malformations, Clinical Dermatology. Published January 1, 2016. Pages 901–922. © 2016.)

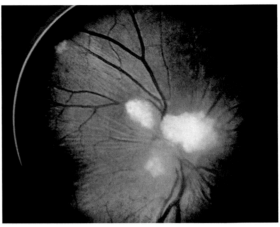

FIG. 10.4 Retinal hamartomas of tuberous sclerosis. (Courtesy Tsao, Hensin; Luo, Su. Neurofibromatosis and Tuberous Sclerosis Complex, Dermatology. Published January 1, 2018. Pages 985–1003.e2. © 2018.)

## Tuberous Sclerosis (Bourneville Syndrome)[11,35,36]

*OMIM*: #191100, #613254

*Description*: Tuberous sclerosis complex is associated with seizures, intellectual disability, cardiac rhabdomyomas, facial angiofibromas, periungual fibromas, shagreen patches, hamartomatous lesions, and a high association with the autism spectrum disorder. A diagnosis may be made by establishing a pathogenic mutation in the associated genes or meeting the clinical diagnostic criteria of 2012 (Table 10.3). A definite diagnosis involves two major features or one major feature with two minor features. (Exception: combination of lymphangioleiomyomatosis and angiomyolipomas without other features does not meet criteria.) A possible diagnosis involves one major feature or one major and one minor feature or more than two minor features.

*Epidemiology*: incidence of 1/6000

*Eye findings*: facial angiofibromas of eyelids, retinal hamartomas (Fig. 10.4)

*Inheritance*: AD (2/3 de novo)

*Known genes or gene locus*: *TSC1* and *TSC2*

## Von Hippel-Lindau Syndrome (Retinal Angiomatosis)[18,19,37]

*OMIM*: #193300

*Description*: Von Hippel-Lindau syndrome is an inherited cancer syndrome, predisposing patients to a variety of tumors, both benign and malignant. Common tumors predisposed by VHL include pheochromocytomas, renal cell carcinomas (clear cell), retinal angiomas and hemangioblastomas (Fig. 10.5), cerebellar hemangioblastomas, and pancreatic tumors.

*Epidemiology*: incidence of 1/36,000

*Eye findings*: retinal angioma, retinal hemangioblastoma

*Inheritance*: AD, most inherited, 20% de novo

*Known genes or gene locus*: *VHL*

## Wyburn-Mason Syndrome[38]

*OMIM*: n/a

*Description*: Wyburn-Mason Syndrome is characterized by congenital arteriovenous malformations typically affecting the eyes, central nervous system, and occasionally skin. Arteriovenous malformations (AVMs) of the CNS can cause seizure, paralysis,

### TABLE 10.3
### Major and Minor Clinical Features of Tuberous Sclerosis

| Major Features | Minor Features |
|---|---|
| >3 angiofibromas or forehead plaque | >3 dental enamel pits |
| >3 hypomelanotic macules | >2 intraoral fibromas |
| >2 ungual fibromas | Nonrenal hamartomas |
| Shagreen patch or multiple collagenomas | Retinal achromic patch |
| Multiple retinal hamartomas | "Confetti" skin lesions |
| >3 Cortical dysplasias | Multiple renal cysts |
| Subependymal nodule(s) | |
| Subependymal giant cell astrocytoma(s) | |
| Cardiac rhabdomyoma | |
| Lymphangioleiomyomatosis | |
| >2 angiomyolipomas | |

**TABLE 10.4**
Neurocutaneous Disorders With Known Gene Associations and Key Ophthalmic Features

| Neurocutaneous Disorders | OMIM | Known Gene | Key Ophthalmic Feature(s) |
|---|---|---|---|
| Ataxia-telangiectasia (louis-bar syndrome) | #208900 | ATM | Oculocutaneous telangiectasias, oculomotor abnormalities |
| Basal cell nevus syndrome | #109400 | PTCH1, PTCH2, SUFU | Periocular basal cell carcinomas |
| Blue rubber bleb nevus syndrome | %112200 | — | Proptosis |
| Cerebral cavernous malformations | #116860 | CCM1 | Retinal cavernous hemangioma |
| Hereditary hemorrhagic telangiectasia (Osler-Rendu-Weber disease) | #187300 | ENG, HHT3, HHT4, GDF2, ACVRL1 | Conjunctival telangiectasia |
| Hypomelanosis of ito (incontinentia pigmenti achromians) | #300337 | (Chromosomal mosaicism) | Strabismus |
| Incontinentia pigmenti | #308300 | IKBKG | Retinal vascular proliferation, retinal detachments |
| Klippel-Trenaunay-Weber syndrome | %149000 | — | Conjunctival telangiectasia, glaucoma |
| Legius syndrome | #611431 | SPRED1 | Hypertelorism |
| Leopard syndrome (Noonan syndrome with multiple lentigines) | #151100 | PTPN11, RAF1, BRAF | Hypertelorism |
| Neurocutaneous melanosis | #249400 | NRAS | Iris melanosis |
| Neurofibromatosis type 1 (von Recklinghausen disease) | #162200 | NF1 | Lisch nodules, optic nerve glioma |
| Neurofibromatosis type 2 | #101000 | NF2 | Posterior subcapsular cataracts, optic nerve sheath meningiomas |
| PHACE association | 606519 | — | Cataract, microphthalmia, optic nerve hypoplasia |
| Schimmelpenning-Feuerstein-Mims syndrome (organoid nevus syndrome, epidermal nevus syndrome, linear sebaceous nevus syndrome) | #163200 | Postzygotic somatic mutations in NRAS, HRAS, KRAS | Eyelid lipodermoid, coloboma |
| Sturge-Weber syndrome (cerebrofacial angiomatosis) | #185300 | Somatic mutations in GNAQ | Diffuse choroidal hemangioma, glaucoma |
| Tuberous sclerosis (Bourneville syndrome) | #191100,#613254 | TSC1, TSC2 | Retinal hamartomas |
| von Hippel-Lindau syndrome (retinal angiomatosis) | #193300 | VHL | Retinal hemangioblastoma |
| Wyburn-Mason syndrome | — | — | Racemose hemangioma of the retina |

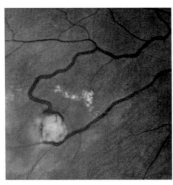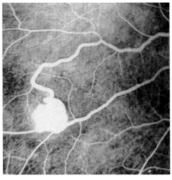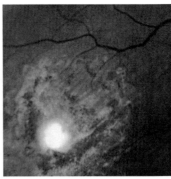

FIG. 10.5 Small capillary hemangioblastoma showing dilated and tortuous feeding vessels in color fundus photo (left). Fluorescein angiogram shows the hyperfluorescent vascular tumor with its feeding and draining vessels (middle). Regression of the lesion after treatment with laser photocoagulation (right). (Courtesy Freund, K. Bailey, MD; Sarraf, David, MD. Oncology The Retinal Atlas. Published December 31, 2016. Pages 763–912. © 2017.)

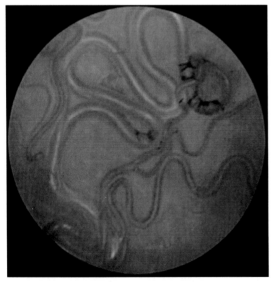

FIG. 10.6 Wyburn-Mason syndrome. Complex arteriovenous malformation of retina. (Courtesy Augsburger, James J.; Bolling, James P.; Corrêa, Zélia M. Phakomatoses, Ophthalmology. Published January 1, 2014. Pages 844–849.e1. © 2014.)

*Epidemiology*: unknown

*Eye findings*: blepharoptosis, cranial nerve palsies, dilated conjunctival vessels, optic atrophy, proptosis, racemose hemangioma of the retina (Fig. 10.6)

*Inheritance*: Unknown

*Known genes or gene locus*: Unknown

## REFERENCES

1. Kerrison JB, Newman NJ. The phacomatoses. *Neurosurg Clin N Am.* 1999;10(4):775–787.
2. Rosser T. Neurocutaneous disorders. *Continuum Lifelong Learn Neurol.* 2018;24(1):96–129. Copyright: © 2018 American Academy of Neurology.
3. Korf BR, Bebin EM. Neurocutaneous disorders in children. *Pediatr Rev.* 2017;38(3):119–128. https://doi.org/10.1542/pir.2015-0118.
4. Edelstein S1, Naidich TP, Newton TH. The rare phakomatoses. *Neuroimaging Clin N Am.* 2004;14(2):185–217.
5. Sabatini C, et al. Treatment of neurofibromatosis type 1. *Curr Treat Options Neurol.* 2015;17(6):355.
6. Friedman JM. Neurofibromatosis 1. In: Adam MP, Ardinger HH, Pagon RA, et al., eds. *GeneReviews® [Internet].* Seattle (WA): University of Washington, Seattle; 1998:1993–2018.
7. Kinori M, Hodgson N, Zeid JL. Ophthalmic manifestations in neurofibromatosis type 1. *Surv Ophthalmol.* 2018;63(4):518–533. https://doi.org/10.1016/j.survophthal.2017.10.007. Epub 2017 Nov 16.
8. Davidson TB, et al. Microdeletion del(22)(q12.2) encompassing the facial development-associated gene, MN1 (meningioma 1) in a child with Pierre-Robin sequence (including cleft palate) and neurofibromatosis 2 (NF2): a case report and review of the literature. *BMC Med Genet.* 2012;13:19.

headache and nuchal rigidity. Hemorrhage of the AVMs may cause severe neurologic deficits or death. Retinal and vitreous hemorrhages, retinal central venous occlusion with risk of rubeosis iridis and secondary glaucoma can occur as complications. Other reported ocular complications include proptosis, cranial nerve palsies, strabismus, amblyopia, gaze paresis, nystagmus, optic atrophy, papilledema, and hemianopias.

9. Rouleau GA, Merel P, Lutchman M, et al. Alteration in a new gene encoding a putative membrane-organizing protein causes neuro-fibromatosis type 2. *Nature*. 1993;363: 515–521.

10. Evans DG. Neurofibromatosis 2. In: Adam MP, Ardinger HH, Pagon RA, et al., eds. *GeneReviews® [Internet]*. Seattle (WA): University of Washington, Seattle; 1998:1993–2018.

11. Leung AK, Robson WL. Tuberous sclerosis complex: a review. *J Pediatr Health Care*. 2007;21(2):108–114.

12. Hodgson N, Kinori M, Goldbaum MH, Robbins SL. Ophthalmic manifestations of tuberous sclerosis: a review. *Clin Exp Ophthalmol*. 2017;45(1):81–86. https://doi.org/10.1111/ceo.12806 [Epub 2016 Sep. 15].

13. Rowley SA. Ophthalmic manifestations of tuberous sclerosis: a population based study. *Br J Ophthalmol*. 2001; 85(4):420–423.

14. Maslin JS, Dorairaj SK, Ritch R. Sturge-weber syndrome (encephalotrigeminal angiomatosis): recent advances and future challenges. *Asia Pac J Ophthalmol (Phila)*. 2014;3(6):361–367.

15. Shirley MD, Tang H, Gallione CJ, et al. Sturge-Weber syndrome and port-wine stains caused by somatic mutation in GNAQ. *N Eng J Med*. 2013;368:1971–1979.

16. Baselga E. Sturge-Weber syndrome. *Semin Cutan Med Surg*. 2004;23(2):87–98.

17. Lavaju P, Mahat P. Management of childhood glaucoma in Sturge Weber syndrome: a challenge. *Nepal J Ophthalmol*. 2015;7(14):194–197. https://doi.org/10.3126/nepjoph.v7i2.14979.

18. Chittiboina P, Lonser RR. Von Hippel-Lindau disease. *Handb Clin Neurol*. 2015;132:139–156.

19. Frantzen C, Klasson TD, Links TP, et al. Von Hippel-Lindau syndrome. In: Adam MP, Ardinger HH, Pagon RA, et al., eds. *GeneReviews® [Internet]*. Seattle (WA): University of Washington, Seattle; 2000:1993–2018.

20. Swift M, Morrell D, Cromartie E, Chamberlin AR, Skolnick MH, Bishop DT. The incidence and gene frequency of ataxia-telangiectasia in the United States. *Am J Hum Genet*. 1986;39(5):573.

21. Teekhasaenee C, Ritch R. Glaucoma in phakomatosis pigmentovascularis. *Ophthalmology*. 1997;104(1):150–157.

22. Gatti R, Perlman S. Ataxia-telangiectasia. In: Adam MP, Ardinger HH, Pagon RA, et al., eds. *GeneReviews® [Internet]*. Seattle (WA): University of Washington, Seattle; 1999:1993–2018.

23. Jacob AG, Driscoll DJ, Shaughnessy WJ, Stanson AW, Clay RP, Gloviczki P. Klippel-Trenaunay syndrome: spectrum and management. *Mayo Clin Proc*. 1998;73(1): 28–36 (Elsevier).

24. Luks VL, Kamitaki N, Vivero MP, et al. Lymphatic and other vascular malformative/overgrowth disorders are caused by somatic mutations in PIK3CA. *J Pediatrics*. 2015;166(4):1048–1054.

25. Moreira Júnior CA, Moreira Neto CA, Amadeu NT, Ghem MRD. Ophthalmological manifestation of the Klippel Trenaunay syndrome. *Rev Bras Oftalmol*. 2016; 75(5):405–408.

26. Mirzaa G, Conway R, Graham Jr JM, et al. PIK3CA-related segmental overgrowth. In: Adam MP, Ardinger HH, Pagon RA, et al., eds. *GeneReviews® [Internet]*. Seattle (WA): University of Washington, Seattle; 2013: 1993–2018.

27. Destro M, D'Amico DJ, Gragoudas ES, et al. Retinal manifestations of neurofibromatosis: diagnosis and management. *Arch Ophthalmol*. 1991;109(5):662–666.

28. Ferner RE, Huson SM, Thomas N, et al. Guidelines for the diagnosis and management of individuals with neurofibromatosis 1. *J Medical Genetics*. 2007;44(2): 81–88.

29. Huson SU, Jones DY, Beck L. Ophthalmic manifestations of neurofibromatosis. *Br J Ophthalmol*. 1987;71(3): 235–238.

30. Bosch MM, Boltshauser E, Harpes P, Landau K. Ophthalmologic findings and long-term course in patients with neurofibromatosis type 2. *Am J Ophthalmol*. 2006;141(6): 1068–1077.

31. Evans DGR, Huson SM, Donnai D, et al. A clinical study of type 2 neurofibromatosis. *QJM Int J Med*. 1992;84(1): 603–618.

32. Evans DGR, Salvador H, Chang VY, et al. Cancer and central nervous system tumor surveillance in pediatric neurofibromatosis 2 and related disorders. *Clin Cancer Res*. 2017; 23(12):e54–e61.

33. Parry DM, Eldridge R, Kaiser-Kupfer MI, Bouzas EA, Pikus A, Patronas N. Neurofibromatosis 2 (NF2): clinical characteristics of 63 affected individuals and clinical evidence for heterogeneity. *Am J Med Genet A*. 1994;52(4): 450–461.

34. Shirley MD, Tang H, Gallione CJ, et al. Sturge–Weber syndrome and port-wine stains caused by somatic mutation in GNAQ. *N Engl J Med*. 2013;368(21): 1971–1979.

35. Evans DG, Howard E, Giblin C, et al. Birth incidence and prevalence of tumor-prone syndromes: estimates from a UK family genetic register service. *Am J Med Genet A*. 2010;152(2):327–332.

36. Northrup H, Krueger DA. International tuberous sclerosis complex consensus group. Tuberous sclerosis complex diagnostic criteria update: recommendations of the 2012 international tuberous sclerosis complex consensus conference. *Pediatr Neurol*. 2013;49(4): 243–254.

37. Lonser RR, Glenn GM, Walther M, et al. Von Hippel-Lindau disease. *Lancet*. 2003;361(9374):2059–2067.

38. Skorin L, Simmons DK. Wyburn-mason syndrome. *Mayo Clin Proc*. 2008;83(2):135 (Elsevier).

# CHAPTER 11

# Genetic Abnormalities of the Retina and Choroid

VIKRAM S. BRAR • MARIAM NASIR • DEV R. SAHNI • JESSICA RANDOLPH • NATARIO L. COUSER

Descriptions of retinal pathology began after the invention of the ophthalmoscope in 1851 by Hermann von Helmholtz, which allowed the examination of the interior of the eye.[2,3] Numerous reports over the subsequent century and a half have described the clinical findings and inheritance patterns of inherited retinal disorders. This group of conditions is extensively heterogeneous; nearly 1 in 3000 persons, or about 2 million worldwide, are affected by one of these disorders, many of which eventually lead to significant visual limitations.[1] Inheritance patterns within the group range from the classic Mendelian inheritance, to mitochondrial or multifactorial (complex) inheritance. In some cases, individuals who are genetic carriers may exhibit retinal findings. Not infrequently, these disorders develop as a result of a de novo mutation. Mutations typically involve proteins functioning in phototransduction or the visual cycle. Inherited retinal diseases may affect the retina and choroid in varied ways and location; some are restricted to the macula, some primarily affect the peripheral retina, while others encompass the entire retina and/or choroid.

The sequencing of the human genome in 2003, along with recent advances in gene identification in the last two decades have significantly advanced our understanding of the pathophysiology of these conditions.[4] Due to these advances, along with ease of surgical accessibility, immune-privileged status, and tight blood-ocular barriers, the retina has been an ideal target for gene therapy.[5]

Retinal gene transfer was first reported in a mouse model of retinitis pigmentosa in 1996.[6] Briard dogs with *RPE65* gene mutations, which have similar clinical characteristics of Leber congenital amaurosis present in humans, became a valuable model for gene therapy.[5,7,8] The Food and Drug Administration approved voretigene neparvovec-rzyl (*Luxturna*, Spark Therapeutics) in 2017 for the treatment of Leber congenital amaurosis, which was the first approval by the FDA in the United States for a disease caused by mutations in a specific gene.[9] Individuals with confirmed biallelic mutations of the *RPE65* gene are eligible for therapy with this novel agent.

Many of the conditions have overlapping clinical characteristics such as night blindness, visual impairment, cataracts, chorioretinal atrophy or degeneration, myopia, and retinal pigment epithelial alterations. Clinical findings may be isolated to the retina and visual systems, although numerous inherited retinal disorders are a part of a syndrome with systemic findings in variety of organ systems. Some conditions characteristically have unique phenotypes that facilitate identifying the correct diagnosis.

Oguchi disease, for example, exhibits the Mizuo-Nakamura phenomenon; there is gray or diffuse yellow coloration of the retina, which is present upon exposure to light but disappears with dark adaptation.[10,11] This phenomenon is a pathognomonic finding for Oguchi disease. Gyrate atrophy, which has the largest incidence in Finland, has a typical pattern of chorioretinal atrophy and a specific identifiable defect in ornithine metabolism.[12,13] The following guide summarizes the clinical features, ocular manifestations, inheritance pattern, and, if known, the gene/loci of select inherited retinal diseases to facilitate diagnosis and in some cases treatment.

## GENETIC DISORDERS
### Abetalipoproteinemia (Bassen-Kornzweig Syndrome)[14,15]
*OMIM*: #200100

*Description*: Abetalipoproteinemia is characterized by the malabsorption of lipid-soluble vitamins, cholesterol, and dietary fats due to the body's inability to produce certain lipoproteins. Other common clinical features include retinal degeneration, neuropathy, coagulopathy, steatorrhea, and developmental delay.

*Epidemiology*: prevalence of 1/1,000,000

*Eye findings*: anisocoria, nystagmus, ptosis, retinal degeneration, pigmentary retinopathy, strabismus

*Inheritance*: AR

*Known genes or gene locus*: MTP

## Age-Related Macular Degeneration[16,17]

*OMIM*: #603075

*Description*: Age-related macular degeneration is a common disorder characterized by gradual deterioration of the macula leading to progressive central vision loss. It has a global prevalence of 170 million.

*Epidemiology*: affects 11 million individuals in the United States

*Eye findings*: choroidal neovascularization, drusen, geographic atrophy, retinal pigment epithelium atrophy

*Inheritance*: Multifactorial

*Known genes or gene locus*: ABCA4, HMCN1, CFH, CFHR3, CFHR1, CF1, C9, C2, CFB, ARMD10, ERCC6, LOC387715, HTRA1, FBLN5, RAX2, C3, APOE, CST3

## Aicardi Syndrome[18–20]

*OMIM*: %304050

*Description*: Aicardi syndrome is a rare disorder that occurs only in females; the disorder is lethal in males. It is characterized by infantile spasms, dysgenesis, or agenesis of the corpus callosum, and chorioretinal lacunae.

*Epidemiology*: incidence of 1/105,000–1/167,000

*Eye findings*: cataract, chorioretinal lacunae, microphthalmia, nystagmus, optic nerve atrophy, optic nerve coloboma, retinal detachment, sparse lateral eyebrows

*Inheritance*: XLD

*Known genes or gene locus*: Unknown

## Aland Island Eye Disease[21,22]

*OMIM*: #300600

*Description*: Aland island eye disease is associated with various ocular defects and is often mistaken for ocular albinism, but there is no misrouting of optic nerve axons.

*Epidemiology*: unknown

*Eye findings*: astigmatism, decreased visual acuity, fundus hypopigmentation, nystagmus, progressive myopia, protan color vision defect

*Inheritance*: XLR

*Known genes or gene locus*: CACNA1F

## Alpers Syndrome[23,24]

*OMIM*: #203700

*Description*: Alpers syndrome or Alpers-Huttenlocher syndrome is characterized by mitochondrial DNA depletion leading to epilepsy, psychomotor retardation, and liver disease. Symptoms usually began between the ages of 2 and 4 years.

*Epidemiology*: prevalence of 1/100,000

*Eye findings*: abnormal visual evoked potential, cortical blindness

*Inheritance*: AR

*Known genes or gene locus*: POLG

## Alström Syndrome[25,26]

*OMIM*: #203800

*Description*: Alström syndrome is an early childhood disease that can affect most organ systems but is characterized mainly by blindness, sensorineural hearing loss, childhood obesity, and type II diabetes. Other possible complications include dilated cardiomyopathy, renal failure, liver failure, and pulmonary dysfunction. The gene mutation has been localized to cilia.

*Epidemiology*: unknown

*Eye findings*: cone-rod dystrophy, cataracts, nystagmus, photophobia, pigmentary retinopathy

*Inheritance*: AR

*Known genes or gene locus*: ALMS1

## Arima Syndrome[27,28]

*OMIM*: %243910

*Description*: Arima syndrome is a rare disease characterized by ocular and brain abnormalities (agenesis of cerebellar vermis), cystic kidney disease, and liver disease.

*Epidemiology*: unknown

*Eye findings*: abnormal eye movements, blepharoptosis, chorioretinal coloboma, extinguished electroretinogram, nystagmus, retinal dystrophy

*Inheritance*: AR

*Known genes or gene locus*: Unknown

## Ayazi Syndrome[29,30]

*OMIM*: #303110

*Description*: Ayazi syndrome, also known as chromosome Xq21 deletion syndrome, is characterized by choroideremia, intellectual disability, congenital deafness, and obesity.

*Epidemiology*: unknown

*Eye findings*: choroideremia, chorioretinal degeneration, strabismus

*Inheritance*: XLR

*Known genes or gene locus*: CHM, POU3F4

*Special notes*: Female carriers often exhibit mild choroideremia and chorioretinal degeneration.

## Bardet-Biedl Syndrome[31,32]

OMIM: #209900

*Description*: Bardet-Biedl syndrome is associated with blindness, obesity, polydactyly, hypogonadism, kidney abnormalities (nephrogenic diabetes insipidus), and intellectual disability. Abnormal cilia account for many of the clinical manifestations.

*Epidemiology*: prevalence of 1/140,000–1/160,000

*Eye findings*: cataracts, pigmentary retinopathy, strabismus

*Inheritance*: AR

*Known genes or gene locus*: CCDC28B, SDCCAG8, ARL6, BBS1, WDPCP, BBS5, LZTFL1, BBS7, BBS12, PTHB1, TMEM67, C8orf37, IFT74, TRIM32, BBIP1, BBS10, CEP290, TTC8, BBS4, BBS2, MKS1, MKKS, IFT27

## Best Macular Dystrophy[33,34]

OMIM: #153700

*Description*: Best macular dystrophy, also called Best disease or Best vitelliform dystrophy, is a childhood-onset dystrophy associated with bilateral macular characteristic egg yolk vitelliform macular lesions.

*Epidemiology*: prevalence of 1/10,000

*Eye findings*: yellow macular lesion, mixed yellow pigmented macular lesion (Fig. 11.1), geographic atrophy, choroidal neovascularization, subretinal gliosis

*Inheritance*: AD

*Known genes or gene locus*: BEST1 (chloride channel on the basolateral surface of the retinal pigment epithelium)

*Special note*: Electrooculogram is abnormal with an Arden (light peak/dark trough) ratio of 1.5 or less, whereas the electroretinogram is normal in patients with Best disease.

## Blau Syndrome[35,36]

OMIM: #186580

*Description*: Blau syndrome is characterized by presentation of erythema or exanthema and symmetric polyarthritis with granulomatous inflammation in children before 3–4 years of age. Between 7 and 12 years of age, patients also develop ocular anomalies. Presentation results from *NOD2* mutations causing gain of function in the caspase recruitment domain 15 protein, leading to subsequent enhancement of proinflammatory cytokines.

*Epidemiology*: incidence of 1/1,670,000

*Eye findings*: anterior uveitis, panuveitis, band keratopathy, cataracts (resulting from granulomatous uveitis), choroiditis, glaucoma, macular edema, optic disc edema, optic disc pallor, peripapillary nodules, retinal detachment

*Inheritance*: AD

*Known genes or gene locus*: NOD2

## Bradyopsia Also Known as Prolonged Electroretinal Response Suppression[37,38]

OMIM: #608415

*Description*: Bradyopsia is a rare condition characterized by a delayed response to luminance which can cause blindness when confronted in sudden bright light. Adaption to dim light can also be delayed in patients also with retinitis pigmentosa or congenital stationary night blindness.

*Epidemiology*: unknown

*Eye findings*: ocular findings indicated normal to subnormal visual acuity which increased in most patients with the use of pinholes due to decreased retinal illuminance. Electroretinogram amplitude findings were reduced for second bright white flash of 0.5 Hz and subsequent flashes indicating rod dysfunction.

*Inheritance*: AR

*Known genes or gene locus*: RGS9, RGS9BP

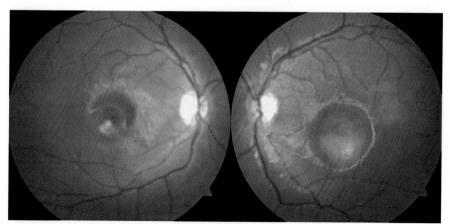

FIG. 11.1 Best disease. Bilateral mixed yellow pigmented macular lesion; right eye (left), left eye (right).

## Choroidal Dystrophy Central Areolar[39,40]

*OMIM*: #215500

*Description*: Choroidal dystrophy central areolar is a macular dystrophy that presents in adults between the ages of 30 and 60 years. It causes progressive vision loss due to macular atrophy and hypopigmentation.

*Epidemiology*: unknown

*Eye findings*: central choriocapillaris atrophy, retinal pigment epithelium atrophy at the central macula

*Inheritance*: AR (choroidal dystrophy central areolar 1), AD (choroidal dystrophy central areolar 2)

*Known genes or gene locus*: CACD1 (choroidal dystrophy central areolar 1), PRPH2 (choroidal dystrophy dentral areolar 2), CACD3 (choroidal dystrophy central areolar 3)

## Choroideremia[41,42]

*OMIM*: #303100

*Description*: Choroideremia is characterized by peripheral atrophy of the retinal pigment epithelium, photoreceptors, and choroidal blood vessels. It usually affects only the periphery and spares the macula, resulting in tunnel vision.

*Epidemiology*: prevalence of 1/50,000−1/100,000

*Eye findings*: peripheral chorioretinal degeneration (Fig. 11.2), night blindness, visual field constriction

*Inheritance*: XLR

*Known genes or gene locus*: CHM

*Special notes*: Female carriers often exhibit asymptomatic peripheral pigmentary changes in the retina.

## Cockayne Syndrome[43,44]

*OMIM*: #216400

*Description*: Cockayne syndrome is evident in the first few years of life and is characterized by microcephaly, failure to thrive, photosensitivity, vision loss, hearing loss, severe dental caries, bone abnormalities, and intellectual disability.

*Epidemiology*: incidence of 1/2,000,000−1/3,000,000

*Eye findings*: cataracts, corneal opacity, decreased lacrimation, hyperopia, iris hypoplasia, microphthalmos, nystagmus, optic atrophy, pigmentary retinopathy, strabismus

*Inheritance*: AR

*Known genes or gene locus*: ERCC8 (type A), ERCC6 (type B)

## Cone-Rod Dystrophy[45–57]

*OMIM*: #304020

*Description*: Cone-rod dystrophy involves loss of both cone and rod functions. In contrast to cone dystrophy, where rod function is reduced later in life, in cone-rod dystrophy, both cone and rod functions show early impairment in function. Patients present with decreased central vision, loss of color vision, and may experience photophobia. Nyctalopia or night blindness may also occur during the disease course due to abnormal rod function. Onset is in early childhood with progression to legal blindness by age 40. Cone-rod dystrophy may be associated with disorders such as Bardet-Biedel syndrome or spinocerebellar ataxia type 7 (SCA7), for example.

*Epidemiology*: prevalence of 1/30,000−1/40,000

*Eye findings*: decreased central vision, central scotoma, dyschromatopsia, macular pigment deposits and atrophy, temporal optic nerve pallor, retinal vascular attenuation, peripheral retinal pigmentary changes

*Inheritance*: AD, AR, XLR

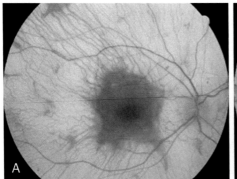 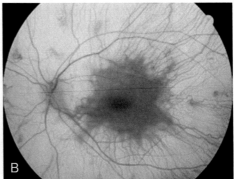

FIG. 11.2 Choroideremia. Chorioretinal atrophy of right **(A)** and left **(B)** eye. (Courtesy MacDonald IM, Russell L. Choroideremia: new findings from ocular pathology and review of recent literature. *Surv Ophthalmol*. May 1, 2009;54(3):401−407. © 2009.)

*Known genes or gene locus*: Several forms with known molecular basis. *ABCA4* is the most prevalent gene involved in AR cone-rod dystrophy. *CRX* and *GUCY2D* are the most prevalent causes of AD cone-rod dystrophy. *RPGR* is responsible for about two-thirds of X-linked forms; the *CACNA1F* gene on chromosome Xp11.23 and an unidentified gene at chromosome Xq27 are also associated with the X-linked form. Additional genes involved with autosomal forms include *ADAM9, AIPL1, C8ORF37, CDHR1, DRAM2, GUCA1A, PITPNM3, POC1B, PROM1, RAB28, RAXL1, RIMS1, RPGRIP1, SEMA4A, TTLL5,* and *UNC119*.

## Congenital Disorder of Glycosylation[58,59]

*OMIM*: #212065

*Description*: Congenital disorder of glycosylation usually presents in infancy and affects many parts of the body. Clinical features are numerous and may include eye abnormalities, hypotonia, neuropathy, retracted nipples, failure to thrive, abnormal liver function, pericardial effusion, blood clotting, and ataxia due to cerebellar hypoplasia.

*Epidemiology*: unknown

*Eye findings*: nystagmus, strabismus, pigmentary retinopathy

*Inheritance*: AR, X-linked

*Known genes or gene locus*: *DDOST, ALG6, PGM1, DPM3, STT3B, RFT1, ALG3, SRD5A3, NUS1, ALG2, DPM2, DOLK, ALG8, ALG9, DPAGT1, STT3A, ATP6V0A2, ALG11, MPI, ALG1, PMM2, MPDU1, DPM1, ALG12, ALG13, SSR4*

## Congenital Stationary Night Blindness (CSNB)/Oguchi Disease[10,60–76]

*OMIM*: #258100 (oguchi disease-1), #610444 (AD 3), #616389 (type 1G), #610445 (AD 1), #163500 (AD2), #615058 (1F-AR), #300071, #257270 (1B-AR), #617024 (type 1H), #613411 (oguchi disease-2), #613216 (1C, AR), #613830(1D, AR), 614565(1E, AR), #310500(1A, X-linked), #300071 (2A, X-linked)

*Description*: Congenital stationary night blindness (CSNB) comprises a heterogenous group of largely nonprogressive retinal disorders arising due to either photoreceptor, bipolar cell signaling, or retinal pigment epithelial dysfunction. Symptoms are variable, ranging from mild to more severe nyctalopia, decreased vision, and high refractive error. CSNB may be divided into two subgroups, comprising those with normal and those with abnormal fundus appearance. Patients with a mostly normal appearing fundus have either Riggs or Schubert-Bornschein subtypes based on ERG findings. The Schubert-Bornschein subtype can be further subclassified into complete and incomplete forms. Patients with abnormal fundus appearance have either fundus albipunctatus or Oguchi disease.

*Epidemiology*: unknown

*Eye findings*: patients with the Riggs and Schubert-Bornschein subtypes of CSNB have a normal fundus appearance; depending on subtype they present with mild disease characterized mainly by nyctalopia in the former, and variable diseases characterized by decreased vision, nyctalopia, nystagmus, and high myopia in the latter. Patients with fundus albipunctatus present with normal visual acuity and visual fields, but also with nyctalopia. Fundus findings are limited to white flecks in the posterior pole and retinal periphery. Patients with Oguchi disease have a fundus appearance characterized by the Mizuo-Nakamura phenomenon, showing a golden yellow fundus normalizing in color after dark adaptation. Symptoms are limited to nyctalopia with normal vision.

*Inheritance*: AD, AR, X-Linked

*Known genes or gene locus*:

CSNB with normal fundus

1. Riggs type
   AD, AR: *GNAT1*
   AR: *SLC24A1*
2. Schubert-Bornschein type
   a. Complete form
      X-linked: *NYX*
      AR: *GRM6, TRPM1, GPR179, LRIT3*
   b. Incomplete form
      X-linked: *CACNA1F*
      AR: *CABP4*

CSNB with abnormal fundus

1. Fundus albipunctatus
   AR: *RDH5, RLBP1*
2. Oguchi disease
   AR: *SAG, GRK1*

## Donnai-Barrow Syndrome[77–79]

*OMIM*: #222448

*Description*: Donnai-Barrow syndrome, also called faciooculoacousticorenal syndrome, is a disorder characterized by facial dysmorphism, agenesis of the corpus callosum, diaphragmatic hernia, exomphalos, variable intellectual disability, ocular abnormalities, and hearing loss.

*Epidemiology*: unknown

*Eye findings*: cataract, downslanting palpebral fissures, hypertelorism, prominent eyes, high myopia, iris coloboma, retinal detachment, retinal dystrophy

*Inheritance*: AR
*Known genes of gene locus*: LRP2

## Doyne Honeycomb Dystrophy (Malattia Leventinese)[80,81]

*OMIM*: #126600
*Description*: Doyne honeycomb dystrophy is characterized by the accumulation of drusen under the retinal pigment epithelium. The drusen enlarge over time and form a honeycomb pattern leading to a decrease in visual acuity due to geographic atrophy and choroidal neovascular membrane.
*Epidemiology*: unknown
*Eye findings*: drusen, photophobia, retinal degeneration, scotoma, choroidal neovascularization
*Inheritance*: AD
*Known genes or gene locus*: EFEMP1

## Ectodermal Dysplasia, Ectrodactyly, and Macular Dystrophy[82–84]

*OMIM*: #225280
*Description*: Ectodermal dysplasia, ectrodactyly, and macular dystrophy or EEM syndrome is a rare disease characterized by ectodermal dysplasia, ectrodactyly, and progressive bilateral macular dystrophy. Common manifestations include hypotrichosis, dental anomalies, and syndactyly.
*Epidemiology*: unknown
*Eye findings*: macular degeneration, pigmentary retinopathy
*Inheritance*: AR
*Known genes or gene locus*: CDH3

## Familial Exudative Vitreoretinopathy[85,86]

*OMIM*: #133780
*Description*: Familial exudative vitreoretinopathy (FEVR) is characterized by peripheral neovascularization due to incomplete development of the vessels in the retina. There is a wide variation in the signs and symptoms among individuals based on the level of severity and risk of ischemia.
*Epidemiology*: unknown
*Eye findings*: retinal detachment, retinal ischemia, retinal neovascularization, strabismus, vitreoretinal traction, vitreous hemorrhage
*Inheritance*: AD (exudative vitreoretinopathy 1, 3, 4, 5, 6, 7), X-linked (exudative vitreoretinopathy 2), AR (exudative vitreoretinopathy 4)
*Known genes or gene locus*: FZD4 (exudative vitreoretinopathy 1), NDP (exudative vitreoretinopathy 2), EVR3 (exudative vitreoretinopathy 3), LRP5 (exudative

vitreoretinopathy 4), TSPAN12 (exudative vitreoretinopathy 5), ZNF408 (exudative vitreoretinopathy 6), CTNNB1 (exudative vitreoretinopathy 7)

## Galactosialidosis[87,88]

*OMIM*: #256540
*Description*: Galactosialidosis is a lysosomal storage disease associated with both β-galactosidase and neuraminidase deficiencies. There are three phenotypic subtypes based on age of onset, with the infantile form resulting in early death. Common clinical features include hepatosplenomegaly, growth retardation, cardiac involvement, and neurologic abnormalities.
*Epidemiology*: unknown
*Eye findings*: cherry-red spot, corneal opacities
*Inheritance*: AR
*Known genes or gene locus*: CTSA

## Gardner Syndrome[89,90]

*OMIM*: #175100
*Description*: Gardner syndrome is a form of familial adenomatous polyposis (FAP) associated with colorectal polyps, osteomas, epidermoid cysts, fibromas, lipomas, and desmoid tumors.
*Epidemiology*: prevalence of 1/1,000,000 in the United States; incidence of FAP estimated 1/7000–22,000
*Eye findings*: compared with routine congenital hypertrophy of retinal pigment epithelium (CHRPE), those associated with Gardner syndrome are atypical in that there are multiple in each eye, and teardrop in shape with the apex directed at the optic nerve. Bear track CHRPE are not associated with this syndrome.
*Inheritance*: AD
*Known genes or gene locus*: APC

## Glutaric Acidemia Type 1[91,92]

*OMIM*: #231670
*Description*: Glutaric acidemia type I is a metabolic disorder caused by a glutaryl-CoA dehydrogenase deficiency leading to neuronal loss, particularly in the basal ganglia. It usually presents in the first year of life and is characterized by macrocephaly, hypotonia, muscle spasms, and developmental delay.
*Epidemiology*: prevalence of 1/30,000–1/40,000
*Eye findings*: nystagmus, optic atrophy, retinal hemorrhage
*Inheritance*: AR
*Known genes or gene locus*: GCDH

## GM1-Gangliosidosis, Type I[93,94]

*OMIM*: #230500

*Description*: GM1-gangliosidosis is a lysosomal storage disease caused by β-galactosidase-1 deficiency, which leads to progressive loss of neurons in the central nervous system. It is divided into three types based on age of onset: infantile (type I), juvenile (type II), and adult (type III). Type I children usually die by 1–2 years of age and can have mild cornea clouding in addition to retinal cherry-red spot and optic nerve involvement. This type presents in infancy and is characterized by neurodegeneration, hepatosplenomegaly, skeletal dysplasia, ataxia, vision loss, developmental delay, coarsening of facial features, and early death. Type III is the mildest form and does not have cherry-red spot. Cornea histology shows corneal epithelial cells with foamy cytoplasm.

*Epidemiology*: prevalence of 1/100,000–1/200,000.

*Eye findings*: cherry-red spot in 50%, corneal clouding, tortuous conjunctival vessels, hypertelorism, nystagmus, optic atrophy, strabismus

*Inheritance*: AR

*Known genes or gene locus*: GLB1

## Goldmann-Favre Syndrome[95,96]

*OMIM*: #268100

*Description*: Goldmann-Favre syndrome is the severe form of enhanced S-cone syndrome that is associated with progressive retinal degeneration, increased number of blue cones in the retina, and a reduced number of green and red cones.

*Epidemiology*: unknown

*Eye findings*: cataracts, nonleaking macular edema, night blindness, pigmentary retinopathy, retinoschisis, vision loss, vitreous degeneration

*Inheritance*: AR

*Known genes or gene locus*: NR2E3

*Special note*: Undetectable electroretinogram

## Gyrate Atrophy[12,13]

*OMIM*: #258870

*Description*: Gyrate atrophy is characterized by progressive loss of cells in the retina due to deficiency of ornithine aminotransferase (causing hyperornithinemia). There are usually no other symptoms besides vision loss, but it could also be associated with hyperammonemia, peripheral neuropathy, and muscle weakness due to the breakdown of type II muscle fibers. Treatment includes maintaining a monitored low arginine diet.

*Epidemiology*: prevalence of 1/50,000 individuals in Finland; less common in other countries

*Eye findings*: cataracts, myopia, night blindness, progressive peripheral scallop-shaped chorioretinal degeneration (Fig. 11.3)

*Inheritance*: AR

*Known genes or gene locus*: OAT

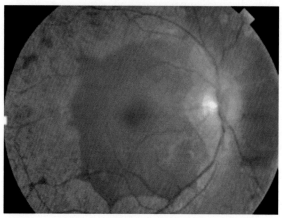

FIG. 11.3 Gyrate atrophy. Characteristic areas of chorioretinal degeneration in the periphery. (Courtesy Lloyd IC. Manchester Royal Eye Hospital; from Ashworth JL, Morris AM. Neurometabolic disease and the eye. In: *Taylor and Hoyt's Pediatric Ophthalmology and Strabismus*; January 1, 2017:664–680.e2. © 2017.)

## Incontinentia Pigmenti (Bloch-Sulzberger Syndrome)[97,98]

*OMIM*: #308300

*Description*: Incontinentia pigmenti, also known as Bloch-Sulzberger syndrome, first presents in early infancy and is characterized by skin, teeth, eye, hair, nail, and neurologic abnormalities. Specific changes include blistering rash in early infancy period, characteristic patterns of clustered pigmented macules ("splashed paint"), skin hyperpigmentation or hypopigmentation, small teeth, pitted fingernails, and alopecia.

*Epidemiology*: unknown; 1000 cases reported in the literature

*Eye findings*: cataract, optic atrophy, microphthalmos, absent/abnormal foveal avascular zone, retinal vascular proliferation due to incomplete vascularization of the retina and nonperfusion, traction retinal detachment, strabismus

*Inheritance*: XLD

*Known genes or gene locus*: IKBKG

*Special note*: It is usually lethal in males early in development due to the complete loss of the IKBKG protein, and thus, it is more commonly found in females.

## Infantile Cerebellar Retinal Degeneration[99,100]

*OMIM*: #614559

*Description*: Infantile cerebellar retinal degeneration usually presents between 2 to 6 months of age and is characterized by hypotonia, athetosis, failure to thrive, seizures, hearing impairment, and vision loss. MRI scans often show progressive cerebral and cerebellar atrophy and dysgenesis of the corpus callosum.

*Epidemiology*: unknown

*Eye findings*: optic atrophy, nystagmus, retinal degeneration, strabismus

*Inheritance*: AR

*Known genes or gene locus*: ACO2

## Jalili Syndrome[101,102]

OMIM: #217080

*Description*: Jalili syndrome is a combination of cone-rod dystrophy and amelogenesis imperfecta. In addition to early progressive vision loss, there is discoloration and abnormal shape of teeth as soon as they appear.

*Epidemiology*: unknown

*Eye findings*: achromatopsia, bull's eye macular lesion, cone-rod dystrophy, night blindness, nystagmus, optic pale disc, photophobia, progressive central vision loss

*Inheritance*: AR

*Known genes or gene locus*: CNNM4

## Juvenile X-Linked Retinoschisis[103,104]

OMIM: #312700

*Description*: Juvenile X-linked retinoschisis is a congenital retinal dystrophy that causes vision loss in males due to the splitting of the inner retinal layers. Vision usually stabilizes during childhood and early adulthood but begins to deteriorate more rapidly during middle adulthood.

*Epidemiology*: prevalence of 1/15,000–1/30,000

*Eye findings*: foveal schisis with nonleaking cystic maculopathy, hyperopia, nystagmus, retinal detachment, peripheral retinoschisis, strabismus, vitreous hemorrhage

*Inheritance*: X-linked recessive

*Known genes or gene locus*: RS1

## Knobloch Syndrome[105,106]

OMIM: #267750

*Description*: Knobloch syndrome is characterized by numerous eye abnormalities and an occipital skull defect. The most common skull defect is an occipital encephalocele, which could be associated with an intellectual disability, but most people with this syndrome exhibit normal intelligence.

*Epidemiology*: unknown

*Eye findings*: cataracts, dislocated lens, high myopia, nystagmus, retinal detachment, vitreoretinal degeneration

*Inheritance*: AR

*Known genes or gene locus*: COL18A1

## Late-Onset Retinal Degeneration[107–109]

OMIM: #605670

*Description*: Late-onset retinal degeneration is characterized by progressive central and peripheral chorioretinal degeneration that usually presents in the sixth decade of life.

*Epidemiology*: unknown

*Eye findings*: drusen, choroidal neovascularization, choroidal atrophy, night blindness, retinal degeneration, choroidal neovascularization

*Inheritance*: AD

*Known genes or gene locus*: C1QTNF5

## Laurence-Moon Syndrome[110,111]

OMIM: #245800

*Description*: Laurence-Moon syndrome is characterized by hypopituitarism, cerebellar ataxia, peripheral neuropathy, spastic paraplegia, and eye abnormalities. It has close similarities to Bardet-Biedl syndrome and Oliver-McFarlane syndrome.

*Epidemiology*: unknown

*Eye findings*: cataracts, choroidal atrophy, nystagmus, pigmentary retinopathy

*Inheritance*: AR

*Known genes or gene locus*: PNPLA6

## Long-Chain 3-Hydroxyacyl-CoA Dehydrogenase Deficiency[112,113]

OMIM: #609016

*Description*: Long-chain 3-hydroxyacyl-coA dehydrogenase (LCHAD) deficiency prevents the conversion of certain fats into energy. It usually presents in infancy and characterized by lethargy, hypoglycemia, hypotonia, muscle atrophy, neuropathy, cardiomyopathy, liver problems, and retinal abnormalities.

*Epidemiology*: prevalence of 1/62,000 in Finland

*Eye findings*: pigmentary retinal degeneration

*Inheritance*: AR

*Known genes or gene locus*: HADHA

## Leber Congenital Amaurosis[114–133]

OMIM: #20400

*Description*: Clinical features of this early onset retinal dystrophy include vision loss, nystagmus, and severe retinal dysfunction. At birth both profound vision loss and pendular nystagmus are fundamental characteristics.

*Epidemiology*: prevalence of 2/100,000–3/100,000

*Eye findings*: cataract, diminished electroretinogram, eye poking (digital ocular reflex), nystagmus, photophobia, nyctalopia, vision loss, pigmentary retinal degeneration (Fig. 11.4)

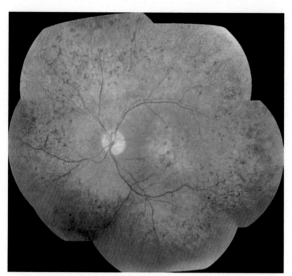

FIG. 11.4 Leber congenital amaurosis; RDH12 -associated disease. Bone spicule pigmentary changes with maculopathy. (Courtesy Michaelides M, Holder GE, Moore AT. Inherited retinal disorders. In: *Taylor and Hoyt's Pediatric Ophthalmology and Strabismus*; January 1, 2017: 462–486.e2. © 2017.)

*Inheritance*: AD, AR

*Known genes or gene locus*: GUCY2D, RPE65, SPATA7, AIPL1, RPGRIP1, CRX, CRB1, NMNAT1, CEP290, IMPDH1, RD3, RDH12, LRAT, TULP1, KCNJ13, GDF6, PRPH2

*Special comment*: The Food and Drug Administration recently approved voretigene neparvovec-rzyl (Luxturna, Spark Therapeutics) for the treatment of Leber congenital amaurosis. Individuals with confirmed biallelic mutations of the *RPE65* gene are eligible for therapy with this novel subretinal injection.

## Leigh Syndrome[134–136]

*OMIM*: #25600

*Description*: Progressive neurodegenerative disorder with focal or bilateral lesions in the central nervous system. The lesions are characterized by gliosis, capillary proliferation, spongiosis, and necrosis. The lesion areas include basal ganglia, cerebellum, thalamus, brainstem, and spinal cord.

*Epidemiology*: incidence of 1/40,000; prevalence varies by population

*Eye findings*: nystagmus, ophthalmoplegia, optic atrophy, pigmentary retinal degeneration

*Inheritance*: Mitochondrial

*Known genes or gene locus*: BCS1L, NDUFA10, SDHA, NDUFS4, NDUFAF2, NDUFAF6, SURF1, COX15, NDUFS3, NDUFS8, FOXRED1, NDUFA9, NDUFA12, COX10, NDUFS7

## Mainzer-Saldino Syndrome[137–139]

*OMIM*: #266920

*Description*: Skeletal ciliopathies characterized by constriction of bones. The thoracic cage, ribs, and tubular bones are involved. The acetabular roof has a trident appearance which is unique to the disorder. There are variable types of this syndrome and polydactyly is sometimes apparent.

*Epidemiology*: unknown

*Eye findings*: bone spicule deposits, night blindness, nystagmus, occasional strabismus, pigmentary retinopathy

*Inheritance*: AR

*Known genes or gene locus*: IFT140

## Mannosidosis[140–142]

*OMIM*: #248510, #248500

*Description*: This condition is a lysosomal storage disorder. The enzyme deficient is lysosomal β-mannosidase. Clinical features include delayed development, seizures, and intellectual disability. Angiokeratomas, peripheral neuropathy, immunosuppression, and hypotonia are other clinical features.

*Epidemiology*: unknown

*Eye findings*: conjunctival vessel tortuosity, epicanthal folds, heavy eyebrows, impaired smooth muscle pursuits, lens opacities, nystagmus, optic atrophy, progressive retinal degeneration, strabismus

*Inheritance*: AR

*Known genes or gene locus*: MANBA, MAN2B1

## Maternally Inherited Diabetes and Deafness[143–146]

*OMIM*: #520000

*Description*: A multiorgan mitochondrial disorder characterized by sensorineural hearing loss and diabetes. Some patients experience cardiomyopathy, seizures, and unsteady gait.

*Epidemiology*: 1% of diabetes cases

*Eye findings*: concentric narrowing of visual fields, external ophthalmoplegia, macular pattern dystrophy, normal visual acuity, pigmentary retinopathy, ptosis

*Inheritance*: Mitochondrial

*Known genes or gene locus*: MTTL1, MTTE, MTTK

## MERRF Syndrome[147,148]

*OMIM*: #545000

*Description*: Mitochondrial syndrome with wide organ involvement. Some characteristics include cerebellar ataxia, myalgia, ptosis, myopathy, polyneuropathy, lactic acidosis, tremor, epilepsy, and dyskinesia.

*Epidemiology*: prevalence of 1/5000

*Eye findings*: optic atrophy, pigmentary retinal changes

*Inheritance*: Mitochondrial

*Known genes or gene locus*: MTTK, MTTL1, MTTH, MTTS1, MTTS2, MTTF

## Methylmalonic Acidemia With Homocystinuria Type CBLC[149–151]

*OMIM*: #277400

*Description*: Clinical disorder characterized by altered cobalamin metabolism. Due to altered metabolism the enzyme methionine synthase is unable to perform synthesis. The missing coenzymes are adenosylcobalamin and methylcobalamin. Some clinical features include failure to thrive, poor feeding, developmental delay, cytopenias, encephalopathy, hypotonia.

*Epidemiology*: incidence of 1/200,000

*Eye findings*: macular degeneration, nystagmus, optic atrophy, pigmentary retinopathy

*Inheritance*: AR

*Known genes or gene locus*: MMACHC

## Mohr-Tranebjaerg Syndrome[152–154]

*OMIM*: #304700

*Description*: Also known as deafness dystonia syndrome, Mohr-Tranebjaerg syndrome is a neurodegenerative syndrome characterized by early onset of hearing loss during childhood, then progressive ataxia and dystonia during adolescence, visual impairment during early adulthood, and dementia from the fourth decade. Although there are more than 90 cases known, not all cases have been reported and the prevalence is unknown.

*Epidemiology*: unknown

*Eye findings*: cortical blindness, abnormal electroretinogram, myopia, photophobia, constricted visual fields

*Inheritance*: XLR

*Known genes or gene locus*: TIMM8A

## Mucopolysaccharidosis Type II (Hunter Syndrome)[155,156]

*OMIM*: #309900

*Description*: Clinical disorder characterized by accumulation of glycosaminoglycans in various organs of the body. The deficient enzyme is lysosomal iduronate-2-sulfatase. Clinical features include severe neurologic degeneration, with also airway abnormalities, cardiomyopathy, and skeletal deformities reported.

*Epidemiology*: prevalence of 1/100,000

*Eye findings*: optic atrophy, ptosis, papilledema, rod-cone pigmentary retinopathy

*Inheritance*: XLR

*Known genes or gene locus*: IDS

## Neuronal Ceroid Lipofuscinosis (Batten Disease)[157–159]

*OMIM*: #204200

*Description*: The neuronal ceroid lipofuscinosis disorders are characterized by accumulation of inclusion bodies which are autoflourescent. Two major subtypes exist, which consist of accumulation of saposins or subunit c of mitochondrial ATPase. Clinical features include progressive neurologic manifestations such as seizures, intellectual disability, and blindness.

*Epidemiology*: incidence of 1/100,000

*Eye findings*: attenuation of retinal blood vessels, night blindness, optic atrophy, pigmentary retinopathy, bull's eye maculopathy, abnormal electroretinogram

*Inheritance*: AD, AR (majority)

*Known genes or gene locus*: CLN3

## Neuropathy, Ataxia, and Retinitis Pigmentosa[157,160–162]

*OMIM*: /#551500

*Description*: Disorder characterized by sensorimotor neuropathy, ataxia, pigmentary retinopathy, and proximal muscle weakness.

*Epidemiology*: prevalence of 1/100,00–9/100,000

*Eye findings*: blindness, night blindness, nystagmus, ophthalmoplegia, optic atrophy, salt and pepper retinopathy, severe vision loss, sluggish pupils, vascular attenuation

*Inheritance*: Mitochondrial

*Known genes or gene locus*: MT-ATP6

## Niemann-Pick Disease Type A, B, C1, C2[163–166]

*OMIM*: #257200 (A), #607616 (B), #257220 (C1/D), #607625 (C2)

*Description*: Disease caused by a deficiency of acid sphingomyelinase. The disorder causes progressive neurodegeneration with type A fatal early and type B with a later onset.

*Epidemiology*: incidence of types A and B combined 1: 250,000. Incidence of type C 1:150,000. Incidence within Ashkenazi Jews is 1:40,000.

*Eye findings*: types A and B: Cherry-red macula (less common in type B), granular appearing macula, intracellular lipid accumulation in retinal neurons/amacrine cells/retinal pigment epithelial cells/receptors, lens with brownish coloration on anterior surface and white spots on posterior capsule, stromal haziness. Type C1: Abnormal saccadic movements, vertical supranuclear gaze palsy. Type C2: Supranuclear palsy.

*Inheritance*: AR

*Known genes or gene locus*: NPC1 (type 1C/D), NPC2 (type C2), SMPD1 (types A and B)

## Norrie Disease[167-170]

*OMIM*: #310600

*Description*: Rare disorder characterized by congenital blindness due to abnormal development and pathology of the neuroretina in males. Intellectual disability, epilepsy, and deafness can also occur. Female carriers can manifest retinal changes or hearing loss.

*Epidemiology*: unknown

*Eye findings*: corneal and vitreous opacities (persistent fetal vasculature), cataracts, iris atrophy, leukocoria, microphthalmia, optic atrophy, pseudoglioma, retinal detachment, retinal dysplasia, sclerocornea, synechiae.

*Inheritance*: XLR

*Known genes or gene locus*: NDP

## North Carolina Macular Dystrophy[171-173]

*OMIM*: 136550

*Description*: Disorder characterized by progressive macular impairment with varying ophthalmologic findings and severity. The disorder is usually symmetric with full penetrance.

*Epidemiology*: prevalence of <1/100,000

*Eye findings*: drusen-like deposits in macula that can progress to atrophy and staphyloma of the retina and choroid, central scotomata, disciform scars in macula, peripheral retinal atrophy, peripheral retinal drusen

*Inheritance*: AD

*Known genes or gene locus*: DHS6S1

## O' Donnell Pappas Syndrome[42,85,174]

*OMIM*: 136520

*Description*: Foveal hypoplasia (FVH) is defined as a lack of foveal depression. This type of hypoplasia can accompany a varying number of phenotypic characteristics such as microphthalmia, achromatopsia and albinism. O' Donnell Papas syndrome in particular is characterized by FVH with presenile cataract and peripheral corneal pannus.

*Epidemiology*: unknown

*Eye findings*: cataracts, congenital nystagmus, FVH, peripheral corneal pannus, presenile cataract

*Inheritance*: AD, AR

*Known genes or gene locus*: PAX6, SLC38A8

## Occult Macular Dystrophy[175,176]

*OMIM*: #613587

*Description*: Hereditary macular dystrophy without visible fundus abnormalities. The disease is classically distinguished by decreased visual acuity with a normal appearing fundus, full-field electroretinograms, and fluorescein angiograms. Abnormal appearing focal macular electroretinograms and multifocal electroretinograms are apparent.

*Epidemiology*: unknown

*Eye findings*: color blindness, dyschromatopsia, progressive decreased vision, reduced focal macular electroretinogram

*Inheritance*: AD

*Known genes or gene locus*: RP1L1

## Oguchi Disease[10,11]

*OMIM*: /#258100, #613411

*Description*: Congenital inherited disease is characterized by normal visual acuity, visual field, and color vision. The disease is nonprogressive, affects the retinal rods, and results in stationary night blindness. The Mizuo-Nakamura phenomenon is pathognomonic for the disease. There is a diffuse gray or yellow coloration of the retina which is present upon exposure to light but disappears with dark adaptation.

*Epidemiology*: unknown

*Eye findings*: A and B waves decreased or absent under lighted conditions, congenital stationary night blindness, golden yellow fundus in light that disappears in dark adaptation (Mizuo-Nakamura phenomenon)

*Inheritance*: AR

*Known genes or gene locus*: SAG, GRK1

## Patterned Dystrophy of Retinal Pigment Epithelium[177,178]

*OMIM*: #169150

*Description*: Macular disorder signified by accumulation of lipofuscin within the retinal pigment epithelium. There are three different patterned types—reticular, macroreticular, and butterfly shaped.

*Epidemiology*: unknown

*Eye findings*: abnormal deposit of pigment in perifoveal pigment epithelium, variable choroidal neovascularization, globular deposits along arcades, loss of central vision, night blindness, rare photophobia, tritan and protan defect (variable), yellow-pigmented material in butterfly shape

*Inheritance*: AD

*Known genes or gene locus*: PRPH2

## Persistent Hyperplastic Primary Vitreous[179–181]

*OMIM*: #221900, %611308

*Description*: Persistent hyperplastic primary vitreous (PHPV) is the abnormal presence of a retrolenticular fibrovascular membrane, typically unilateral, due to a failure of the primary vitreous to completely regress in utero.

*Epidemiology*: unknown

*Eye findings*: retrolenticular fibrovascular membrane, cataract, leukocoria, strabismus, glaucoma, microphthalmia, retinal detachment

*Inheritance*: AR; AD has also been reported

*Known genes or gene locus*: ATOH7 (AR)

## Progressive Bifocal Chorioretinal Atrophy[182,183]

*OMIM*: %600790

*Description*: Disorder characterized by progressive chorioretinal atrophy. The disorder presents in two distinct phases at birth and then early in the neonatal period. The atrophic lesions are first present temporally and then present in the nasal region.

*Epidemiology*: prevalence of <1/1,000,000

*Eye findings*: chorioretinal dystrophy, macular and nasal progressive lesions (atrophic), myopia, nystagmus, poor vision, progressive bifocal chorioretinal atrophy, retinal detachment

*Inheritance*: AD

*Known genes or gene locus*: Unknown

## Pseudoxanthoma Elasticum[184,185]

*OMIM*: #264800

*Description*: Inherited disorder with predilection for pathologic changes in the skin, vascular walls, and Bruch's membrane. Common findings include plucked chicken skin, gastrointestinal bleeds, and cardiac abnormalities. The disorder is characterized by accumulation of elastic fibers which are mineralized and fragmented.

*Epidemiology*: prevalence of 1/100,000–9/100,000

*Eye findings*: angioid streaks (Fig. 11.5), atrophy of retinal pigment epithelium and outer retina, central vision loss, choroidal neovascularization, colloid bodies, hyperpigmented spots (paired-owl's eyes) macular degeneration, optic head drusen, peau d'orange retinal changes

*Inheritance*: AR

*Known genes or gene locus*: ABCC6

## Refsum Disease[186,187]

*OMIM*: #266500

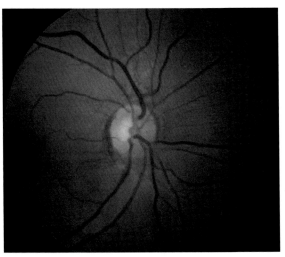

FIG. 11.5 Pseudoxanthoma elasticum. Angioid streaks, right eye.

*Description*: Disorder characterized by both anosmia and early-onset retinitis pigmentosa. The pathology is caused by abnormal lipid metabolism, which results in elevated phytanic acid. Other accompanying clinical characteristics include neuropathy, cerebellar ataxia, deafness, and ichthyosis.

*Epidemiology*: prevalence of 1–9/1,000,000

*Eye findings*: cataracts, constricted visual fields, degenerative maculopathy, night blindness, optic atrophy, pigmentary retinopathy

*Inheritance*: AR

*Known genes or gene locus*: PHYH, PEX7

## Retinal Vasculopathy With Cerebral Leukodystrophy[188,189]

*OMIM*: 192315

*Description*: Disease characterized by central nervous system degeneration, stroke, motor, and cognitive difficulties. The pathology also involves the microvessels of the brain with resultant leukodystrophy and retinal vasculopathy.

*Epidemiology*: unknown

*Eye findings*: decreased visual acuity, macular edema, microangiopathic telangiectasia, microaneurysms, retinal vasculopathy, retinal exudates, retinal hemorrhages

*Inheritance*: AD

*Known genes or gene locus*: TREX1

*Special note*: Hereditary vascular retinopathy (HVR), cerebroretinal vasculopathy (CRV), and hereditary endotheliopathy, retinopathy, nephropathy, and stroke (HERNS) were previously considered to be distinct conditions, but they are now believed to be variations of retinal vasculopathy with cerebral leukodystrophy.

## Retinitis Pigmentosa[190–199]

OMIM: #268000

*Description*: Group of heterogeneous pathologic disorders affecting the retina. Early symptoms include night vision loss and decreased central vision. The "bone spicule" appearance is a characteristic of the disorder. This represents dark pigmented clumps within the fundus.

Promising studies investigating the safety and efficacy of a variety of management/treatment strategies for patients affected by retinitis pigmentosa have been either recently performed or underway. These include studies investigating CRISPR/Cas9 gene editing, vitamin A supplementation, gene therapy, stem cells, retinal prosthesis and nerve growth factor (NGF) eye drops.

*Epidemiology*: prevalence of 1/3000–1/5000

*Eye findings*: attenuated retinal vessels (Fig. 11.6), cataracts, constricted visual fields including notably ring scotoma, cystoid macular edema, dyschromatopsia, night blindness, photopsia, pigmentary retinopathy (Fig. 11.6), posterior subcapsular cataracts, waxy pallor of optic disc (Fig. 11.6)

*Inheritance*: AD, AR, XLR

*Known genes or gene locus*:

AR: *SPATA7, LRAT, TULP1, RP1, RHO, CRB1, TULP1, ABCA4, RPE65, EYS, CERKL, FAM161A, SEMA4A, PRCD, NR2E3, MERTK, USH2A, PDE6B, PROM1, PDE6A, RGR, CNGB1, IDH3B, SAG, CNGA1, TTC8, RDH12, C2ORF71, ARL6, IMPG2, PDE6G, ZNF513, DHDDS, CLRN1, MAK, C8ORF37, CDHR1, RBP3, NEK2, SLC7A14, KIZ, IFT172, ZNF408,* *HGSNAT, BBS2, AGBL5, POMGT1, REEP6, ARHGEF18, HK1, IFT140, IFT43*

AD: *AIPL1, RP1, RHO, PRPH2, RP9, IMPDH1, PRPF31, PRPF8, CA4, PRPF3, ABCA4, NRL, FSCN2, TOPORS, SNRNP200, SEMA4A, NR2E3, KLHL7, RGR, GUCA1B, BEST1, PRPF6, PRPF4*

X-Linked: *RP2, OFD1, RPGR*

Digenic mutations in the *PRPH2* and *ROM1* genes

Syndromic mitochondrial form by mutation in *MTTS2*

## Retinoblastoma[200–202]

OMIM: #180200

*Description*: Disorder characterized by early-onset embryonic malignant neoplasms of immature retinal cell origin. It can be unilateral or bilateral, and if present with a pineal or parasellar tumor, it is called trilateral retinoblastoma. Commonly presents with leukocoria or strabismus.

*Epidemiology*: incidence of 1/15,000–1/28,000

*Eye findings*: white or yellow tumor extending from the retina (Fig. 11.7), anisocoria, heterochromia, hyphema, pseudohypopyon, intraocular inflammation, glaucoma, leukocoria, neovascularization of iris, orbital cellulitis, proptosis, retinal calcification, retinal detachment, retinoma, red painful eye, spontaneous globe perforation, strabismus, tearing, vitritis, vitreous hemorrhage

*Inheritance*: AD, sporadic

*Known genes or gene locus*: RB1

## Revesz Syndrome[203–205]

OMIM: #268130

*Description*: Telomere disorder within a spectrum of dyskeratosis congenita. Characteristics include bone

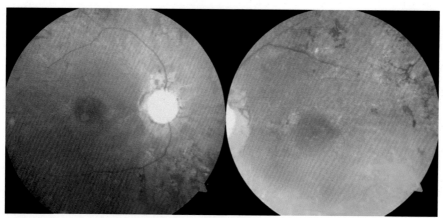

FIG. 11.6 Retinitis pigmentosa. Attenuated retinal vessels, waxy pallor of optic disc cataracts, and pigmentary retinopathy; right eye (left), left eye (right). (Courtesy Dr. Jessica Randolph, Virginia Commonwealth University School of Medicine.)

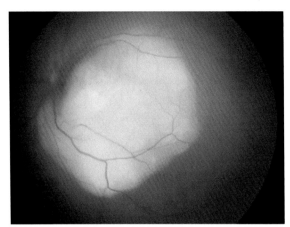

FIG. 11.7 Retinoblastoma. White or yellow tumor extending from the retina, left eye.

marrow failure and integumentary changes such as reticulate skin pigmentation, nail dystrophy, and oral leukoplakia.

*Epidemiology*: prevalence of <1/1,000,000
*Eye findings*: bilateral subretinal masses, conjunctival scarring, corneal opacification, exudative retinopathy, leukocoria, megalocornea, nystagmus, ectropion, entropion, trichiasis
*Inheritance*: AD
*Known genes or gene locus*: TINF2

## Rhyns Syndrome[206,207]
*OMIM*: #602152
*Description*: Disease characterized by a tetrad of retinitis pigmentosa, hypopituitarism, nephronophthisis, and skeletal dysplasia.
*Epidemiology*: prevalence of <1/1,000,000
*Eye findings*: enopthalmos, ptosis, pigmentary retinopathy
*Inheritance*: Presumed AR
*Known genes or gene locus*: Unknown

## Roifman Syndrome[208,209]
*OMIM*: #616651
*Description*: Disorder characterized by the pentad of phenotypic and immunologic manifestations of growth retardation, spondyloepiphyseal dysplasia, cognitive delay, facial dysmorphism, and antibody deficiency.
*Epidemiology*: prevalence of <1/1,000,000
*Eye findings*: arteriolar attenuation, downslanting palpebral fissures, ERGs completely extinguished, long eyelashes, long palpebral fissures, narrow palpebral fissures, prominent eyelashes, retinal dystrophy, refractive error, strabismus, wrinkling of inner limiting membrane

*Inheritance*: AR
*Known genes or gene locus*: RNU4ATAC

## Sandhoff Disease (GM2-Gangliosidosis, Type II)[210–212]
*OMIM*: #268800
*Description*: Disorder characterized by neurodegenerative abnormalities with accumulation of GM2-gangliosides within neurons. Both Tay-Sachs and Sandhoff diseases are clinically indistinguishable. Some additional characteristics include developmental retardation, doll-like faces, dementia, and blindness.
*Epidemiology*: prevalence of 1/130,000
*Eye findings*: blindness, cherry-red spot, optic atrophy
*Inheritance*: AR
*Known genes or gene locus*: HEXB

## Senior-Loken Syndrome[213,214]
*OMIM*: #266900
*Description*: Disorder characterized by features of Leber congenital amaurosis and nephronophthisis.
*Epidemiology*: prevalence of 1/1,000,000
*Eye findings*: arteriolar narrowing, bone corpuscle pigment clumping, flat electroretinogram, hyperopia, nystagmus, photophobia, sectoral pigmentary retinopathy, tapetoretinal degeneration
*Inheritance*: AR
*Known genes or gene locus*: NPHP1, NPHP4 SDCCAG8, WDR19, CEP290, IQCB1

## Sialidosis Type 1[215,216]
*OMIM*: #256550
*Description*: Also known as cherry-red spot myoclonus syndrome, sialidosis type I is a neuraminidase deficiency that causes lysosomal storage of sialylated glycopeptides and oligosaccharides. It is the less severe form of sialidosis, and manifestations can include myoclonus, gait disturbance, ataxia, tremors, seizures, and cherry-red spot eye abnormality.
*Epidemiology*: unknown
*Eye findings*: cherry-red spot eye abnormality, reduced visual acuity, impaired color vision, night blindness
*Inheritance*: AR
*Known genes or gene locus*: NEU1

## Sialidosis Type 2[217,218]
*OMIM*: #256550
*Description*: A disorder in which neuraminidase deficiency causes lysosomal storage of sialylated glycopeptides and oligosaccharides, leading to serious health problems affecting many organs and tissues, including the nervous system. The disorder is the more severe

form of sialidosis and is further divided into juvenile and infantile forms. It can include manifestations such as muscular hypotonia, hepatosplenomegaly, seizures, and abnormal bone development.

*Epidemiology*: unknown
*Eye findings*: cherry-red spot, corneal opacity
*Inheritance*: AR
*Known genes or gene locus*: NEU1

## Sickle Cell Anemia[219,220]

OMIM: #603903

*Description*: Disorder characterized by multisystem involvement due to polymerization of hemoglobin with resultant sickle-shaped red blood cells, vaso-occlusion, chronic anemia and vasculopathy.

*Epidemiology*: incidence of 1/500 in African Americans and 1/1000-1/1400 in Hispanics.

*Eye findings*: acute proptosis, angioid streaks, anterior uveitis (granulomatous), arteriovenous anastomoses, comma-shaped vessels in conjunctiva, hyphemas, thinning of temporal retina, retinal vascular occlusions, "sea fan" neovascularization, retinal and vitreous hemorrhages, thrombosis of central retinal artery or vein, traction retinal detachments
*Inheritance*: AR
*Known genes or gene locus*: HBB

## Snowflake Vitreoretinal Degeneration[221–223]

OMIM: #603208

*Description*: Progressive and developmental eye disorder affecting multiple tissues within the eye.

*Epidemiology*: prevalence of <1/1,000,000

*Eye findings*: attenuation of arterioles, cataract, corneal guttae, fibrillar degeneration, gel liquefaction, miniscule yellow-white retinal dots, occasional optically empty vitreous cavity, perivascular sheathing, thickened cortical vitreous, waxy pallor of optic nerve.
*Inheritance*: AD
*Known genes or gene locus*: KCNJ13

## Sorsby Fundus Dystrophy[224–226]

OMIM: #136900

*Description*: Disorder characterized by macular atrophy with subretinal gliosis due to early multifocal choroidal neovascularization. Peripheral vision loss can occur later in life.

*Epidemiology*: prevalence of 1/220,000

*Eye findings*: atrophy of the retinal pigment epithelium and choriocapillaris, choroidal atrophy, choroidal neovascular membrane with hemorrhage (recurrent), pigment dispersion with ocular hypertension/glaucoma, night blindness (responsive to treatment with vitamin A), progressive macular atrophy, pseudodrusen,

retinal edema, retinal exudates, severe visual loss, subretinal gliosis
*Inheritance*: AD
*Known genes or gene locus*: TIMP3

## Spondyloepiphyseal Dysplasia[227,228]

OMIM: #183900

*Description*: Chondrodysplasia characterized by dwarfism, skeletal abnormalities, and vision and hearing problems.

*Epidemiology*: unknown

*Eye findings*: hypertelorism, myopia, vitreoretinal degeneration, retinal detachment
*Inheritance*: AD
*Known genes or gene locus*: COL2A1

## Stargardt Disease/Fundus Flavimaculatus[229–231]

OMIM: #248200, #600110, #603786

*Description*: This disease is one of the most common causes of childhood macular dystrophy and progressive form of juvenile macular degeneration. Pathology caused by an accumulation of lipofuscin in the retinal pigment epithelium. About 70% may have a "dark" or "silent" choroid on fluorescein angiography.

*Epidemiology*: prevalence of 1/8000–1/10,000

*Eye findings*: macular pisciform flecks (Fig. 11.8A), "beaten-bronze" appearance of the macula, atrophy of retinal pigment epithelium centrally, peripheral pigment clumping, photophobia, progressive macular atrophy, prolonged dark adaptation, later disease onset and scattered flecks with fundus flavimaculatus, temporal pallor of optic nerve, vision loss, yellow pisciform round linear subretinal lipofuscin deposits, silent choroid on fluorescein angiography (Fig. 11.8B)
*Inheritance*: AR (typically), AD
*Known genes or gene locus*: ABCA4 (majority cases), ELOVL4, PROM1

## Stickler Syndrome[171,232–235]

OMIM: #108300, #604841, #184840, #614134, #614284, #609508

*Description*: Disorder characterized by a conglomerate of skeletal, auditory, ocular, and orofacial abnormalities. Accompanying features that have been sporadically described include midline clefting, flat midface, spondyloepiphyseal dysplasia, sensorineural hearing loss, early-onset osteoarthritis, and Pierre Robin sequence.

*Epidemiology*: incidence of 1/7500-1/9000. Type 1 most common.

*Eye findings*: blindness, peripheral cataracts/lenticular opacities (Fig. 11.9), optically empty vitreous, decreased

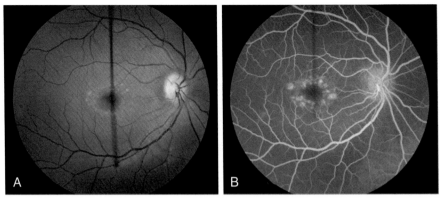

FIG. 11.8 Stargardt disease. Color photograph of yellowish pisciform flecks **(A)**, and characteristic dark choroid and staining of pisciform lesions on fluorescein angiograph **(B)**. (Courtesy Duker, Jay S. *Stargardt Disease, Atlas of Retinal OCT: Optical Coherence Tomography*; January 1, 2018:149−151. © 2018.)

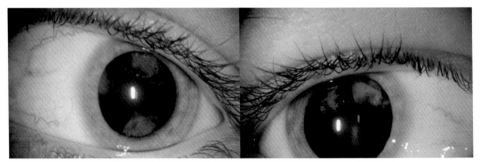

FIG. 11.9 Bilateral peripheral cataracts; right eye (left), left eye (right). (Courtesy Dr. Scott Lambert, Stanford University School of Medicine.)

EOG, decreased visual field, glaucoma, retinal hypopigmentation in a tessellated pattern, myopia, posterior vitreous detachments, ring scotoma, retinal detachment and vitreoretinal degeneration, no ocular signs (type III). Of note, nonprogressive axial myopia and vitreous degeneration in a nonbeaded pattern (unlike type 1) are distinguishing features for type 2. Can also see paravascular radial lattice retinopathy. Type IV is distinguished by lack of cataracts, presence of myopia, and vitreoretinal degeneration.

*Inheritance*: AD (types I, II, III), AR (types IV, V)

*Known genes or gene locus*: COL2A1, COL11A1, COL11A2, COL9A1, COL9A2

## Tay-Sachs Disease (GM2-Gangliosidosis, Type I)[211,236,237]

*OMIM*: #272800

*Description*: Progressive neurodegenerative disorder characterized by developmental delay, paralysis, dementia, and blindness with death occurring at 2−3 years of age normally.

*Epidemiology*: unknown; more common in Ashkenazi

*Eye findings*: blindness, interrupted saccades, macular pallor with prominence of fovea centralis (cherry red spot), optic atrophy

*Inheritance*: AR

*Known genes or gene locus*: HEXA

## Usher Syndrome[238−243]

*OMIM*: #276900

*Description*: Usher syndrome is characterized by sensorineural hearing deficiencies at birth with later development of retinitis pigmentosa.

*Epidemiology*: prevalence of 3.2/100,000−6.2/100,000

*Eye findings*: cataracts, hyperfluorescent areas of fundus, hypermetropic astigmatism (type 3), pigmentary retinopathy, severely reduced ERG, peripheral vision loss

*Inheritance*: AR

*Known genes or gene locus*: USH2A, CLRN1, ADGRV1, HARS, WHRN, USH1K, PCDH15, CDH23, PDZD7, USH1C, MYO7A, USH1H, C1B2, SANS, USH1E

## Van Den Bosch Syndrome[244]

*OMIM*: %314500

*Description*: Disorder characterized by a pentad of skeletal deformity, anhidrosis, mental deficiency, choroideremia, and acrokeratosis verruciformis.

> *Epidemiology*: prevalence of <1/1,000,000
> *Eye Findings*: choroideremia
> *Inheritance*: XLR
> *Known genes or gene locus*: Unknown

## Vici Syndrome[245-248]

*OMIM*: #242840

*Description*: Disorder characterized by a variety of clinical manifestations including agenesis of corpus callosum, variable immunodeficiency, cataracts, cardiomyopathy, and pigmentary alterations. Accompanying neurodegenerative defects make universal developmental delay, failure to thrive, and microcephaly.

> *Epidemiology*: prevalence of <1/1,000,000
> *Eye findings*: bilateral or unilateral cataracts, mild ptosis, ocular albinism, optic neuropathy, nystagmus, retinal hypopigmentation
> *Inheritance*: AR
> *Known genes or gene locus*: EPG5

## Vitelliform Macular Dystrophy[33,178,249-251]

*OMIM*: #153700

*Description*: Disorder characterized by large deposits of egg yolk or vitelliform deposits in the subretinal space. The lesions are lipofuscin deposits, similar to pattern dystrophy.

> *Epidemiology*: unknown
> *Eye findings*: central yellow submacular (typically subfoveal) accumulation of lipofuscin, macular atrophy, choroidal neovascularization, decreased visual acuity, diffuse fine hard drusen in macula and paracentral area, metamorphosia, photophobia
> *Inheritance*: AD
> *Known genes or gene locus*: IMPG2 (type 5), IMPG1 (type 4), PRPH2 (type 3), BEST1 (type 2)

## Vitreoretinochoroidopathy Dominant[204,252,253]

*OMIM*: #193220

*Description*: Vitreoretinal disease characterized by a variety of ocular manifestations and classic chorioretinal hypo and hyperpigmentation.

> *Epidemiology*: unknown

> *Eye findings*: acute and chronic glaucoma, chorioretinal hypopigmentation and hyperpigmentation, concentric visual field reduction, cystoid macular edema, diffuse retinal vascular incompetence, dyschromatopsia, fibrillary vitreous with pleocytosis, pigmentary retinopathy, peripapillary atrophy, preretinal white dots, presenile cataracts, reduced light/dark ratio, retinal detachment, microphthalmia, neovascularization, nystagmus, small corneas and shallow anterior chambers, strabismus
> *Inheritance*: AD
> *Known genes or gene locus*: BEST1

## Wagner Syndrome[254-258]

*OMIM*: #143200

*Description*: Rare disorder characterized by vitreoretinal degeneration. Approximately, 300 cases have been described. Distinct from other vitreoretinopathies by nyctalopia, anterior segment dysgenesis, and tractional retinal detachment.

> *Epidemiology*: unknown
> *Eye findings*: optically empty vitreous with veils, retinal degeneration. In older patients with this condition, chorioretinal atrophy, peripheral tractional retinal detachment, and cataract.
> *Inheritance*: AD
> *Known genes or gene locus*: VCAN

## Wolfram Syndrome[259-263]

*OMIM*: #222300, #604928, #598500

*Description*: Wolfram syndrome is a neurodegenerative disease that is associated with childhood-onset diabetes insipidus, diabetes mellitus, optic atrophy, and deafness (DIDMOAD)

> *Epidemiology*: unknown
> *Eye findings*: cataract, diabetic retinopathy, glaucoma, microspherophakia, nystagmus, optic atrophy, paracentral scotomas, peripheral constriction, pigmentary retinopathy, ptosis
> *Inheritance*: AR; there is also a mitochondrial form (#598500)
> *Known genes or gene locus*: WFS1, CISD2

## REFERENCES

1. Sahel JA, Marazova K, Audo I. Clinical characteristics and current therapies for inherited retinal degenerations. *Cold Spring Harb Perspect Med*. 2014;5:a017111.
2. Keeler CR. 150 years since Babbage's ophthalmoscope. *Arch Ophthalmol*. 1997;115(11):1456–1457.
3. Wheeler JR. *Br J Ophthalmol*. 1946;30(5):264.
4. Francis PJ. Genetics of inherited retinal disease. *J R Soc Med*. 2006;99(4):189–191.

5. Samiy N. Gene therapy for retinal diseases. *J Ophthal Vis Res.* 2014;9(4):506−509. https://doi.org/10.4103/2008-322X.150831.

6. Bennett J, Tanabe T, Sun D, et al. Photoreceptor cell rescue in retinal degeneration (rd) mice by in vivo gene therapy. *Nat Med.* 1996;2:649−654.

7. Le Meur G, Stieger K, Smith AJ, et al. *Gene Ther.* 2007; 14(4):292−303 [Epub 2006 Oct 5].

8. Acland GM, Aguirre GD, Ray J, et al. Gene therapy restores vision in a canine model of childhood blindness. *Nat Genet.* 2001;28:92−95.

9. Feuerstein A. *FDA Approves First Gene Therapy Targeting Rare Form of Inherited Blindness. Biotech.* December 19, 2017. Retrieved from https://www.statnews.com/2017/12/19/gene-therapy-blindness-fda-approval/.

10. Nakamura M, Yamamoto S, Okada M, Ito S, Tano Y, Miyake Y. Novel mutations in the arrestin gene and associated clinical features in Japanese patients with Oguchi's disease. *Ophthalmology.* 2004;111:1410−1414.

11. Waheed NK, Qavi AH, Malik SN, et al. A nonsense mutation in S-antigen (p.glu306ter) causes Oguchi disease. *Mol Vis.* 2012;18:1253−1259.

12. Kaiser-Kupfer M, Kuwabara T, Uga S, Takki K, Valle D. Cataracts in gyrate atrophy: clinical and morphologic studies. *Invest Ophthal Vis Sci.* 1983;24:432−436.

13. Takki K, Simell O. Genetic aspects in gyrate atrophy of the choroid and retina with hyperornithinaemia. *Br J Ophthal.* 1974;58:907−916.

14. Illingworth DR, Connor WE, Miller RG. Abetalipoproteinemia: report of two cases and review of therapy. *Arch Neurol.* 1980;37:659−662.

15. Scanu AM, Aggerbeck LP, Kruski AW, Lim CT, Kayden HJ. A study of the abnormal lipoproteins in abetalipoproteinemia. *J Clin Invest.* 1974;53:440−453.

16. de Jong PTVM. Age-related macular degeneration. *N Eng J Med.* 2006;355:1474−1485.

17. Imamura Y, Noda S, Hashizume K, et al. Drusen, choroidal neovascularization, and retinal pigment epithelium dysfunction in SOD1-deficient mice: a model of age-related maculardegeneration. *Proc Nat Acad Sci.* 2006;103:11282−11287.

18. Dennis J, Bower BD. The Aicardi syndrome. *Dev Med Child Neurol.* 1972;14:382−390.

19. Donnenfeld AE, Packer RJ, Zackai EH, Chee CM, Sellinger B, Emanuel BS. Clinical, cytogenetic, and pedigree findings in 18 cases of Aicardi syndrome. *Am J Med Genet.* 1989;32:461−467.

20. Couser NL, Masood MM, Aylsworth AS, Stevenson RE. Ocular manifestations in the X-linked intellectual disability syndromes. *Ophthal Genet.* 2017;38(5):401−412.

21. Schwartz M, Rosenberg T. Aland eye disease: linkage data. *Genomics.* 1991;10:327−332.

22. van Dorp DB, Eriksson AW, Delleman JW, et al. Aland eye disease: no albino misrouting. *Clin Genet.* 1985;28: 526−531.

23. Davidzon G, Mancuso M, Ferraris S, et al. POLG mutations and Alpers syndrome. *Ann Neurol.* 2005;57:921−924.

24. Harding BN. Progressive neuronal degeneration of childhood with liver disease (Alpers-Huttenlocher syndrome): a personal review. *J Child Neurol.* 1990;5:273−287.

25. Khan AO, Bifari IN, Bolz HJ. Ophthalmic features of children not yet diagnosed with Alstrom syndrome. *Ophthalmology.* 2015;122:1726−1727.

26. Marshall JD, Beck S, Maffei P, Naggert JK. Alstrom syndrome. *Eur J Hum Genet.* 2007;15:1193−1202.

27. Dekaban AS. Hereditary syndrome of congenital retinal blindness (Leber), polycystic kidneys and maldevelopment of the brain. *Am J Ophthal.* 1969;68:1029−1037.

28. Matsuzaka T, Sakuragawa N, Nakayama H, Sugai K, Kohno Y, Arima M. Cerebro-oculo-hepato-renal syndrome (Arima's syndrome): a distinct clinocopathological (sic) entity. *J Child Neurol.* 1986;1:338−346.

29. Ayazi S. Choroideremia, obesity, and congenital deafness. *Am J Ophthal.* 1981;92:63−69.

30. Nussbaum RL, Lesko JG, Lewis RA, Ledbetter SA, Ledbetter DH. Isolation of anonymous DNA sequences from within a submicroscopic X chromosomal deletion in a patient with choroideremia, deafness, and mental retardation. *Proc Nat Acad Sci.* 1987;84:6521−6525.

31. Croft JB, Swift M. Obesity, hypertension, and renal disease in relatives of Bardet-Biedlsyndrome sibs. *Am J Med Genet.* 1990;36:37−42.

32. Mykytyn K, Nishimura DY, Searby CC, et al. Evaluation of complex inheritance involving the most common Bardet-Biedl syndrome locus (BBS1). *Am J Hum Genet.* 2003;72:429−437.

33. Leroy BP. Bestrophinopathies. In: Traboulsi EI, ed. *Genetic Diseases of the Eye.* 2nd ed. New York: Oxford Univ. Press; 2012:426−436.

34. Mullins RF, Kuehn MH, Faidley EA, Syed NA, Stone EM. Differential macular and peripheral expression of bestrophin in human eyes and its implications for Best disease. *Invest ophthal Vis Sci.* 2007;48:3372−3380.

35. Sfriso P, Caso F, Tognon S, Galozzi P, Gava A, Punzi L. Blau syndrome, clinical and genetic aspects. *Autoimmun Rev.* 2012;12:44−51.

36. Sarens IL. Blau syndrome-associated uveitis: preliminary results from an international prospective interventional case series. *Am J Ophthalmol.* 2017.

37. Kooijman AC, Houtman A, Damhof A, van Engelen JP. Prolonged electro-retinal response suppression (PERRS) in patients with stationary subnormal visual acuity and photophobia. *Doc Ophthalmol.* 1991;78(3-4): 245−254.

38. Nishiguchi KM, Sandberg MA, Kooijman AC, et al. Defects in RGS9 or its anchor protein R9AP in patients with slow photoreceptor deactivation. *Nature.* 2004; 427(6969):75−78.

39. Boon CJ, Klevering BJ, Cremers FP, et al. Central areolar choroidal dystrophy. *Ophthalmology.* 2009;116:771−782.

40. Krill AE, Archer D. Classification of the choroidal atrophies. *Am J Ophthal.* 1971;72:562−585.

41. Ohba N, Isashiki Y. Clinical and genetic features of choroideremia. *Jpn J Ophthal.* 2000;44:317.

42. Perez-Cano HJ, Garnica-hayashi RE, Zenteno JC. CHM gene molecular analysis and X-chromosome inactivation pattern determination in two families with choroideremia. *Am J Med Genet*. 2009;149A:2134–2140.

43. Mahmoud AAH, Yousef GM, Al-Hifzi I, Diamandis EP. Cockayne syndrome in three sisters with varying clinical presentation. *Am J Med Genet*. 2002;111:81–85.

44. Moyer DB, Marquis P, Shertzer ME, Burton BK. Cockayne syndrome with early onset of manifestations. *Am J Med Genet*. 1982;13:225–230.

45. Hamel CP. Cone rod dystrophies. *Orphanet J Rare Dis*. 2007;2:1–7.

46. Roosing S, Thiadens AA, Hoyng CB, Klaver CC, den Hollander AI, Cremers FP. Causes and consequences of inherited cone disorders. *Prog Retin Eye Res*. 2014;42:1–26.

47. Talib M, van Schooneveld MJ, Thiadens AA, et al. Clinical and genetic characteristics of male patients with RPGR-associated retinal dystrophies: a Long-Term Follow-Up Study. *Retina*. 2018:1–14.

48. Moore AT. Cone and cone-rod dystrophies. *J Med Genet*. 1992;29:289–290.

49. Hittner HM, Murphree AL, Garcia CA, Justice Jr J, Chokshi DB. Dominant cone-rod dystrophy. *Doc Ophthal*. 1975;39:29–52.

50. Ferrell RE, Hittner HM, Chakravarti A. Autosomal dominant cone-rod dystrophy: a linkage study with 17 biochemical and serological markers. *Am J Med Genet*. 1981;8:363–369.

51. Papaioannou M, Bessant D, Payne A, et al. A new family of Greek origin maps to the CRD locus for autosomal dominant cone-rod dystrophy on 19q. *J Med Genet*. 1998;35:429–431.

52. Itabashi T, Wada Y, Sato H, Kawamura M, Shiono T, Tamai M. Novel 615delC mutation in the CRX gene in a Japanese family with cone-rod dystrophy. *Am J Ophthal*. 2004;138:876–877.

53. Bergen AAB, Pinckers AJLG. Localization of a novel X-linked progressive cone dystrophy gene to Xq27: evidence for genetic heterogeneity. *Am J Hum Genet*. 1997; 60:1468–1473 [Note: Erratum: *Am J Hum Genet* 1997; 61:471].

54. Yang Z, Peachey NS, Moshfeghi DM, et al. Mutations in the RPGR gene cause X-linked cone dystrophy. *Hum Mol Genet*. 2002;11:605–611.

55. Hong H-K, Ferrell RE, Gorin MB. Clinical diversity and chromosomal localization of X-linked cone dystrophy (COD1). *Am J Hum Genet*. 1994;55:1173–1181.

56. Holopigian K, Seiple W, Greenstein VC, Hood DC, Carr RE. Local cone and rod system function in progressive cone dystrophy. *Invest Ophthal Vis Sci*. 2002;43:2364–2373.

57. Hauke J, Schild A, Neugebauer A, et al. A novel large in-frame deletion within the CACNA1F gene associates with a cone-rod dystrophy 3-like phenotype. *PLoS One*. 2013; 8:e76414.

58. Carchon H, Van Schaftingen E, Matthijs G, Jaeken J. Carbohydrate-deficient glycoprotein syndrome type Ia (phosphomannomutase deficiency). *Biochim Biophys Acta*. 1999;1455:155–165.

59. de Lonlay P, Seta N, Barrot S. A broad spectrum of clinical presentations in congenital disorders of glycosylation I: a series of 26 cases. *J Med Genet*. 2001;38:14–19.

60. Zeitz C, Robson AG. Audo I. Congenital stationary night blindness: an analysis and update of genotype-phenotype correlations and pathogenic mechanisms. *Prog Retin Eye Res*. 2015;45:58–110.

61. Dryja TP, Hahn LB, Reboul T, Arnaud B. Missense mutation in the gene encoding the alpha subunit of rod transducin in the Nougaret form of congenital stationary night blindness. *Nat Genet*. 1996;13:358–365.

62. Riazuddin SA, Shahzadi A, Zeitz C, et al. A mutation in SLC24A1 implicated in autosomal-recessive congenital stationary night blindness. *Am J Hum Genet*. 2010;87: 523–531.

63. Pusch CM, Zeitz C, Brandau O, et al. The complete form of X-linked congenital stationary night blindness is caused by mutations in a gene encoding a leucine-rich repeat protein. *Nat Genet*. 2000;26:324–327.

64. Bech-Hansen NT, Naylor MJ, Maybaum TA, et al. Mutations in NYX, encoding the leucine-rich proteoglycan nyctalopin, cause X-linked complete congenital stationary night blindness. *Nat Genet*. 2000; 26:319–323.

65. Zeitz C, van Genderen M, Neidhardt J, et al. Mutations in GRM6 cause autosomal recessive congenital stationary night blindness with a distinctive scotopic 15-Hz flicker electroretinogram. *Invest Ophthal Vis Sci*. 2005;46: 4328–4335.

66. Dryja TP, McGee TL, Berson EL, et al. Night blindness and abnormal cone electroretinogram ON responses in patients with mutations in the GRM6 gene encoding mGluR6. *Proc Nat Acad Sci*. 2005;102:4884–4889.

67. van Genderen MM, Bijveld MMC, Claassen YB, et al. Mutations in TRPM1 are a common cause of complete congenital stationary night blindness. *Am J Hum Genet*. 2009;85:730–736.

68. Li Z, Sergouniotis PI, Michaelides M, et al. Recessive mutations of the gene TRPM1 abrogate ON bipolar cell function and cause complete congenital stationary night blindness in humans. *Am J Hum Genet*. 2009;85: 711–719.

69. Audo I, Kohl S, Leroy BP, et al. TRPM1 is mutated in patients with autosomal-recessive complete congenital stationary night blindness. *Am J Hum Genet*. 2009;85: 720–729.

70. Audo I, Bujakowska K, Orhan E, et al. Whole-exome sequencing identifies mutations in GPR179 leading to autosomal-recessive complete congenital stationary night blindness. *Am J Hum Genet*. 2012;90:321–330 [Note: Erratum: *Am J Hum Genet* 2012;91:209].

71. Peachey NS, Ray TA, Florijn R, et al. GPR179 is required for depolarizing bipolar cell function and is mutated in autosomal-recessive complete congenital

stationary night blindness. *Am J Hum Genet.* 2012;90:
331−339.

72. Strom TM, Nyakatura G, Apfelstedt-Sylla E, et al. An L-type calcium-channel gene mutated in incomplete X-linked congenital stationary night blindness. *Nat Genet.* 1998;19:260−263.

73. Bech-Hansen NT, Naylor MJ, Maybaum TA, et al. Loss-of-function mutations in a calcium-channel alpha-1-subunit gene in Xp11.23 cause incomplete X-linked congenital stationary night blindness. *Nat Genet.* 1998;19:264−267.

74. Yamamoto H, Simon A, Eriksson U, Harris E, Berson EL, Dryja TP. Mutations in the gene encoding 11-cis retinol dehydrogenase cause delayed dark adaptation and fundus albipunctatus. *Nat Genet.* 1999;22:188−191.

75. Gonzalez-Fernandez F, Kurz D, Bao Y, et al. 11-cis Retinal dehydrogenase mutations as a major cause of the congenital night-blindness disorder known as fundus albipunctatus. *Mol Vis.* 1999;5:41.

76. Fuchs S, Nakazawa M, Maw M, Tamai M, Oguchi Y, Gal A. A homozygous 1-base pair deletion in the arrestin gene is a frequent cause of Oguchi disease in Japanese. *Nat Genet.* 1995;10:360−362.

77. Donnai D, Barrow M. Diaphragmatic hernia, exomphalos, absent corpus callosum, hypertelorism, myopia, and sensorineural deafness: a newly recognized autosomal recessive disorder? *Am J Med Genet.* 1993;47: 679−682.

78. Kantarci S, Al-Gazali L, Hill RS, et al. Mutations in LRP2, which encodes the multiligand receptor megalin, cause Donnai-Barrow and facio-oculo-acoustico-renal syndromes. *Nat Genet.* 2007;39:957−959.

79. Schowalter DB, Pagon RA, Kalina RE, McDonald R. Facio-oculo-acoustico-renal (FOAR) syndrome: case report and review. *Am J Med Genet.* 1997;69:45−49.

80. Matsumoto M, Traboulsi EI. Dominant radial drusen and Arg345Trp EFEMP1 mutation. *Am J Ophthal.* 2001;131: 810−812.

81. Pearce WG. Doyne's honeycomb retinal degeneration: clinical and genetic features. *Br J Ophthal.* 1968;52:73−78.

82. Kjaer KW, Hansen L, Schwabe GC, et al. Distinct CDH3 mutations cause ectodermal dysplasia, ectrodactyly, macular dystrophy (EEM syndrome). *J Med Genet.* 2005;42: 292−298.

83. Ohdo S, Hirayama K, Terawaki T. Association of ectodermal dysplasia, ectrodactyly, and macular dystrophy: the EEM syndrome. *J Med Genet.* 1983;20:52−57.

84. Senecky Y, Halpern GJ, Inbar D, Attias J, Shohat M. Ectodermal dysplasia, ectrodactylyand macular dystrophy (EEM syndrome) in siblings. *Am J Med Genet.* 2001; 101:195−197.

85. Ober RR, Bird AC, Hamilton AM, Sehmi K. Autosomal dominant exudative vitreoretinopathy. *Br J Ophthal.* 1980;64:112−120.

86. Ranchod TM, Ho LY, Drenser KA, Capone Jr A, Trese MT. Clinical presentation of familial exudative vitreoretinopathy. *Ophthalmology.* 2011;118:2070−2075.

87. Kleijer WJ, Hoogeveen A, Verheijen FW, et al. Prenatal diagnosis of sialidosis with combined neuraminidase and beta-galactosidase deficiency. *Clin Genet.* 1979;16: 60−61.

88. Loonen MCB, Reuser AJJ, Visser P, Arts WFM. Combined sialidase (neuraminidase) and beta-galactosidase deficiency: clinical, morphological and enzymological observations in a patient. *Clin Genet.* 1984;26:139−149.

89. Blair NP, Trempe CL. Hypertrophy of the retinal pigment epithelium associated with Gardner's syndrome. *Am J Ophthal.* 1980;90:661−667.

90. Hockey KA, Mulcahy MT, Montgomery P, Levitt S. Deletion of chromosome 5q and familial adenomatous polyposis. *J Med Genet.* 1989;26:61−62.

91. Kolker S, Christensen E, Leonard JV, et al. Guideline for the diagnosis and management of glutaryl-CoA dehydrogenase deficiency (glutaric aciduria type I). *J Inherit Metab Dis.* 2007;30:5−22.

92. Tsai F, Lee H, Wang A, et al. Experiences during newborn screening for glutaric aciduria type 1: diagnosis, treatment, genotype, phenotype, and outcomes. *J Chin Med Assoc JCMA.* 2017;80(4):253−261.

93. Giugliani R, Dutra JC, Pereira MLS, et al. GM(1) gangliosidosis: clinical and laboratory findings in eight families. *Hum Genet.* 1985;70:347−354.

94. Hoogeveen AT, Reuser AJJ, Kroos M, Galjaard H. GM1-gangliosidosis: defective recognition site on beta-galactosidase precursor. *J Biol Chem.* 1986;261:5702−5704.

95. Bernal S, Solans T, Gamundi MJ, et al. Analysis of the involvement of the NR2E3 gene in autosomal recessive retinal dystrophies. *Clin Genet.* 2008;73:360−366.

96. Jacobson SG, Roman AJ, Roman MI, Gass JDM, Parker JA. Relatively enhanced S cone function in the Goldmann-Favre syndrome. *Am J Ophthal.* 1991;111:446−453.

97. Minic S, Trpinac D, Obradovic M. Incontinentia pigmenti diagnostic criteria update. *Clin Genet.* 2014; 85:536−542.

98. Spallone A. Incontinentia pigmenti (Bloch-Sulzberger syndrome): seven case reports from one family. *Br J Ophthal.* 1987;71:629−634.

99. Metodiev MD, Gerber S, Hubert L, et al. Mutations in the tricarboxylic acid cycle enzyme, aconitase 2, cause either isolated or syndromic optic neuropathy with encephalopathy and cerebellar atrophy. *J Med Genet.* 2014;51: 834−838.

100. Spiegel R, Pines O, Ta-Shma A, et al. Infantile cerebellar-retinal degeneration associated with a mutation in mitochondrial aconitase, $ACO_2$. *Am J Hum Genet.* 2012;90: 518−523.

101. Jalili IK. Cone-rod dystrophy and amelogenesis imperfecta (Jalilisyndrome): phenotypes and environs. *Eye.* 2010;24:1659−1668 [Note: Erratum: *Eye* 2010;24: 1734−1735].

102. Parry DA, Mighell AJ, El-Sayed W, et al. Mutations in CNNM4 cause Jalili syndrome, consisting of autosomal-recessive cone-rod dystrophy and amelogenesis imperfecta. *Am J Hum Genet.* 2009;84:266−273.

103. Pimenides D, George NDL, Yates JRW, et al. X-linked retinoschisis: clinical phenotype and RS1 genotype in 86 UK patients. *J Med Genet.* 2005;42:e35.

104. Sikkink SK, Biswas S, Parry NRA, Stanga PE, Trump D. X-linked retinoschisis: an update. *J Med Genet.* 2007;44: 225–232.

105. Czeizel AE, Goblyos P, Kustos G, Mester E, Paraicz E. The second report of Knobloch syndrome. *Am J Med Genet.* 1992;42:777–779.

106. Keren B, Suzuki OT, Gerard-Blanluet M, et al. CNS malformations in Knobloch syndrome with splice mutation in COL18A1 gene. *Lett Am J Med Genet.* 2007;143A: 1514–1518.

107. Hayward C, Shu X, Cideciyan AV, et al. Mutation in a short-chain collagen gene, CTRP5, results in extracellular deposit formation in late-onset retinal degeneration: a genetic model for age-related macular degeneration. *Hum Mol Genet.* 2003;12:2657–2667.

108. Jacobson SG, Cideciyan AV, Sumaroka A, Roman AJ, Wright AF. Late-onset retinal degeneration caused by C1QTNF5 mutation: sub-retinal pigment epithelium deposits and visual consequences. *JAMA Ophthalmol.* 2014; 132(10):1252–1255.

109. Milam AH, Curcio CA, Cideciyan AV, et al. Dominant late-onset retinal degeneration with regional variation of sub-retinal pigment epithelium deposits, retinal function, and photoreceptor degeneration. *Ophthalmology.* 2000;107:2256–2266.

110. Bowen P, Ferguson-Smith MA, Mosier D, Lee CSN, Butler HG. The Laurence-Moon syndrome. Association with hypogonadotrophic hypogonadism and sex-chromosome aneuploidy. *Arch Intern Med.* 1965;116: 598–604.

111. Farag TI, Teebi AS. Bardet-Biedl and Laurence-Moon syndromes in a mixed Arab population. *Clin Genet.* 1988;33: 78–82.

112. Jackson S, Bartlett K, Land J, et al. Long-chain 3-hydroxyacyl-CoA dehydrogenase deficiency. *Pediat Res.* 1991;29:406–411.

113. Rocchiccioli F, Wanders RJA, Aubourg P, et al. Deficiency of long-chain 3-hydroxyacyl-CoA dehydrogenase: a cause of lethal myopathy and cardiomyopathy in early childhood. *Pediat Res.* 1990;28:657–662.

114. Chung DC, Traboulsi EI. Leber congenital amaurosis: clinical correlations with genotypes, gene therapy trials update, and future directions. *J AAPOS.* 2009;13:587–592.

115. Kumaran N, Moore AT, Weleber RG, Michaelides M. Leber congenital amaurosis/early-onset severe retinal dystrophy: clinical features, molecular genetics and therapeutic interventions. *Br J Ophthalmol.* July 8, 2017. https://doi.org/10.1136/bjophthalmol-2016-309975.

116. Perrault I, Rozet JM, Gerber S, et al. Leber congenital amaurosis. *Mol Genet Metab.* 1999;68(2):200–208 (review).

117. Camuzat A, Rozet J-M, Dollfus H, et al. Evidence of genetic heterogeneity of Leber's congenital amaurosis (LCA) and mapping of LCA1 to chromosome 17p13. *Hum Genet.* 1996;97:798–801.

118. Hanein S, Perrault I, Gerber S, et al. Leber congenital amaurosis: comprehensive survey of the genetic heterogeneity, refinement of the clinical definition, and genotype-phenotype correlations as a strategy for molecular diagnosis. *Hum Mutat.* 2004;23:306–317.

119. Wiszniewski W, Lewis RA, Stockton DW. Potential involvement of more than one locus in trait manifestation for individuals with Leber congenital amaurosis. *Hum Genet.* 2011;129:319–327.

120. Yano S, Oda K, Watanabe Y, et al. Two sib cases of Leber congenital amaurosis with cerebellar vermis hypoplasia and multiple systemic abnormalities. *Am J Med Genet.* 1998;78:429–432.

121. Camuzat A, Dollfus H, Rozet J-M, et al. A gene for Leber's congenital amaurosis maps to chromosome 17p. *Hum Mol Genet.* 1995;4:1447–1452.

122. Khan AO, Al-Mesfer S, Al-Turkmani S, Bergmann C, Bolz HJ. Genetic analysis of strictly defined Leber congenital amaurosis with (and without) neurodevelopmental delay. *Brit J Ophthal.* 2014;98:1724–1728.

123. Khanna H, Davis EE, Murga-Zamalloa CA, et al. A common allele in RPGRIP1L is a modifier of retinal degeneration in ciliopathies. *Nat Genet.* 2009;41:739–745.

124. Lambert SR, Sherman S, Taylor D, Kriss A, Coffey R, Pembrey M. Concordance and recessive inheritance of Leber congenital amaurosis. *Am J Med Genet.* 1993;46: 275–277.

125. Cremers FPM, van den Hurk JAJM, den Hollander AI. Molecular genetics of Leber congenital amaurosis. *Hum Mol Genet.* 2002;11:1169–1176.

126. Francois J. Leber's congenital tapetoretinal degeneration. *Int Ophthal Clin.* 1968;8:929–947.

127. Gillespie FD. Congenital amaurosis of Leber. *Am J Ophthal.* 1966;61:874–880.

128. Milam AH, Barakat MR, Gupta N, et al. Clinicopathologic effects of mutant GUCY2D in Leber congenital amaurosis. *Ophthalmology.* 2003;110:549–558.

129. Riess O, Weber B, Noeremolle A, Shaikh RA, Hayden MR, Musarella MA. Linkage studies and mutation analysis of the PDEB gene in 23 families with Leber congenital amaurosis. *Hum Mutat.* 1992;1:478–485.

130. Sohocki MM, Bowne SJ, Sullivan LS, et al. Mutations in a new photoreceptor-pineal gene on 17p cause Leber congenital amaurosis. *Nat Genet.* 2000;24:79–83.

131. Zernant J, Kulm M, Dharmaraj S, et al. Genotyping microarray (disease chip) for Leber congenital amaurosis: detection of modifier alleles. *Invest Ophthal Vis Sci.* 2005; 46:3052–3059.

132. Schappert-Kimmijser J, Henkes HE, Van den Bosch J. Amaurosis congenita (leber). *Arch Ophthal.* 1959;61: 211–218.

133. Schroeder R, Mets MB, Maumenee IH. Leber's congenital amaurosis: retrospective review of 43 cases and a new fundus finding in two cases. *Arch Ophthal.* 1987;105: 356–359.

134. Sudo A, Honzawa S, Nonaka I, Goto Y. Leigh syndrome caused by mitochondrial DNA G13513A mutation: frequency and clinical features in Japan. *J Hum Genet.* 2004;49:92–96.

135. Ugalde C, Triepels RH, Coenen MJH, et al. Impaired complex I assembly in a Leigh syndrome patient with a novel missense mutation in the ND6 gene. *Ann Neurol.* 2003; 54:665–669.

136. Van den Bosch BJC, Gerards M, Sluiter W, et al. Defective NDUFA9 as a novel cause of neonatally fatal complex I disease. *J Med Genet.* 2012;49:10–15.

137. Beals RK, Weleber RG. Conorenal dysplasia: a syndrome of cone-shaped epiphysis, renal disease in childhood, retinitis pigmentosa and abnormality of the proximal femur. *Am J Med Genet.* 2007;143:2444–2447.

138. Perrault I, Saunier S, Hanein S, et al. Mainzer-Saldino Syndrome is a ciliopathy caused by IFT140 mutations. *Am J Hum Genet.* 2012;90:864–870.

139. Schmidts M, Vodopiutz J, Christou-Savina S, et al. Mutations in the gene encoding IFT dynein complex component WDR34 cause Jeune asphyxiating thoracic dystrophy. *Am J Hum Genet.* 2013;93:932–944.

140. Bedilu R, Nummy KA, Cooper A, et al. Variable clinical presentation of lysosomal beta-mannosidosis in patients with null mutations. *Mol Genet Metab.* 2002;77:282–290.

141. Cooper A, Sardharwalla IB, Roberts MM. Human beta-mannosidase deficiency. *Lett N Eng J Med.* 1986;315:1231.

142. Malm D, Nilssen Ø. Alpha-Mannosidosis. In: Adam MP, Ardinger HH, Pagon RA, et al., eds. *GeneReviews® [Internet].* Seattle (WA): University of Washington, Seattle; 2001:1993–2018.

143. Ballinger SW, Shoffner JM, Hedaya EV, et al. Maternally transmitted diabetes and deafness associated with a 10.4 kb mitochondrial DNA deletion. *Nat Genet.* 1992; 1:11–15.

144. Guillausseau P-J, Massin P, Dubois-LaForgue D, et al. Maternally inherited diabetes and deafness: a multicenter study. *Ann Intern Med.* 2001;134:721–728.

145. Murphy R, Turnbull DM, Walker M, Hattersley AT. Clinical features, diagnosis and management of maternally inherited diabetes and deafness (MIDD) associated with the 3243A>G mitochondrial point mutation. *Diabet Med.* 2008;25(4):383–399. https://doi.org/10.1111/j.1464-5491.2008.02359.x [Epub 2008 Feb 18. Review].

146. Reardon W, Ross RJM, Sweeney MG, et al. Diabetes mellitus associated with a pathogenic point mutation in mitochondrial DNA. *Lancet.* 1992;340:1376–1379.

147. DiMauro S. Mitochondrial diseases. *Biochim Biophys Acta.* 2004;1658(1–2):80–88 [review].

148. Finsterer J, Zarrouk-Mahjoub S. Management of epilepsy in MERRF syndrome. *Seizure J Br Epilepsy Assoc.* n.d.;50:166–170.

149. Brandstetter Y, Weinhouse E, Splaingard ML, Tang TT. Cor pulmonale as a complication of methylmalonic acidemia and homocystinuria (cbl-C type). *Am J Med Genet.* 1990;36:167–171.

150. Carrillo N, Adams D, Venditti CP. *Disorders of Intracellular Cobalamin Metabolism.* February 25, 2008.

151. Van Hove JLK, Van Damme-Lombaerts R, Grunewald S, et al. Cobalamin disorder cbl-C presenting with late-

152. Roesc K, Hynds PJ, Varga R, Tranebjaerg L, Koehler CM. The calcium-binding aspartate/glutamate carriers, citrin and aralar1, are new substrates for the DDP1/TIMM8a-TIMM13 complex. *Hum Molec Genet.* 2004;13:2101–2111.

153. Ujike H, Tanabe Y, Takehisa Y, Hayabara T, Kuroda S. A family with X-linked dystonia-deafness syndrome with a novel mutation of the DDP gene. *Arch Neurol.* 2001; 58:1004–1007.

154. Mohr J, Mageroy K. Sex-linked deafness of a possibly new type. *Acta Genet Stat Med.* 1960;10:54–62.

155. Huang C-T, Chu S-Y, Lee Y-C. Optical coherence tomography of chorioretinopathy caused by mucopolysaccharidoses. *Ophthalmology.* 2015;122:1535–1537.

156. Wraith JE, Scarpa M, Beck M, et al. Mucopolysaccharidosis type II (Hunter syndrome): a clinical review and recommendations for treatment in the era of enzyme replacement therapy. *Eur J Pediat.* 2008;167:267–277.

157. Bras J, Verloes A, Schneider SA, Mole SE, Guerreiro RJ. Mutation of the Parkinsonism gene ATP13A2 causes neuronal ceroid-lipofuscinosis. *Hum Mol Genet.* March 2, 2012.

158. Mole SE, Williams RE, Goebel HH. Correlations between genotype, ultrastructural morphology and clinical phenotype in the neuronal ceroid lipofuscinoses. *Neurogenetics.* 2005;6:107–126.

159. Wisniewski KE, Kida E, Patxot OF, Connell F. Variability in the clinical and pathological findings in the neuronal ceroid lipofuscinoses: review of data and observations. *Am J Med Genet.* 1992;42:525–532.

160. Claeys KG, Abicht A, Hausler M, et al. Novel genetic and neuropathological insights in neurogenic muscle weakness, ataxia, and retinitis pigmentosa (NARP). *Muscle Nerve.* 2016;54(2):328–333.

161. Kerrison JB, Biousse V, Newman NJ. Retinopathy of NARP syndrome. *Arch Ophthal.* 2000;118:298–299.

162. Lopez-Gallardo E, Solano A, Herrero-Martin MD, et al. NARP syndrome in a patient harbouring an insertion in the MT-ATP6 gene that results in a truncated protein. *J Med Genet.* 2009;45:64–67.

163. McGovern MM, Aron A, Brodie SE, Desnick RJ, Wasserstein MP. Natural history of Type A Niemann-Pick disease: possible endpoints for therapeutic trials. *Neurology.* 2006;66(2):228–232.

164. Schuchman EH. The pathogenesis and treatment of acid sphingomyelinase-deficient Niemann-Pick disease. *J Inherit Metab Dis.* 2007;30(5):654–663 [review].

165. Verot L, Chikh K, Freydière E, Honorè R, Vanier MT, Millat G. Niemann-Pick C disease: functional characterization of three NPC2 mutations and clinical and molecular update on patients with NPC2. *Clin Genet.* 2007; 71(4):320–330.

166. Vanier MT, Millat G. Niemann-Pick disease type C. *Clin Genet.* 2003;64(4):269–281 [review].

167. Anderson SR, Warburg M. Norrie's disease. *Arch Ophthal.* 1961;66:614–618.

168. Lev D, Weigl Y, Hasan M, et al. A novel missense mutation in the NDP gene in a child with Norrie disease and

severe neurological involvement including infantile spasms. *Am J Med Genet.* 2007;143A:921−924.

169. Michaelides M, Luthert PJ, Cooling R, Firth H, Moore AT. Norrie disease and peripheral venous insufficiency. *Br J Ophthalmol.* 2004;88(11):1475 [Erratum in *Br J Ophthalmol* 2005;89(5):645].

170. Ohba N, Yamashita T. Primary vitreoretinal dysplasia resembling Norrie's disease in a female: association with X autosome chromosomal translocation. *Br J Ophthal.* 1986;70:64−71.

171. Ang A, Poulson AV, Goodburn SF, Richards AJ, Scott JD, Snead MP. Retinal detachment and prophylaxis in type 1 Stickler syndrome. *Ophthalmology.* 2008;115(1):164−168.

172. Bowne SJ, Sullivan LS, Wheaton DK, et al. North Carolina macular dystrophy (MCDR1) caused by a novel tandem duplication of the PRDM13 gene. *Mol Vis.* 2016;22:1239−1247.

173. Pauleikhoff D, Sauer CG, Muller CR, Radermacher M, Merz A, Weber BHF. Clinical and genetic evidence for autosomal dominant North Carolina macular dystrophy in a German family. *Am J Ophthal.* 1997;124:412−415.

174. Recchia FM, Carvalho-Recchia CA, Trese MT. Optical coherence tomography in the diagnosis of foveal hypoplasia. *Arch Ophthal.* 2002;120:1587−1588.

175. Piao C-H, Kondo M, Tanikawa A, Terasaki H, Miyake Y. Multifocal electroretinogram in occult macular dystrophy. *Invest Ophthal Vis Sci.* 2000;41:513−517.

176. Tsunoda K, Usui T, Hatase T, et al. Clinical characteristics of occult macular dystrophy in family with mutation of RP1L1 gene. *Retina.* 2012;32:1135−1147.

177. Vaclavik V, Tran HV, Gaillard M-C, Schorderet DF, Munier FL. Pattern dystrophy with high intrafamilial variability associated with Y141C mutation in the peripherin/RDS gene and successful treatment of subfoveal CNV related to multifocal pattern type with anti-VEGF (ranibizumab) intravitreal injections. *Retina.* 2012;32:1942−1949.

178. Yang Z, Li Y, Jiang L, et al. A novel RDS/peripherin gene mutation associated with diverse macular phenotypes. *Ophthal Genet.* 2004;25:133−145.

179. Lin AE, Biglan AW, Garver KL. Persistent hyperplastic primary vitreous with vertical transmission. *Ophthal Paediat Genet.* 1990;11:121−122.

180. Prasov L, Masud T, Khaliq S, et al. ATOH7 mutations cause autosomal recessive persistent hyperplasia of the primary vitreous. *Hum Mol Genet.* 2012;21:3681−3694.

181. Khan K, Logan CV, McKibbin M, et al. Next generation sequencing identifies mutations in atonal homolog 7 (ATOH7) in families with global eye developmental defects. *Hum Mol Genet.* 2012;21:776−783.

182. Douglas AA, Waheed I, Wyse CT. Progressive bifocal chorio-retinal atrophy: a rare familial disease of the eyes. *Br J Ophthal.* 1968;52:742−751.

183. Kelsell RE, Godley BF, Evans K, et al. Localization of the gene for progressive bifocal chorioretinal atrophy (PBCRA) to chromosome 6q. *Hum Mol Genet.* 1995;4:1653−1656.

184. Finger RP, Issa PC, Ladewig MS, et al. Pseudoxanthoma elasticum: genetics, clinical manifestations and therapeutic approaches. *Surv Ophthalmol.* 2009;54:272−285.

185. Orssaud C, Roche O, Dufier J-L, Germain DP. Visual impairment in pseudoxanthoma elasticum: a survey of 40 patients. *Ophthal Genet.* 2015;36:327−332.

186. Rüether K, Baldwin E, Casteels M, et al. Adult Refsum disease: a form of tapetoretinal dystrophy accessible to therapy. *Surv Ophthalmol.* 2010;55(6):531−538.

187. Wanders RJA, Waterham HR, Leroy BP. Refsum disease. In: Pagon RA, Adam MP, Ardinger HH, et al., eds. *GeneReviews® [Internet].* Seattle (WA): University of Washington, Seattle; 2006:1993−2017.

188. Ophoff RA, DeYoung J, Service SK, et al. Hereditary vascular retinopathy, cerebroretinal vasculopathy, and hereditary endotheliopathy with retinopathy, nephropathy, and stroke map to a single locus on chromosome 3p21.1-p21.3. *Am J Hum Genet.* 2001;69:447−453.

189. Richards A, van den Maagdenberg AMJM, Jen JC. C-terminal truncations in human 3-prime-5-prime DNA exonuclease TREX1 cause autosomal dominant retinal vasculopathy with cerebral leukodystrophy. *Nat Genet.* 2007;39:1068−1070.

190. Kaiser PK, Friedman NJ, Pineda II R. *The Massachusetts Eye and Ear Infirmary Illustrated Manual of Ophthalmology.* 2nd ed. Philadelphia: Saunders; 2004:407−408.

191. Veltel S, Gasper R, Eisenacher E, Wittinghofer A. The retinitis pigmentosa 2 gene product is a GTPase-activating protein for Arf-like 3. *Nat Struct Mol Biol.* 2008;15:373−380.

192. *RETINITIS PIGMENTOSA. Online Mendelian Inheritance in Man (OMIM)*; April 11, 2018. https://www.omim.org/entry/268000.

193. Falsini B, Iarossi G, Chiaretti A, et al. NGF eye-drops topical administration in patients with retinitis pigmentosa, a pilot study. *J Transl Med.* 2016;14:8.

194. Peng Y-Q, Tang L-S, Yoshida S, Zhou Y-D. Applications of CRISPR/Cas9 in retinal degenerative diseases. *Int J Ophthalmol.* 2017;10(4):646−651.

195. Huang XF. Current pharmacological concepts in the treatment of the retinitis pigmentosa. *Adv Exp Med Biol.* 2018;1074:439−445. https://doi.org/10.1007/978-3-319-75402-4-54.

196. Berson EL, Weigel-DiFranco C, Rosner B, Gaudio AR, Sandberg MA. Association of vitamin A supplementation with disease course in children with retinitis pigmentosa. *JAMA Ophthalmol.* 2018;136(5):490−495. https://doi.org/10.1001/jamaophthalmol.2018.0590.

197. Weiss JN, Levy S. Stem cell ophthalmology treatment study: bone marrow derived stem cells in the treatment of retinitis pigmentosa. *Stem Cell Investig.* 2018;5:18. https://doi.org/10.21037/sci.2018.04.02.

198. Finn AP, Grewal DS, Vajzovic L. Argus II retinal prosthesis system: a review of patient selection criteria, surgical considerations, and post-operative outcomes. *Clin Ophthalmol.* 2018;12:1089−1097. https://doi.org/10.2147/OPTH.S137525.

199. DiCarlo JE, Mahajan VB, Tsang SH. Gene therapy and genome surgery in the retina. *J Clin Invest.* 2018;128(6): 2177–2188. https://doi.org/10.1172/JCI120429.

200. Balmer A, Zografos L, Munier F. Diagnosis and current management of retinoblastoma. *Oncogene.* 2006;25: 5341–5349.

201. Hanahan D, Weinberg RA. The hallmarks of cancer. *Cell.* 2000;100:57–70.

202. Shields CL, Honavar S, Shields JA, Demirci H, Meadows AT. Vitrectomy in eyes with unsuspected retinoblastoma. *Ophthalmology.* 2000;107:2250–2255.

203. Gupta MP, Talcott KE, Kim DY, Agarwal S, Mukai S. Retinal findings and a novel TINF2 mutation in revesz syndrome: clinical and molecular correlations with pediatric retinal vasculopathies. *Ophthal Genet.* 2017;38(1): 51–60.

204. Traboulsi EI, Payne JW. Autosomal dominant vitreoretinochoroidopathy. Report of the third family. *Arch Ophthalmol.* 1993;111(2):194–196 [review].

205. Trivedi MG, Rai PJ, Shirwadkar SP, et al. Ocular findings of revesz syndrome in a 12-year-old girl. *J Pediatr Ophthalmol Strabismus.* 2016;53(2):128.

206. Di Rocco M, Picco P, Arslanian A, et al. Retinitis pigmentosa, hypopituitarism, nephronophthisis, and mild skeletal dysplasia (RHYNS): a new syndrome? *Am J Med Genet.* 1997;73:1–4.

207. Hedera P, Gorski JL. Retinitis pigmentosa, growth hormone deficiency, and acromelic skeletal dysplasia in two brothers: possible familial RHYNS syndrome. *Am J Med Genet.* 2001;101(2):142–145.

208. Farach LS, Little ME, Duker AL, et al. The expanding phenotype of RNU4ATAC pathogenic variants to lowry wood syndrome. *Am J Med Genet A.* 2017.

209. Merico D, Roifman M, Braunschweig U, et al. Compound heterozygous mutations in the noncoding RNU4ATAC cause Roifman syndrome by disrupting minor intron splicing. *Nat Commun.* 2015;6:8718 [Note: Electronic Article].

210. Brownstein S, Carpenter S, Polomeno RC, Little JM. Sandhoff's disease (GM2 gangliosidosis type 2). Histopathology and ultrastructure of the eye. *Arch Ophthalmol.* 1980;98(6):1089–1097.

211. Chen H, Chan AY, Stone DU, Mandal NA. Beyond the cherry-red spot: ocular manifestations of sphingolipid-mediated neurodegenerative and inflammatory disorders. *Surv Ophthalmol.* 2014;59(1):64–76.

212. Moon JG, Shin MA, Pyo H, Choi SU, Kim HK. An infantile case of sandhoff disease presenting with swallowing difficulty. *Ann Rehabil Med.* 2017;41(5):892–896.

213. Aggarwal HK, Jain D, Yadav S, Kaverappa V, Gupta A. Senior-loken syndrome with rare manifestations: a case report. *Eurasian J Med.* 2013;45(2):128–131.

214. Ronquillo CC, Bernstein PS, Baehr W. Senior-Loken Syndrome: a syndromic form of retinal dystrophy associated with nephronophthisis. *Vis Res.* July 19, 2012 [Epub ahead of print].

215. Bonten EJ, Arts WF, Beck M, et al. Novel mutations in lysosomal neuraminidase identify functional domains and determine clinical severity in sialidosis. *Hum Mol Genet.* 2000;9:2715–2725.

216. Federico A, Cecio A, Apponi Battini G, Michalski JC, Strecker G, Guazzi GC. Macular cherry-red spot and myoclonus syndrome: juvenile form of sialidosis. *J Neurol Sci.* 1980;48:157–169.

217. Canafoglia L, Robbiano A, Pareyson D, et al. Expanding sialidosis spectrum by genome-wide screening: NEU1 mutations in adult-onset myoclonus. *Neurology.* 2014; 82:2003–2006.

218. Franceschetti S, Uziel G, Di Donato S, Caimi L, Avanzini G. Cherry-red spot myoclonus syndrome and alpha-neuraminidase deficiency: neurophysiological, pharmacological and biochemical study in an adult. *J Neurol Neurosurg Psychiatry.* 1980;43(10):934–940.

219. Lim JI. Ophthalmic manifestations of sickle cell disease: update of the latest findings. *Curr Opin Ophthalmol.* 2012;23(6):533–536.

220. Rees DC, Williams TN, Gladwin MT. Sickle cell disease. *Lancet.* 2010;376:2018–2031.

221. Gheiler M, Pollack A, Uchenik D, Godel V, Oliver M. Hereditary snowflake vitreoretinal degeneration. *Birth Defects Orig Art Ser.* 1982;XVIII(6):577–580.

222. Hejtmancik JF, Jiao X, Li A, et al. Mutations in KCNJ13 cause autosomal-dominant snowflake vitreoretinal degeneration. *Am J Hum Genet.* 2008;82:174–180.

223. Jiao X, Ritter III R, Hejtmancik JF, Edwards AO. Genetic linkage of snowflake vitreoretinal degeneration to chromosome 2q36. *Invest Ophthal Vis Sci.* 2004;45:4498–4503.

224. Christensen DRG, Brown FE, Cree AJ, Ratnayaka JA, Lotery AJ. Sorsby fundus dystrophy - a review of pathology and disease mechanisms. *Exp Eye Res.* 2017;165:35–46.

225. Gliem M, Muller PL, Mangold E, et al. Reticular pseudodrusen in sorsby fundus dystrophy. *Ophthalmology.* 2015; 122(8):1555–1562.

226. Menassa N, Burgula S, Empeslidis T, Tsaousis KT. Bilateral choroidal neovascular membrane in a young patient with sorsby fundus dystrophy: the value of prompt treatment. *BMJ Case Rep.* 2017;2017. https://doi.org/10.1136/bcr-2017-220488.

227. Fraser GR, Friedmann AI, Maroteaux P, Glen-Bott AM, Mittwoch U. Dysplasia spondyloepiphysaria conge- nita and related generalized skeletal dysplasia among children with severe visual handicaps. *Arch Dis Child.* 1969; 44(236):490–498.

228. Chan D, Taylor TKF, Cole WG. Characterization of an arginine 789 to cysteine substitution in alpha-1(II) collagen chains of a patient with spondyloepiphyseal dysplasia. *J Biol Chem.* 1993;268(20):15238–15245.

229. Collison FT, Fishman GA. Visual acuity in patients with Stargardt disease after age 40. *Retina.* October 24, 2017. https://doi.org/10.1097/IAE.0000000000001903 [Epub ahead of print].

230. Fujinami K, Zernant J, Chana RK, et al. Clinical and molecular characteristics of childhood-onset Stargardt disease. *Ophthalmology*. October 10, 2014 [Epub ahead of print].

231. Tanna P, Strauss RW, Fujinami K, Michaelides M. Stargardt disease: clinical features, molecular genetics, animal models and therapeutic options. *Br J Ophthalmol*. August 4, 2016 [review].

232. Ang A, Ung T, Puvanachandra N, et al. Vitreous phenotype: a key diagnostic sign in Stickler syndrome types 1 and 2 complicated by double heterozygosity. *Am J Med Genet A*. 2007;143(6):604–607.

233. Baker S, Booth C, Fillman C, et al. A loss of function mutation in the COL9A2 gene cause autosomal recessive Stickler syndrome. *Am J Med Genet*. 2011;155A:1668–1672.

234. Richards AJ, Laidlaw M, Whittaker J, et al. High efficiency of mutation detection in type 1 stickler syndrome using a two-stage approach: vitreoretinal assessment coupled with exon sequencing for screening COL2A1. *Hum Mutat*. 2006;27(7):696–704 [Erratum in: *Hum Mutat* 2006; 27(11):1156].

235. Van Camp G, Snoeckx RL, Hilgert N, et al. A new autosomal recessive form of Stickler syndrome is caused by a mutation in the COL9A1 gene. *Am J Hum Genet*. 2006;79(3):449–457.

236. Fernandes Filho JA, Shapiro BE. Tay-Sachs disease. *Arch Neurol*. 2004;61(9):1466–1468 [review].

237. Rucker JC, Shapiro BE, Han YH, et al. Neuro-ophthalmology of late-onset Tay-Sachs disease (LOTS). *Neurology*. 2004;63:1918–1926.

238. Blanco-Kelly F, Jaijo T, Aller E, et al. Clinical aspects of Usher syndrome and the USH2A gene in a Cohort of 433 patients. *JAMA Ophthalmol*. November 6, 2014 [Epub ahead of print].

239. Eisenberger T, Slim R, Mansour A, et al. Targeted next-generation sequencing identifies a homozygous nonsense mutation in ABHD12, the gene underlying PHARC, in a family clinically diagnosed with Usher syndrome type 3. *Orphanet J Rare Dis*. 2012;7(1):59.

240. Geng R, Geller SF, Hayashi T, et al. Usher syndrome IIIA gene clarin-1 is essential for hair cell function and associated neural activation. *Hum Mol Genet*. 2009;18(15): 2748–2760 [Epub 2009 May 3].

241. Moller CG, Kimberling WJ, Davenport SLH, et al. Usher syndrome: an otoneurologic study. *Laryngoscope*. 1989; 99:73–79.

242. Pakarinen L, Tuppurainen K, Laippala P, Mäntyjärvi M, Puhakka H. The ophthalmological course of Usher syndrome type III. *Int Ophthalmol*. 1995–1996;19(5): 307–311.

243. Smith RJ, Berlin CI, Hejtmancik JF, et al. Clinical diagnosis of the Usher syndromes. Usher syndrome consortium. *Am J Med Genet*. 1994;50(1):32–38.

244. Van den Bosch J. A new syndrome in three generations of a Dutch family. *Ophthalmologica*. 1959;137:422–423.

245. Byrne S, Dionisi-Vici C, Smith L, Gautel M, Jungbluth H. Vici syndrome: a review. *Orphanet J Rare Dis*. 2016; 11:21.

246. Finocchi A, Angelino G, Cantarutti N, et al. Immunodeficiency in Vici syndrome: a heterogeneous phenotype. *Am J Med Genet*. 2012;158A:434–439.

247. McClelland V, Cullup T, Bodi I, et al. Vici syndrome associated with sensorineural hearing loss and evidence of neuromuscular involvement on muscle biopsy. *Am J Med Genet*. 2010;152A:741–747.

248. Said E, Soler D, Sewry C. Vici syndrome—a rapidly progressive neurodegenerative disorder with hypopigmentation, immunodeficiency and myopathic changes on muscle biopsy. *Am J Med Genet A*. 2012;158A(2): 440–444.

249. Benhamou N, Souied EH, Zolf R, Coscas F, Coscas G, Soubrane G. Adult-onset foveomacular vitelliform dystrophy: a study by optical coherence tomography. *Am J Ophthal*. 2003;135:362–367.

250. Manes G, Meunier I, Avila-Fernandez A. Mutations in IMPG1 cause vitelliform macular dystrophies. *Am J Hum Genet*. 2013;93:571–578.

251. Yamaguchi K, Yoshida M, Kano T, Itabashi T, Yoshioka Y, Tamai M. Adult-onset foveomacular vitelliform dystrophy with retinal folds. *Jpn J Ophthal*. 2001; 45:533–537.

252. Michaelides M, Urquhart J, Holder GE, et al. Evidence of genetic heterogeneity in MRCS (microcornea, rod-cone dystrophy, cataract and posterior staphyloma) syndrome. *Am J Ophthal*. 2006;141:418–420.

253. Reddy MA, Francis PJ, Berry V, et al. A clinical and molecular genetic study of a rare dominantly inherited syndrome (MRCS) comprising of microcornea, rod-cone dystrophy, cataract, and posterior staphyloma. *Br J Ophthal*. 2003;87:197–202.

254. Graemiger RA, Niemeyer G, Schneeberger SA, Messmer EP. Wagner vitreoretinal degeneration. Follow-up of the original pedigree. *Ophthalmology*. 1995; 102(12):1830–1839.

255. Kloeckener-Gruissem B, Bartholdi D, Abdou M-T, Zimmermann DR, Berger W. Identification of the genetic defect in the original Wagner syndrome family. *Mol Vis*. 2006;12:350–355.

256. Miyamoto T, Inoue H, Sakamoto Y, et al. Identification of a novel splice site mutation of the CSPG2 gene in a Japanese family with Wagner syndrome. *Invest Ophthalmol Vis Sci*. 2005;46(8):2726–2735.

257. Mukhopadhyay A, Nikopoulos K, Maugeri A, et al. Erosive vitreoretinopathy and Wagner disease are caused by intronic mutations in CSPG2/versican that result in an imbalance of splice variants. *Invest Ophthal Vis Sci*. 2006; 47:3565–3572.

258. Ronan SM, Tran-Viet KN, Burner EL, Metlapally R, Toth CA, Young TL. Mutational hot spot potential of a novel base pair mutation of the CSPG2 gene in a family

with Wagner syndrome. *Arch Ophthalmol.* 2009;127(11): 1511−1519.

259. Cano A, Rouzier C, Monnot S, et al. French Group of Wolfram Syndrome, Vialettes B. Identification of novel mutations in WFS1 and genotype-phenotype correlation in Wolfram syndrome. *Am J Med Genet A.* 2007; 143A(14):1605−1612.

260. Chaussenot A, Bannwarth S, Rouzier C, et al. Neurologic features and genotype-phenotype correlation in Wolfram syndrome. *Ann Neurol.* 2011;69:501−508.

261. Inoue H, Tanizawa Y, Wasson J, et al. A gene encoding a transmembrane protein is mutated in patients with diabetes mellitus and optic atrophy (Wolfram syndrome). *Nat Genet.* 1998;20(2):143−148.

262. Rando TA, Horton JC, Layzer RB. Wolfram syndrome: evidence of a diffuse neurodegenerative disease by magnetic resonance imaging. *Neurology.* 1992;42:1220−1224.

263. Wragg R, Dias RP, Barrett T, McCarthy L. Bladder dysfunction in Wolfram syndrome is highly prevalent and progresses to megacystis. *J Pediatr Surg.* November 14, 2017. https://doi.org/10.1016/j.jpedsurg.2017.11.025 [Epub ahead of print].

## FURTHER READING

1. Chulz JB, Klockgether T, Dichgans J, Seibel P, Reichmann H. Mitochondrial gene mutations and diabetes mellitus. *Lett Lancet.* 1993;341:438−439.

2. Cipriani V, Silva RS, Arno G, et al. Duplication events downstream of IRX1 cause North Carolina macular dystrophy at the MCDR3 locus. *Sci Rep.* 2017;7:7512.

3. O'Donnell Jr FE, Pappas HR. Autosomal dominant foveal hypoplasia and presenile cataracts: a new syndrome. *Arch Ophthal.* 1982;100:279−281.

4. Perez Y, Gradstein L, Flusser H, et al. Isolated foveal hypoplasia with secondary nystagmus and low vision is associated with a homozygous SLC38A8 mutation. *Eur J Hum Genet.* 2014;22:703−706.

5. Savage SA, Giri N, Baerlocher GM, Orr N, Lansdorp PM, Alter BP. TINF2, a component of the shelterin telomere protection complex, is mutated in dyskeratosis congenita. *Am J Hum Genet.* 2008;82:501−509.

6. Schrijver-Wieling I, van Rens GHMB, Wittebol-Post D, et al. Retinal dystrophy in long chain 3-hydroxy-acyl-CoA dehydrogenase deficiency. *Br J Ophthal.* 1997;81:291−294.

7. Sorr EM, Goldberg RE. Vitelliform dystrophy in a 64-year-old man. *Am J Ophthal.* 1976;82:256−258.

# Resources

SARA FARD • NATARIO L. COUSER

**Website:** American Academy of Ophthalmology (AAO) Recommendations for Genetic Testing of Inherited Eye Diseases
**Description:** AAO task force's 2014 recommendations for ophthalmic genetic testing.
**URL:** https://www.aao.org/clinical-statement/recommen dations-genetic-testing-of-inherited-eye-d

**Website:** American Board of Genetic Counseling
**Description:** The organization in charge of giving credential certification in the field of genetic counseling in the United States and Canada.
**URL:** http://www.abgc.net/home/

**Website:** American College of Medical Genetics
**Description:** An organization composed of various individuals with specializations in genetics focused on the practice of medical genetics.
**URL:** https://www.acmg.net/

**Website:** American Society of Human Genetics
**Description:** Professional organization for specialist in human genetics.
**URL:** http://www.ashg.org/

**Website:** Atlas of Genetics and Cytogenetics in Oncology and Haematology
**Description:** Online encyclopedia and database atlas of genes, cytogenetics, and cancer diseases that includes an overview of eye tumors.
**URL:** http://atlasgeneticsoncology.org//Tumors/EyeTum OverviewID5272.html

**Website:** Children's Craniofacial Association
**Description:** Educational resource and patient support for craniofacial syndromes.
**URL:** https://ccakids.org/

**Website:** Clinical Trials Database
**Description:** A database that contains clinical studies of human participants from around the world.
**URL:** http://www.clinicaltrials.gov/

**Website:** Diseases Database
**Description:** Diseases Database is a cross-referenced index and search portal of internal medical disorders, symptoms and signs, congenital and inherited disorders, infectious diseases and organisms, drugs and medications, and common hematological and biochemical investigation abnormalities. This database resembles an online standard medical textbook, with definitions, explanations and links to web resources.
**URL:** http://www.diseasesdatabase.com/

**Website:** Dolan DNA Learning Center
**Description:** This website, with hands-on programs, links to educational and bioinformatics websites, and other resources including libraries and online 3D simulations, designed to enhance understanding of genes in education. Hosted by the Cold Spring Harbor Laboratory.
**URL:** https://www.dnalc.org/

**Website:** Eye Wiki Genetic Eye Diseases
**Description:** List of select genetic eye conditions in AAO's online eye encyclopedia written and maintained by eye physicians and surgeons.
**URL:** http://eyewiki.aao.org/Genetic_Eye_Diseases

**Website:** Face2Gene by FDNA
**Description:** A search and reference application that utilizes facial dysmorphology novel analysis technology to detect dysmorphic features from facial photos.
**URL:** http://www.fdna.com/

**Website:** From the Blueprint to You
**Description:** A website with genetic education resources for teachers, including the booklet, "From the Blueprint to You," that explores the world of genetics; DNA; the Human Genome Project; the ethical, legal, and social implications of genetic research; and the future of genomics. Hosted by the National Human Genome Research Institute.
**URL:** https://www.genome.gov/12511466/from-the-blueprint-to-you/

**Website:** GeneCards
**Description:** Comprehensive database containing information on known and predicted human genes.
**URL:** http://www.genecards.org/

**Website:** GeneEd: Genetics, Education, Discovery

**Description:** A website with illustrations and animations, designed to facilitate learning about cell biology, DNA, genes and chromosomes, inheritance patterns, epigenetics, genetic conditions, evolution, biostatistics, biotechnology, DNA forensics, and top issues in genetics. Hosted by the National Library of Medicine.

**URL:** https://geneed.nlm.nih.gov/

**Website:** GeneReviews

**Description:** Publications consisting of standardized and clinical information for the diagnoses, management, and treatment of patients with inherited conditions.

**URL:** http://www.ncbi.nlm.nih.gov/books/NBK1116/advanced/

**Website:** Genetic Alliance

**Description:** Nonprofit health advocacy group with a network of numerous disease advocacy organizations that has a focus of promoting health in genetic research and technology.

**URL:** http://www.geneticalliance.org/

**Website:** Genetic and Rare Disease Information Center (GARD)

**Description:** A database that is part of the NIH that provides useful information about genetic and rare diseases.

**URL:** http://rarediseases.info.nih.gov/gard

**Website:** Genetic Centers, Clinics, and Departments

**Description:** A website designed to facilitate the identification of genetic counselors, centers, clinics and departments, both nationally and internationally. Hosted by the Genetics Education Center at the University of Kansas Medical Center.

**URL:** http://www.kumc.edu/gec/prof/genecntr.html

**Website:** Genetics Home Reference

**Description:** A website that provides information about genetic variations.

**URL:** http://ghr.nlm.nih.gov/

**Website:** Hereditary Ocular Disease, University of Arizona

**Description:** A database of hereditary ocular diseases for patients and clinicians.

**URL:** http://disorders.eyes.arizona.edu/

**Website:** HUGO Gene Nomenclature Committee (HGNC)

**Description:** Authority that assigns the nomenclature standards for human genes.

**URL:** http://www.genenames.org/

**Website:** Human Genome Epidemiology Network (HuGENet)

**Description:** An international collaboration on public health genomics, useful for sharing population-based human genome epidemiologic information, hosted by Centers for Disease Control (CDC).

**URL:** http://www.cdc.gov/genomics/hugenet/default.htm

**Website:** Human Genome Project Education Resources

**Description:** A collection of publications, teaching aids, and additional internet resources, hosted by the Human Genome Program of the US Department of Energy.

**URL:** https://web.ornl.gov/sci/techresources/Human_Genome/map.shtml

**Website:** Human Genome Resources

**Description:** Comprehensive one-stop genomic information center, hosted by the National Center for Biotechnology Information. Allows for genome data viewing of all autosomal, sex, and mitochondrial chromosomes.

**URL:** www.ncbi.nlm.nih.gov/genome/guide/human/

**Website:** Human Genome Variation Society (HGVS)

**Description:** Maintains genomic variation data and nomenclature information on sequence variants.

**URL:** http://www.hgvs.org/

**Website:** Hunt for missing heritability: challenges and opportunities for novel locus discovery in non-European populations

**Description:** Webinar to explore common and rare genetic variants in populations other than the European cohort, including African, Asian, and other ancestries, in search for novel susceptibility genes.

**URL:** webinar.sciencemag.org/webinar/archive/hunt-missing-heritability

**Website:** International Society for Genetic Eye Diseases and Retinoblastoma (ISGEDR)

**Description:** Professional organization with a goal of promoting shared information, collaborations, and the dissemination of scientific knowledge of genetic diseases of the eye and retinoblastoma.

**URL:** https://isgedr.com/

**Website:** Learn Genetics

**Description:** A website designed to teach individuals about genetics, including basic genetics, pigeon breeding, variation and selection with respect to time, epigenetics and genetic science, among other topics including human health, cell biology, neuroscience, plants, ecology, and science tools. Hosted

by the Genetic Science Learning Center at the University of Utah.
URL: http://learn.genetics.utah.edu/

**Website:** Life Sciences Core Facilities
**Description:** A website designed to provide information on a wide range of scientific and technical services available to researchers in the fields of genetics and life sciences at large. Hosted by the Weizmann Institute of Science.
URL: http://www.weizmann.ac.il/Biological_Services/

**Website:** Mastermind genome search
**Description:** Mastermind is a search engine designed to accelerate variant curation by searching through millions of articles and providing possible disease-gene-variant relationships. Mastermind does not draw conclusions about the clinical significance of these individual variants, but instead provides the user with all the necessary evidence to do so on their own.
URL: https://mastermind.genomenon.com/

**Website:** Matchmaker Exchange
**Description:** A website designed to find genetic etiologies for rare diseases through standardized application programming interfaces and procedural conventions. At Matchmaker Exchange, teams, and projects work toward a federated platform to match similar phenotypic and genotypic profiles. Hosted by the Matchmaker Exchange project, which launched in 2013.
URL: http://www.matchmakerexchange.org/

Website: MedGen
**Description:** Published material related to human medical genetics.
URL: http://www.ncbi.nlm.nih.gov/medgen/

**Website:** MitoAction
**Description:** MitoAction is a nonprofit organization, started in 2005, that is aimed at improving the quality of life of individuals and families affected by mitochondrial disease.
URL: www.mitoaction.org/support

**Website:** Mitochondrial Medicine Society
**Description:** Website for the Mitochondrial Medicine Society, founded in 2000, that represents a group of international physicians, researchers, and clinicians promoting the identification, management, and treatment strategies for mitochondrial diseases.
URL: www.mitosoc.org/

**Website:** My Family Health Portrait
**Description:** Tool used to create a family health history.
URL: https://familyhistory.hhs.gov/FHH/html/index.html

**Website:** National Center for Biotechnology Information (NCBI)
**Description:** Formed as a division of the National Library of Medicine in 1988, which now serves as a central hub for providing numerous databases, tools, and educational resources of biomedical information.
URL: http://www.ncbi.nlm.nih.gov/

**Website:** National Human Genome Research Institute Glossary
**Description:** Contains terms and concepts used in the study of genetics for the public.
URL: http://www.genome.gov/Glossary/

**Website:** National Institutes of Health Genetic Testing Registry (GTR)
**Description:** Serves as a centralized location for providers to submit genetic test information.
URL: http://www.ncbi.nlm.nih.gov/gtr/

**Website:** National Newborn Screening and Global Resource Center (NNSGRC)
**Description:** Contains information on newborn screening, state contacts, general resources and provides information sheets that describe the proper steps to follow after receiving a screening report.
URL: http://genes-r-us.uthscsa.edu/resources.htm

**Website:** National Ophthalmic Disease Genotyping and Phenotyping Network (eyeGENE)
**Description:** National Eye Institute research initiative allowing researchers access to DNA samples, clinical data, and patients interested in research.
URL: https://www.nei.nih.gov/eyegene/

**Website:** National Organization for Rare Disorders (NORD)
**Description:** An organization that provides support to those with rare disease by providing funding, research, education, and networking.
URL: http://www.rarediseases.org/

**Website:** National Society of Genetic Counselors
**Description:** An organization composed of trained genetic counselors and other health professionals dedicated to the promotion of genetic counseling.
URL: http://www.nsgc.org/

**Website:** OMIM (Online Mendelian Inheritance in Man)
**Description:** A database of human genes and genetic phenotypes.
URL: http://www.omim.org/

**Website:** Orphanet
**Description:** Provides information about rare diseases and treatments.

URL: http://www.orpha.net/consor/cgi-bin/index.php

**Website:** Pediatric Ophthalmology Education Center
**Description:** AAO pediatric ophthalmology resource center.
**URL (Main page):** https://www.aao.org/pediatric-ophthalmology-strabismus
**URL (Genetic Eye Specific):** https://www.aao.org/pediatric-ophthalmology-strabismus-listing?subspecialty=pediatric-ophthalmology-strabismus&subtopic=Genetic_Eye_Diseases

**Website:** Pedigree Nomenclature
**Description:** A standard used in the design of pedigrees to provide consistent information to research and health professionals as well as those in training.
**URL:** http://www.ncbi.nlm.nih.gov/pubmed/18792771 (Bennett RL et al., Standardized human pedigree nomenclature: update and assessment of the recommendations of the National Society of Genetic Counselors, J Genet Couns. 2008 Oct; 17(5): 424–33, doi: 10.1007/s10897-008-9169-9. Epub 2008 Sep 16.)

**Website:** Scitable
**Description:** A complementary science library for personal learning, with a focus on genetics specifically. Hosted by *Nature* publishing group.
**URL:** www.nature.com/scitable

**Website:** Stanford at The Tech
**Description:** A website designed to help clear misunderstandings about genetics, where individuals can submit questions to a geneticist, explore online exhibits, visit the video gallery, and read pertinent articles. Hosted by the Tech Museum of Innovation, supported by the Department of Genetics at Stanford School of Medicine.
**URL:** http://genetics.thetech.org/

**Website:** Tokyo Medical University Genetics Study Group

**Description:** An animated website designed to enhance understanding of how chromosome abnormalities occur, hosted by the Tokyo Medical University Genetics Study Group.
**URL:** http://www.tokyo-med.ac.jp/genet/index-e.htm

**Website:** Understanding Gene Testing
**Description:** An informative tutorial on genes and genetic testing, with many illustrations to enhance understanding. Hosted by the National Cancer Institute at the US Department of Health and Human Services.
**URL:** http://www.accessexcellence.org/AE/AEPC/NIH/

**Website:** United Mitochondrial Disease Foundation (UMDF)
**Description:** The UMDF's mission is to promote support, research, and education for the identification and treatment of mitochondrial disorders.
**URL:** www.umdf.org/

**Website:** Unique
**Description:** Provides resources and support for families of children who have rare chromosome disorders.
**URL:** http://www.rarechromo.org/html/home.asp

**Website:** Your Genes Your Health
**Description:** An illustrative guide to genetic disorders, with details on disease etiology, inheritance, diagnosis, treatment, and prognosis. Hosted by the Cold Spring Harbor Laboratory.
**URL:** www.ygyh.org

**Website:** Your Genome
**Description:** A website designed to enhance understanding of broad genetic concepts, including DNA, genes, and genomes, with multiple facts, videos, and glossary terms as useful resources.
**URL:** www.yourgenome.org

# Eye Genetic Disorders by Clinical Sign

SARA FARD • NATARIO L. COUSER

1. Almond-shaped palpebral fissures
   CK syndrome
   Cohen syndrome
   Hunter-Mcalpine craniosynostosis syndrome
   Prader-Willi syndrome

2. Blepharophimosis
   Blepharophimosis, ptosis, and epicanthus
     inversus (BPES)
   Cerebrooculofacioskeletal syndrome
   Craniosynostosis-mental retardation syndrome
     of Lin and Gettig
   Dubowitz syndrome
   Ectrodactyly-ectodermal dysplasia-clefting
     (EEC) syndrome
   Frontofacionasal dysplasia
   Goldenhar syndrome (hemifacial microsomia)
   Kaufman oculocerebrofacial syndrome
   Nablus masklike facial syndrome
   Schwartz-Jampel syndrome
   Syndromic microphthalmia 2 (oculofacio-
     cardiodental syndrome)
   Syndromic microphthalmia 9 (Matthew-Wood
     syndrome)
   Waardenburg syndrome

3. Blue sclera
   Axenfeld-Rieger syndrome
   Brittle cornea syndrome
   Dubowitz syndrome
   Ehlers-Danlos syndrome
   Goldberg-Shprintzen megacolon syndrome
   Hallermann-Streiff syndrome
   Kabuki syndrome
   Mevalonic aciduria
   Neonatal progeroid syndrome
   Oculocerebral syndrome with hypopigmentation
   Osteogenesis imperfecta
   Roberts syndrome
   Russell-Silver syndrome
   Turner syndrome

4. Deep-set eyes
   Alagille syndrome
   Avellino corneal dystrophy (combined
     granular-lattice corneal dystrophy)
   Barth syndrome
   Beckwith-Wiedemann syndrome
   Cerebrooculofacioskeletal syndrome
   Christianson syndrome
   Cornelia de Lange syndrome
   Lowe oculocerebrorenal syndrome
   Mental retardation, X-linked with
     cerebellar hypoplasia and distinctive
     facial appearance
   Micro syndrome
   Moyamoya disease, syndromic
   Muscular dystrophy-dystroglycanopathy, Type
     A (MDDGA)
   Short syndrome

5. Downslanting palpebral fissures
   Agenesis of the corpus callosum with mental
     retardation, ocular coloboma, and
     micrognathia
   Antley-Bixler syndrome (ABS)
   Apert syndrome
   Baraitser-Winter syndrome
   Beare-Stevenson cutis gyrata syndrome
   Beckwith-Wiedemann syndrome
   Carpenter syndrome
   Cat eye syndrome
   Char syndrome
   Charge syndrome
   Chondrodysplasia punctata 2 X-linked
     dominant
   Cohen syndrome
   Coloboma and micrognathia
   Cornelia de Lange syndrome
   Craniosynostosis-mental retardation syndrome
     of Lin and Gettig
   Cri du chat syndrome

Cutis laxa, Debre type
DiGeorge syndrome
Fine-Lubinsky syndrome
Goldberg-Shprintzen megacolon syndrome
Hallermann-Streiff syndrome
Lacrimo-auriculo-dento-digital syndrome
Mevalonic aciduria
Miller syndrome
Muenke syndrome
Nager acrofacial dysostosis
Native American myopathy
Neurofibromatosis-Noonan syndrome
Noonan syndrome
Oculoauriculofrontonasal syndrome
Oral-facial-digital syndrome
Pfeiffer syndrome
Pontocerebellar hypoplasia
Roberts syndrome
Roifman syndrome
Rubinstein-Taybi syndrome (broad thumb-hallux syndrome)
Shprintzen-Goldberg craniosynostosis
Simpson-Golabi-Behmel syndrome
Sotos syndrome
Temtamy syndrome
Treacher Collins syndrome
Wolf-Hirschhorn syndrome (Wittwer syndrome)

Methylmalonic aciduria and homocystinuria, CB1F type
MICPCH syndrome
Microcephaly microcornea syndrome, Seemanova type
Moebius syndrome
Neurofibromatosis-Noonan syndrome
Noonan syndrome
Oculodentodigital dysplasia
Opitz trigonocephaly syndrome
PEHO syndrome (progressive encephalopathy with edema, hypsarrhythmia, and optic atrophy)
Pontocerebellar hypoplasia
Prieto syndrome
Rhizomelic chondrodysplasia punctata type 1
Rubinstein-Taybi syndrome (broad thumb-hallux syndrome)
Simpson-Golabi-Behmel syndrome
Syndromic microphthalmia 14
Triple X syndrome
Turner syndrome
Williams syndrome
Wolf-Hirschhorn syndrome (Wittwer syndrome)
Zellweger syndrome—peroxisome biogenesis disorder 1A (PBD1A)

6. Epicanthal folds
   Baraitser-Winter syndrome
   Beckwith-Wiedemann syndrome
   Cantu syndrome
   Carpenter syndrome
   Cat eye syndrome
   Cerebrooculonasal syndrome
   Chime syndrome
   Craniosynostosis-mental retardation syndrome of Lin and Gettig
   Cri du chat syndrome
   CK syndrome
   Down syndrome
   Duane-radial ray syndrome
   Dubowitz syndrome
   Edwards syndrome
   Ehlers-Danlos syndrome
   Hypomelanosis of Ito
   Jacobsen syndrome
   Joubert syndrome
   Juberg-Marsidi syndrome
   Kaufman oculocerebrofacial syndrome
   Leopard syndrome
   Mannosidosis
   Marinesco-Sjogren syndrome

7. Hypertelorism
   Alagille syndrome
   Antley-Bixler syndrome (ABS)
   Apert syndrome
   Axenfeld-Rieger syndrome
   Baller-Gerold syndrome
   Baraitser-Winter syndrome
   Barber Say syndrome
   Basal cell nevus syndrome
   Beare-Stevenson syndrome
   Beckwith-Wiedemann syndrome
   Cat eye syndrome
   Cerebrooculonasal syndrome
   Char syndrome
   Charge syndrome
   Chime syndrome
   Coach syndrome
   Congenital disorder of glycosylation, type Iq
   Cornelia de Lange syndrome
   Craniometaphyseal dysplasia
   Craniosynostosis—Adelaide and Philadelphia types
   Craniosynostosis-mental retardation syndrome of Lin and Gettig

Cri du chat syndrome
Crouzon syndrome
Crouzon syndrome with Acanthosis nigricans
    (crouzonodermoskeletal syndrome)
Beare-Stevenson cutis gyrata syndrome
DiGeorge syndrome
Donnai-Barrow syndrome
Duane-radial ray syndrome
Edwards syndrome
Fraser syndrome
Fine-Lubinsky syndrome
Frontofacionasal dysplasia
Gaucher disease type 1
GM1 gangliosidosis, type I
Gomez-Lopez-Hernandez syndrome
    (cerebello-trigeminal-dermal dysplasia)
Hamamy syndrome
Hypomelanosis of Ito
Jackson-Weiss syndrome
Jacobsen syndrome
Juberg-Marsidi syndrome
Lacrimo-auriculo-dento-digital syndrome
Leopard syndrome
Marshall syndrome
Meckel syndrome
Micpch syndrome
Microcephaly microcornea syndrome, Seema-
    nova type
Moebius syndrome
Molybdenum cofactor deficiency
Moyamoya disease, syndromic
Muenke syndrome
Neonatal progeroid syndrome
Neurofibromatosis-Noonan syndrome
Noonan syndrome
Oculoauriculofrontonasal syndrome
Oral-facial-digital syndrome
Opitz syndrome
Peters plus syndrome (Krause-Kivlin
    syndrome)
Pfeiffer syndrome
POR (cytochrome P450 oxidoreductase)
    deficiency with Antley-Bixler phenotype
Prieto syndrome
Rhizomelic chondrodysplasia punctata type 1
Roberts syndrome
Saethre-Chotzen syndrome
Shprintzen-Goldberg craniosynostosis
    syndrome
Simpson-Golabi-Behmel syndrome
Spondyloepiphyseal dysplasia
Sotos syndrome

Tarp syndrome
Temtamy syndrome
Treacher collins syndrome
Triple X syndrome
Triploidy
Turner syndrome
Waardenburg syndrome
Wolf-Hirschhorn syndrome (Wittwer
    syndrome)
XYY syndrome

8. Hypotelorism
    Craniosynostosis, Boston type
    Craniosynostosis-mental retardation syndrome
        of Lin and Gettig
    Craniotelencephalic dysplasia
    Hereditary neuralgic amyotrophy
    Holoprosencephaly
    Martsolf syndrome
    Meckel syndrome
    Mental retardation, X-linked with cerebellar
        hypoplasia and distinctive facial appearance
    Oculodentodigital dysplasia
    Patau syndrome
    Schilbach-Rott syndrome
    Syndromic microphthalmia 3
        (microphthalmia and esophageal atresia
        syndrome)
    Williams syndrome

9. Synophrys
    Beckwith-Wiedemann syndrome
    Cornelia de Lange syndrome
    Goldberg-Shprintzen megacolon syndrome
    Mucopolysaccharidosis type IIIA (Sanfilippo
        syndrome A)
    Mucopolysaccharidosis type IIIB (Sanfilippo
        syndrome B)
    Mucopolysaccharidosis type IIIC (Sanfilippo
        syndrome C)
    Mucopolysaccharidosis type IIID (Sanfilippo
        syndrome D)
    Proud syndrome
    Waardenburg syndrome

10. Sparse eyebrows or eyelashes
    Aicardi syndrome
    Cerebrooculonasal syndrome
    Dubowitz syndrome
    Dyskeratosis congenita
    Ectrodactyly-ectodermal dysplasia-clefting
        (EEC) syndrome
    Hays-Wells syndrome

Kabuki syndrome
Kaufman oculocerebrofacial syndrome
Keratosis follicularis spinulosa decalvans
Neonatal progeroid syndrome
Renpenning syndrome (mental retardation,
    X-linked, Renpenning type)
Syndromic microphthalmia 3
    (microphthalmia and esophageal atresia
    syndrome)
Treacher Collins syndrome

11. Telecanthus
    Axenfeld-Rieger syndrome
    Barber Say syndrome
    Blepharophimosis, ptosis, and epicanthus
        inversus (BPES)
    Charge syndrome
    Cornelia de Lange syndrome
    Cutis laxa, Debre type
    Dubowitz syndrome
    Frontofacionasal dysplasia
    Goldberg-Shprintzen megacolon syndrome
    Gomez-Lopez-Hernandez syndrome
        (cerebello-trigeminal-dermal dysplasia)
    Kaufman oculocerebrofacial syndrome
    Lacrimo-auriculo-dento-digital syndrome
    Native American myopathy
    Opitz syndrome

Oral-facial-digital syndrome
Short syndrome
Shprintzen-Goldberg craniosynostosis
    syndrome
Wolf-Hirschhorn syndrome (Wittwer
    syndrome)

12. Upslanting palpebral fissures
    Alagille syndrome
    CK syndrome
    Craniosynostosis-mental retardation syndrome
        of Lin and Gettig
    DiGeorge syndrome
    Down syndrome
    Juberg-Marsidi syndrome
    Kaufman oculocerebrofacial syndrome
    Microcephaly microcornea syndrome, Seema-
        nova type
    Neonatal progeroid syndrome
    Opitz trigonocephaly syndrome
    Peters plus syndrome (Krause-Kivlin
        syndrome)
    Prader-Willi syndrome
    Renpenning syndrome (mental retardation,
        X-linked, Renpenning type)
    Rhizomelic chondrodysplasia punctata type 1
    Triple X syndrome
    Wieacker-Wolff syndrome

# Glossary

MAHEER MASOOD • GURJAS S. BAJAJ • NATARIO L. COUSER

**Ablepharon** - Absent eyelids.

**Adeno-associated virus (AAV) vectors** - Vectors derived from adeno-associated viruses and the most frequently used delivery systems in ocular gene therapy.

**Advanced maternal age (AMA)** - A designation given to a woman who gives birth at or over the age of 35.

**Alacrima** - Deficiency or absence of tear production.

**Alleles** - A variant of a gene located at a certain locus.

**Amino acid sequence** - Refers to the order of amino acids in a polypeptide chain.

**Amino acids** - A class of biological molecules characterized by an amine and carboxylic group along with a particular functional group. They are the main building blocks of proteins and have other important biological functions.

**Aneuploidy** - The state in which one or more extra or missing chromosomes are present.

**Aniridia** - Absence of an iris.

**Ankyloblepharon** - The interrupted, partial, or complete fusion of the upper and lower eyelids by webs of skin.

**Anomaly** - An anatomical departure from the phenotype present in the reference population.

**Anophthalmia** - The unilateral or bilateral absence of ocular tissue secondary to the abnormal development of the optic vesicle.

**Association** - Unrelated pattern of anomalies in occurrence more often than expected by chance.

**Autosomal dominant (AD) inheritance** - An inheritance pattern in which only one copy of the mutated gene within a nonsex chromosome is needed to get the disease.

**Autosomal recessive (AR) inheritance** - An inheritance pattern in which two mutated genes, one mutated gene from each parent within the nonsex chromosomes, is needed to get the disease. The effects of those particular inherited chromosomes.

**Autosome** - A chromosome that is numbered and not considered a sex chromosome.

**Blepharitis** - Inflammation of eyelids.

**Blepharophimosis** - Horizontally narrow palpebral fissure.

**Blepharoptosis** - Abnormal relaxation of upper eyelid.

**Carrier testing** - A form of genetic testing used on individuals who may not present with any genetic disorder but are at risk of passing down the trait due to being a carrier. This usually relates to being a carrier of an autosomal recessive or X-linked disorder.

**Central dogma of molecular biology** - Describes the flow of genetic material in that DNA encodes for RNA (transcription), which in turn then encodes for proteins (translation). Exceptions to the classic dogma are now known to exist.

**Chalazion** - Benign, typically painless, inner eyelid nodule due to a blocked oil gland.

**Chromosomal karyotype** - A photographic representation of an individual cell's chromosomes that is used to analyze the number and structure of the chromosomes.

**Chromosomal microarray** - Evaluates the genome in high resolution by using arrayed small DNA pieces to provide a locus by locus measurement of DNA copy number variation at numerous loci simultaneously.

**Chromosome translocation** - An abnormality that involves the exchange of genetic material of nonhomologous chromosomes. Translocations can involve the exchange of equal amounts of material (balanced) or involve additional or missing material (unbalanced).

**Chromosome** - An organized and packed structure of DNA, RNA, and proteins located within a cell.

**Cicatricial lagophthalmos** - Inability to close eyelids due to scarring.

**Clinical genetic testing** - Genetic testing performed to discover information for the patient and family involved.

**Clinical Laboratory Improvement Amendments (CLIA)** - US federal regulatory standards that were first established in 1988 that requires certification for any lab prior to performing clinical diagnostic testing on human samples. The Center for Disease Control (CDC), Center for Medicaid Services (CMS), and the Food and Drug Administration (FDA) play a role in the function of CLIA.

**Cloning** - A process that consists of creating identical copies of the DNA, a cell, or an organism.

**Coloboma** - A unilateral or bilateral incomplete closure of the embryonic optic fissure resulting in a defect in uveal structures and/or optic nerve. Defects are typically located in the inferior or inferonasal portion of the globe.

**Consanguinity** - Used to describe genetic relatedness between individuals due to a common ancestor of origin.

Consultand - The person in the family who presents for a genetic counseling evaluation regarding a known or potential inherited condition.

Corectopia - Displacement of the pupil.

Craniosynostosis - Refers to the premature fusion of the fibrous sutures of the skull during infancy, resulting in malformation of the skull.

Dacryocystitis - Infection of the lacrimal sac.

De novo (sporadic) mutation - An altered gene that appears in the germline or fertilized egg that was not manifested in the family lineage.

Deletion - Change in the DNA sequence involving a portion of the DNA being removed.

Deoxyribonucleic acid (DNA) - A biological molecule, generally double stranded, that encodes the genetic information of an organism.

Direct-to-consumer genetic testing through physician - Genetic testing marketed directly to consumers and physicians, and requires the physician to order the test.

Direct-to-consumer genetic testing - Genetic testing marketed and sold directly to consumers without the involvement of healthcare professionals.

Disease - Condition involving abnormal cognitive or physical function.

Distichiasis - Abnormal eyelashes growing from duct of meibomian gland at eyelid margin.

Duplication - Change in the DNA sequence involving an extra copy or copies of a portion of the DNA.

Dystopia canthorum - Lateral displacement of inner canthus.

Ectropion - Outward turned eyelids.

Entropion - Inward turned eyelids.

Epiblepharon - Inward turning of eyelashes.

Epiphora - Excessive tearing.

Esotropia - Inward misalignment of the eyes.

Euryblepharon - Increased vertical separation of palpebral fissure.

Exome - The part of the genome that corresponds to the complete set of exons.

Exons - Sequences in the DNA that corresponds to protein coding regions.

Exotropia - Outward misalignment of the eyes.

Fluorescence in situ hybridization (FISH) - Uses a targeted approach to analyze a specific sequence of a chromosome. The technique consists of using a specific probe DNA that is labeled and is hybridized to a sample DNA of interest. Recording of the labeled hybridization, or lack of, can then be analyzed.

Frameshift mutation - Change in the DNA sequence, either an insertion or deletion, not a multiple of three, which causes a shift in the reading frame.

Gene locus - The exact location of a gene on a chromosome.

Gene therapy - The experimental process of inserting genes for the purpose of treatment.

Genes - A sequence of DNA that corresponds to a unit of hereditary information, usually coding for a protein.

Genetic counselor - A health professional specialized in the area of genetics and counseling about various genetic information to individuals.

Genetic Information Nondiscrimination Act of 2008 (GINA) - Legislation passed by the US Congress that prohibits employers and health insurance agencies from using genetic information in decisions.

Geneticist - An individual specialized in the study of genetics, which is composed of genes, heredity, and variation.

Genome browser - An online site that contains a collection of genomic data information.

Genome-wide association study (GWAS) - A technique that is used to study genetic markers across complete sets of DNA in different people to find genetic variation in a particular trait.

Genotype - The genetic makeup of an individual usually referring to a specific set of alleles or traits.

Germinal mutation - A change in the DNA sequence in the germline and therefore can be passed on to the next generation.

Germline - The cell line in which the gametes are formed from.

Goniodysgenesis - Malformed ocular drainage angle.

Hemizygosity - State when only one copy of a gene is present in a diploid cell.

Human genome project - An international research study that sequenced the entire human genome and determined the genes that are encoded.

Hypertelorism - Abnormally large spacing between the eyes.

Hypohydrosis - Diminished sweating response.

Hypotelorism - Abnormally small spacing between the eyes.

Hypotrichosis - Abnormal hair loss.

Incidence - How many individuals are diagnosed as having a particular condition over a certain period.

Incomplete penetrance - Refers to the presence of a gene change that is not phenotypically expressed in some individuals but is expressed in others.

Insertion - Change in the DNA sequence involving an additional amount of DNA added in a new location.

Introns - Noncoding sequence found in DNA that is usually excised before translation.

Keratoconjunctivitis sicca - Dryness of cornea and conjunctiva.

Lacrimal mucocele - Lacrimal duct cyst extending into nose.

Lisch nodules - Dome-shaped melanocytic hamartomas on the iris.

Loss of heterozygosity (LOH) - Presence of only one copy of an allele, such as the loss of a portion of a chromosome within tumor tissue.

Madarosis - Loss of eyelashes.

Malformation - A nonprogressive congenital anomaly.

Massively parallel sequencing - High-throughput DNA sequencing that allows for numerous strands of DNA to be sequenced in a parallel fashion. Also called next-generation sequencing.

Megalocornea - Horizontal cornea length exceeding 13 mm or 12 mm in the newborn.

Meiosis - A form of cell division consisting of two nuclear divisions of a diploid cell resulting in the formation of haploid gametes.

Mendelian genetics - Genetic inheritance pattern proposed by Gregor Mendel that is composed of three main laws. The Law of Segregation states that allele segregation results in one allele per gamete. The Law of Independent Assortment states genes from different traits segregate independently. The Law of Dominance states that alleles may be dominant or recessive, and dominant alleles overshadow recessive alleles.

Microblepharon - Vertical shortening of eyelids.

Microcoria - Pupils less than 2 mm in diameter bilaterally.

Microcornea - A small cornea, measuring less than 10 mm in diameter in adults or less than 9 mm horizontally in newborns.

Microdeletion syndromes - A group of disorders affecting multiple genes, resulting from deletions of a chromosome segment spanning less than 5 Mb.

Microphakia - Abnormally small lens.

Microphthalmia - A small, disorganized globe that is two standard deviations below the age-adjusted mean axial length.

Missense mutation - Change in the DNA sequence involving a single base pair which causes an amino acid being substituted for another.

Mitochondrial inheritance - A form of inheritance from the genetic material located within the mitochondria. This form of inheritance is maternal and is always inherited by the progeny due to being part of the ovum.

Mitosis - A form of cell division in which somatic cells produce identical daughter cells.

Mosaicism - The presence of two or more cell populations in one individual that differ in their chromosomal genotype.

Multifactorial inheritance - A combination of various genetic and environmental factors that contribute to the development of a trait.

Mutation - A change in the DNA sequence of a gene.

Nanophthalmos - A small eye, typically with no other associated structural ocular defects.

Negative predictive value - The chance a person who tested negative does not have the condition.

Neurocutaneous - Pertaining to the skin and the nervous system.

Newborn screening - Testing performed on newborn babies to detect for a wide variety of disorders.

Next-generation sequencing - See Massively parallel sequencing.

Noninvasive prenatal testing (NIPT) - Test that uses cell-free circulating fetal DNA in maternal blood during pregnancy to screen for fetal chromosome anomalies.

Nonsense mutation - Change in the DNA sequence involving a single base pair that results in a premature stop codon, which leads to a shortened protein.

Nucleic acid sequence - Refers to the arrangement of letters that make up the nucleotide order in RNA and DNA.

Nucleotide - A nitrogenous base attached to a phosphate group and a pentose sugar molecule. A ribonucleotide, the main unit of RNA, is composed of a phosphate group, a ribose sugar, and a nitrogenous base (adenine [A], cytosine [C], guanine [G], or uracil [U]). A deoxyribonucleotide, the main unit in DNA, is composed of a phosphate group, deoxyribose sugar, and a nitrogenous base (adenine [A], cytosine [C], guanine [G], or thymine [T]).

Obligate carrier - Individual that must be a carrier of the genetic mutation of concern based on the known disorder inheritance pattern and family history obtained.

Ovum - A mature female haploid gamete.

Panel tests - Used to assess for mutations in multiple genes.

Pathogenic variant - Mutation that predisposes an individual to a specific disease.

Pedigree - A genetic representation of a family lineage that demonstrates various inheritance patterns in the family tree.

Personalized medicine - A form of medical practice that uses an individual's genetic makeup to guide treatment.

Peters anomaly - Cleavage of the anterior chamber with central corneal opacity.

Pharmacogenetics - A branch of pharmacology that studies the genetic responses to drug treatments.

Phenotype - The observable physical representation of an expressed gene.

Polymerase chain reaction (PCR) - Technique that allows a short sequence of DNA or RNA to be amplified.

Positive predictive value - The chance a person who tested positive has the condition.

Posterior embryotoxon - Displacement of Schwalbe's line anterior to limbus in cornea.

Prevalence - Total number within a population who have a condition at a particular time, often expressed as a percentage.

Proband - An individual who is being studied in genetics studies. Usually refers to the first affected family member with a genetic disorder or trait that begins the study of the family.

Proteins - A class of biological molecules that are composed of chains of amino acids.

Reflex testing - Automatic subsequent testing that takes place after an initial testing result.

Repeat expansion - Change in the DNA sequence involving consecutive repeated portions of short amounts of DNA.

Research genetic testing - Genetic testing performed as part of a research study to advance our knowledge of understanding genetic diseases, genes, and testing methods which may or may not provide immediate beneficial information to the patient or family involved.

Ribonucleic acid (RNA) - Biological macromolecule, generally single stranded, which primarily conveys information from DNA to control protein synthesis.

Sanger (dideoxy) sequencing - A technique for DNA sequence analysis that uses dideoxy nucleotides that will terminate the growing chain.

Sensitivity - How often a test will read positive for a person who has the condition (true positives).

Sequencing - The process of determining the sequence of a part of the genome.

Silent mutation - Change in the DNA sequence that does not actually change the protein sequence; translation of the same protein occurs.

Single gene tests - Analyzes a single gene in a sample DNA of interest to determine any abnormalities or absence of that single gene.

Single nucleotide polymorphism (SNP) - A form of DNA sequence variation in which a single nucleotide differs in a particular genome location in at least 1% within the population.

Somatic mutation - A change in the DNA that occurs after the conception period, therefore not passed on to the next generation.

Somatic - Any cell of the body excluding the gametes.

Specificity - How often a test will read negative for a person who does not have the condition (true negatives).

Sperm - A haploid male reproductive cell used in fertilization.

Spherophakia - Abnormally small and spherical lens.

Splice site mutation - Change in the DNA sequence that involves the location where intron splicing occurs.

Strabismus - Misalignment of the eyes.

Stye - Bacterial infection of the oil gland in eyelid.

Substitution - Change in the DNA sequence that replaces one base for another base.

Syndrome - Causally related pattern of anomalies.

Synophrys - Unibrow.

Uniparental disomy - A genetic inheritance situation in which both members of a chromosomal pair or both segments of chromosome are inherited from one parent and neither is inherited from the other parent.

Variant of uncertain significance (VUS) - A variation in a gene sequence in which the association of the variation with any disease is unknown.

Whole exome sequencing - A technique used to analyze the entire coding sequence, exons, of a DNA sample of interest. The DNA sample is compared with a control sample by detecting any changes in nucleotide sequences.

Whole genome sequencing - A technique that determines the entire DNA sequence in a genome.

X-linked dominant (XLD) inheritance - A form of inheritance in which a dominant gene is carried on an X chromosome and requires one copy to be expressed.

X-linked recessive (XLR) inheritance - A form of inheritance in which a recessive gene is carried on an X chromosome. Only requires one copy to be expressed in a male and two copies to be expressed in a female.

Zygote - A diploid cell formed from the fusion of a sperm cell and an ovum.

# Index

---

*Note:* Page numbers followed by "f" indicate figures, "t" indicate tables.

Printed in the United States
By Bookmasters